Living Kidney Donation

Krista L. Lentine · Beatrice P. Concepcion
Edgar V. Lerma

Editors

Living Kidney Donation

Best Practices in Evaluation, Care and Follow-up

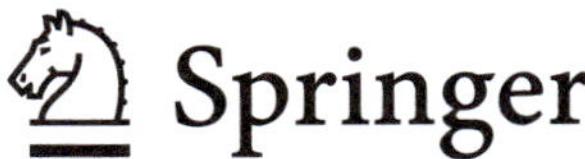

Springer

Editors
Krista L. Lentine
Center for Abdominal Transplantation
Division of Nephrology
Saint Louis University School of Medicine
St. Louis
MO
USA

Beatrice P. Concepcion
Division of Nephrology and Hypertension
Department of Medicine
Vanderbilt University Medical Center
Nashville
TN
USA

Edgar V. Lerma
Section of Nephrology
Department of Medicine
University of Illinois at Chicago
Chicago
IL
USA

ISBN 978-3-030-53620-6   ISBN 978-3-030-53618-3   (eBook)
https://doi.org/10.1007/978-3-030-53618-3

This Springer imprint is published by the registered company Springer Nature Switzerland AG
The registered company address is: Gewerbestrasse 11, 6330 Cham, Switzerland

A short dedication is insufficient to articulate my gratitude to all the professionals, patients, family members, and friends who inspire, motivate, and uplift the commitment to living donor care that infuses the inception, design, and realization of this book.

But, in brief:

To my mentors, coworkers, and collaborators in St. Louis, across the United States, and internationally – for working together to address knowledge gaps in living donation and transplant practices, in pursuit of the most robust evidence for our patients.

To the staff and volunteers at organizations including KDIGO, ASN, AST, NKF, OPTN/UNOS, and the SRTR – for the opportunities to partner in developing policy, guidance, education, and tools to support and optimize living donor evaluation, risk assessment, removal of disincentives, and follow-up.

To Mid-America Transplant – for the Jane A. Beckman endowed chair gift that helps support my time for writing, and for the model of excellence in transplant-related operations and practice.

To this book's chapter authors and my co-editors, Bea and Edgar – for the countless hours in drafting, editing, and polishing to ensure that this book provides the highest-quality content to serve practitioners and their patients.

*To my immediate and extended family – for their tremendous
patience, encouragement, and support that elevate me above
obstacles in achieving my best work.*

*Most of all, to the living donors and candidates, transplant
patients, and families I have the privilege of engaging with in
clinical settings, and through committees and advocacy groups –
for entrusting your care and offering continual reminders of the
awe-inspiring altruism of organ donors and the bravery, hope,
and gratitude of those who seek and receive transplants.*

Krista L. Lentine, MD, PhD, FASN

*Thank you to my co-editors Krista Lentine and Edgar Lerma
who poured not only their expertise into this book but also
countless hours of their time to organize, review, and edit the
material. It was an honor working with both of you. Thank you
to the chapter authors, all experts in the field, for your excellent
contributions. I have learned so much from all of you.*

*Thank you to my mentors, colleagues, trainees, and friends at
the University of the Philippines College of Medicine, Rush
University Medical Center, and Vanderbilt University Medical
Center. Thank you for the excellent education and training that I
received, for continuing to push me to learn, and for being
inspiring role models. Special thanks to Roger Rodby and Hal
Helderman.*

*Thank you to the Vanderbilt kidney transplant team – our
transplant nephrologists and surgeons, nurse practitioners, pre-,
post-, and living donor coordinators, RNs, LPNs, pharmacists,
PSS staff, social workers, RDs, financial coordinators. I am
proud to be your colleague. Thank you for your dedication and
hard work, and for your camaraderie and friendship. You
continuously inspire me to be the best physician that I can be.*

*Thank you to my family – my parents, siblings, in-laws, aunts,
uncles, cousins, nephews, and nieces – for always being there
for me. Thank you for believing in me and supporting me
through all the years away from home. Thank you especially to
my sister Carla Concepcion-Crisol for keeping me grounded,
being a sounding board and imparting your wisdom
whenever needed.*

A very special thank you to my husband Jody Junia and our son Juan Carlos for your unconditional love and unwavering support. Thank you for allowing me the time to pursue my academic interests and spend numerous extra hours at work. You are my world and I am so blessed to have you both.

Lastly, thank you to all organ donors and donors' families who have given the gift of life. I am blessed and privileged to witness transplantation transform lives for the better. This book is dedicated to you.

Beatrice P. Concepcion, MD, MS, FASN

To all my mentors, and friends, at the University of Santo Tomas Faculty of Medicine and Surgery in Manila, Philippines, and Northwestern University Feinberg School of Medicine in Chicago, IL, who have, in one way or another, influenced and guided me to become the physician that I am.

To all the medical students, interns, and residents at Advocate Christ Medical Center and Macneal Hospital, whom I have taught or learned from, especially those who eventually decided to pursue Nephrology as a career.

To my parents and my brothers, without whose unwavering love and support through the good and bad times, I would not have persevered and reached my goals in life.

Most especially, to my two lovely and precious daughters, Anastasia Zofia and Isabella Ann, whose smiles and laughter constantly provide me unparalleled joy and happiness; and my very loving and understanding wife Michelle, who has always been supportive of my endeavors both personally and professionally, and who sacrificed a lot of time and exhibited unwavering patience as I devoted a significant amount of time and effort to this project. Truly, they provide me with motivation and inspiration.

Edgar V. Lerma, MD, FASN

Patients' Foreword

We are the patients, the family members, the donors—the people whom you treat, think about, and write about. Although we have different perspectives on living donation, we unequivocally agree that the act is transformative for donors, recipients, families, and society. Not one of us had a direct or ideal path leading up to this life-changing surgery, but we're all advocates for supporting opportunities to share the gift of life through living donation. The medical aspects of donor evaluation, surgery, and long-term risk assessment have made great strides in the more than half century since the first living donor transplantation was performed in Boston. But living donation and transplantation are far more than medical experiences: they are emotional, familial, financial, and social. We hope that reading our stories provides a memorable personalized framework for the academic discussions of these topics that follow throughout this new clinical handbook.

Kevin Fowler: My family has endured the multi-generational burden of autosomal dominant polycystic kidney disease (ADPKD). When I was a young child, my mother shared stories of her father's struggle with the disease. My grandfather never knew he had ADPKD until he was admitted to a hospital in the late 1950s when he didn't feel well. Shortly after admission, he learned that he was in the final stages of kidney failure. At that time, kidney transplantation was very limited, and hemodialysis was not yet available as a treatment option.

After my grandfather's death, all of his three daughters, including my mom, were diagnosed with ADPKD. While the disease progression varied with each sister, all three eventually progressed to end-stage kidney disease (ESKD), and all of them died on hemodialysis. Owing to a variety of circumstances, not one of them was given the opportunity to receive a kidney transplant. This experience created a dark cloud hanging over my life as I wondered if I would face the same patient journey.

As a husband and father with two young children, I finally made the decision to determine whether I had inherited ADPKD. I asked my primary care physician to conduct an ultrasound, and the test confirmed my worst fears—I was diagnosed with ADPKD that day. I'd always thought that if I had the disease, dialysis would be my fate. Because of my fear of dialysis, I'd never explored the various ESKD treatment options. Fortunately, by talking with a physician friend, I found a nephrologist who changed our family narrative.

On my first appointment with the nephrologist, he told me that I would be able to avoid dialysis completely through preemptive living donor kidney transplantation. That began a family journey to identify a living donor. I thank my wife for serving as a living donor champion—her advocacy in sharing my need for an organ donor helped find the living donor who was a good match, and whose generous gift meant there was no need for me to start dialysis.

Since my preemptive living donor transplant in 2004, I have been an active participant in life. I have seen both of my children enter college, and one will be graduating this year. Moreover, I have been able to work the entire time and even start a business because I was given the best treatment option for ESKD.

Unfortunately, this experience is not the norm for many people with kidney failure, partly because many kidney patients are not fully educated about all of their treatment options or how to effectively share their need for an organ donor with their social network. Also, many healthy, otherwise willing individuals may never have the experience of living donation because they encounter barriers to pursuing or completing the donation process.

Randee Bloom: My son was only 22 when he volunteered to risk his life to save that of his father. Medical facts about his surgery collided with the emotions of love and fear when he faced this momentous decision, suddenly realizing that his choice had the potential to save a life. At the same time, he needed to face formidable challenges, including the risks to his own health at the time of the donation and for many decades to come.

As a family, we were very motivated to make donation and transplantation happen, but we learned firsthand that living donors can face important challenges and struggles. Having major surgery when you're not already sick is not a normal occurrence. It's hard for anyone to "go under the knife," but doing so while you are perfectly well takes true courage. Even after the donor overcomes these fears, they face many logistical problems. Our son lived nearly 1,000 miles from our transplant center at the time. He had to take significant time off from work and other obligations to fly to the center—at considerable expense—several times before the surgery, for laboratory and diagnostic testing, as well as hours of required interviews and highly focused physical and psychosocial examinations. Also, to obtain the care he needed for a successful recovery, he lived at our home for a month.

Our son committed to the US-mandated postdonation follow-up for 2 years. Our transplant center helpfully arranged for him to have several of his lab tests completed at a facility near his home. Although the mandatory period has passed, we view my son's commitment to long-term health monitoring as an important part of the donation process. Efforts to coordinate and facilitate postdonation follow-up are vital in ensuring all living donors have access to the long-term care they need and deserve.

Donating an organ can personally cost the living donor thousands of dollars. It is painful to think that giving the incredible gift of life is simply too expensive for many Americans to manage. Imagine having to choose between having a job and having a father. A more robust support program with policies and resources to cover all out-of-pocket expenses, including lost wages, transportation costs, and coverage for personal and family care, can make all the difference in helping potential living donors turn their desire into action.

I have learned from my son and many other living donors of the gratitude that can accompany the opportunity to save a life. Our son demonstrated strengths he says he didn't know he had, and his sisters' love and admiration blossomed from their gratitude. Our family's surprise in learning that my husband needed an organ transplant also brought the realization that health should never be taken for granted. Educating patients, families, and communities about the benefits of living donation and living donor transplantation, reducing financial disincentives to donation, and supporting optimal care throughout the donation process, including follow-up, should be seen as benefiting the health care for all of us.

Heather Hunt: We walk into transplant hospitals hoping to learn everything we need to know to lead us to a "yes." Instead, we learn there is no systematic collection of long-term data about the living donors who came before us to help inform our decisions.

Some of us take a leap of faith and donate anyway. I had to ask myself whether I would donate to my sister if it meant my life would, hypothetically, be shortened or adversely affected over time. At the time, I had to ask that question in the absence of robust data that told another story. For me, the answer was easy: a shorter life with my sister would be much better than a longer one without her.

Long-term data across a variety of postdonation outcomes would go a long way to moderating the unscientific, hypothetical trade-offs some of us use in deciding whether to donate. Leaving us to wonder about our long-term prospects may be causing too many to shy away, needlessly, from donating. Imagine how many more people would say yes to living donation if they could make decisions based on robust long-term outcome data rather than on leaps of faith.

We wonder if long-term outcome data is not a priority because living donation is an elective surgery. After all, we could walk away if we're uneasy about what we don't know. But long-term outcomes of other elective surgeries are examined; literature on the long-term risks of plastic surgery, for example, is plentiful.

We wonder how much easier our conversations with our parents and spouses and children about our desire to donate would be if the answer to their questions about the long-term implications was not "they didn't study that yet."

We wonder what our signatures on informed consent forms really mean when not informed by ranges of probabilities for lifetime risks.

Although recent years have brought important advances in the science of postdonation risk assessment, such as through cohort studies at certain centers or creative database linkage analyses, there is more to learn—and long-term registries will help. Even if it takes decades, studying us over our lifetimes will help future potential donors and families wonder less.

Long-term study will also guide future candidate selection and shared decision-making. If data demonstrate small and manageable lifetime risks, that could increase potential donor confidence and the number of living donor transplants. If data demonstrate that individuals with certain characteristics face prohibitive risks, then deciding when donation should not move forward is the right outcome, too.

Study us. And help more donor candidates and living donors (and thus transplant recipients) in the future.

Carol Offen: Who are we? We're loved ones: mothers and fathers, wives and husbands and partners, daughters and sons, sisters and brothers. We're also caring friends, neighbors, and members of your community. And some of us are just average, empathetic people who simply saw a need—even in someone we don't know—and wanted to help.

What we're *not* are saints, super-heroes, or natural risk takers, Thanks for the praise, but that's not what it's all about. Please don't perpetuate the idea that someone needs to be superhuman to step up to save a life by undergoing a comparatively low-risk surgery. That attitude may intimidate some potential living donors.

Bravery has little to do with it. Personally, I'm a wimp: I faint at flu shots. But when my adult son's kidneys were failing, and I was the only healthy family member with a compatible blood type to come forward for donor evaluation, I ultimately donated to him in 2006 (paired donation was in its infancy in those days). My son didn't have any risk factors for kidney disease, and we had no family history; all he had was a strep infection that caused his IgA nephropathy. We want people to understand that what happened to our families can happen to any family.

My son and I are both doing well some 14 years out. The benefits for donors don't lend themselves to quantification like our recipients' do—and our benefits can't be measured in a blood test or lab report—but they are just as real.

For family members and couples, the benefits of living donation and transplantation are nothing short of dramatic: as in seeing your child, who's been pale and listless for months or years on dialysis, gradually become his old self again (if only my son could have had a preemptive transplant like Kevin!); a partner who wasn't interested in intimacy since starting dialysis now discovering a new bond; a spouse or parent whose ability to work was limited, resuming a full-time schedule—or even launching a new career—to substantially improve the family's finances; and couples that have shied away from socializing due to the patient's lack of energy being able to enjoy evenings out again. Donors/caregivers, who now have more time, reduced stress, and no doubt improved sleep, surely reap benefits in mood and overall outlook.

For anyone who donates an organ—even to a stranger—such benefits are common. Knowing that you've given someone a chance at a healthy, productive life is an extraordinary and gratifying feeling. Through online donor-support groups, I've been struck by how life changing the experience has felt for most of us, including even the few who later have had complications or whose recipient lost their transplant or later passed away.

That's why, when evaluating people as potential donors, we want transplant teams to give weight to the immeasurable benefits that flow to living donors every day. Of course, we want you to zealously protect our health and definitely give us all the information we need for truly *informed* consent, but we also want you to respect our ability—and yes, our right—to then weigh the risks and benefits in making an informed donation decision (when risks are not deemed prohibitive by the transplant program).

Despite the challenges, we firmly believe that far more people would consider living donation if only they had more information and support. Inform us, support us, study us, and trust us. Together we can save more lives.

<table>
<tr><td>Chapel Hill, NC, USA</td><td>Carol Offen</td></tr>
<tr><td>St. Louis, MO, USA</td><td>Kevin Fowler</td></tr>
<tr><td>West Bloomfield, MI, USA</td><td>Randee Bloom, RN, PhD</td></tr>
<tr><td>Cape Cod, MA, USA</td><td>Heather Hunt, JD</td></tr>
</table>

Preface

Since the advent of the first successful living kidney donation in 1954, living donor transplantation has evolved into the definitive treatment of choice for kidney failure, offering kidney patients the best chance of long-term dialysis-free survival, with a better quality of life, at lowest costs to the healthcare system. Currently, more than 30,000 living persons across the world donate a kidney each year to help a family member, friend, or even a stranger overcome the burden of kidney failure. In 2019, the US federal government formalized unprecedented attention on increasing opportunities for living donor transplantation in the "Advancing American Kidney Health" Executive Order. Despite the tremendous benefits to transplant recipients and society, until recently, the outcomes and optimal care of donors themselves were relatively understudied. Fortunately, things are changing, including landmark developments in living donor risk assessment, policy, and guidance. The book arose from a need to synthesize advances in the field of living donor care into an accessible resource for contemporary practitioners. Organized into 16 main chapters, this book offers guidance on the full range of clinical scenarios encountered in living kidney donation, grounded in the latest and emerging evidence.

Recognition of the critical importance of perspectives of comparison for drawing inferences about donor health outcomes exemplifies one recent milestone in improving donor risk assessment. While general population comparisons can have value as one context, because donors are carefully evaluated and selected, methodologies to assemble control groups of healthy nondonors who would otherwise meet donor selection criteria have been a breakthrough in facilitating estimates of the attributable risks of donation. The critical importance of incorporating such new evidence across living donor care—from risk assessment and informed consent, to specific evaluation domains and follow-up—permeates all chapters of this book as the foundation for optimal evaluation and informed patient choice.

Inconsistencies in prior guidance also highlighted a critical need to strengthen the underlying framework for living donor selection. The year 2017 marked the publication of the first international Kidney Disease: Improving Global Outcomes (KDIGO) living donor guideline and a new framework for evaluating and selecting donor candidates based on the long-term risk of adverse outcomes estimated from *simultaneous* consideration of a profile of demographic and health characteristics. The rationale for an integrated risk-based approach includes: (1) balancing ethical principles of autonomy and justice versus nonmaleficence, which requires consistent decision-making for all donor candidates; (2) supporting consistent, transparent decision-making by integrating multiple parameters into absolute risk estimates, to avoid the inconsistencies that may result from considering parameters in isolation (i.e., relative risk thresholds for individual parameters). To operationalize the approach, the guideline development methodology included partnering with the Chronic Kidney Disease Prognosis Consortium to develop an online tool for projecting 15-year and lifetime risks of kidney failure (a central outcome of interest for donors) based on predonation demographic and health factors. This and other tools for risk projection in the absence of donation and postdonation are now freely available online, and strategies for application to donor candidate evaluation and education are discussed throughout this book.

While current advances are critically important in grounding a new paradigm for donor candidate evaluation and selection, we recognize that such new tools comprise a starting point. Ongoing efforts are needed to improve the precision and generalizability of risk projection, including consideration of additional factors such as genetic and familial traits, and to incorporate tailored prediction of the risk impact of donation. Specific chapters of this book examine the latest information related to use of novel genetic risk markers in donor candidate evaluation, innovations and next steps for risk estimation tools, and related ethical considerations. Use of apolipoprotein L1 (*APOL1*) genotyping as a recently identified precision medicine tool for the risk stratification of African ancestry donor candidates, and associated controversies and limitations, are discussed in several chapters. A chapter dedicated to follow-up considers new and emerging strategies to strengthen the collection of long-term postdonation outcomes data and continually build the evidence for informing future donor candidates and donors.

Non-white racial and ethnic groups are challenged by higher kidney disease burden and need for transplantation, but face clear disparities in access to living donor transplantation. Contributing factors are likely multifactorial, and while appropriate medical risk-based donor exclusions may contribute, there are deficiencies in the education of kidney patients and the community about opportunities for living donation and transplantation, and financial barriers that may prevent donation in otherwise willing, healthy persons. Advocacy initiatives and policies to remove disincentives to donation, support efficiency, innovation and program sustainability, and advance an equitable system of practice are explored in dedicated chapters. We are privileged that this book is introduced by a Patients' Foreward, wherein four individuals articulate what the experience of living donation and the gift of transplantation means to patients and families, and frame the vital need to continue optimizing living donor care, communication, and the patient experience.

This book would not exist without the efforts and insights of the chapter authors, whom we thank for sharing their expertise and working collaboratively to present a harmonized vision for strengthening the safety, protection, informed choice, and follow-up care of all living donors. We thank Margaret Moore and her colleagues at Springer for appreciating the value of our vision, and their support in helping transform our initial ideas into reality.

We hope that general and transplant physicians, as well as related allied health professionals, will look to this book as a comprehensive resource addressing the spectrum of clinical topics encountered in living donor care. However, we also recognize and celebrate the current pace of rapidly evolving evidence. Empirical studies including formal evaluations of education, removal of disincentives, practice efficiency, and risk evaluation and communication are feasible and necessary to honor the life-saving gift of living donors and improve opportunities for healthy, willing persons to safely give the gift of life to patients in need. We look forward to incorporating future evidence and the feedback of readers and the community into the next edition. Until then, we sincerely hope that all readers enjoy this book and benefit as much from reading the content as we did in preparing and writing it.

St. Louis, MO, USA   Krista L. Lentine
Nashville, TN, USA   Beatrice P. Concepcion
Chicago, IL, USA   Edgar V. Lerma

Contents

1 Rationale and Landscape of Living Kidney Donation in Contemporary Practice 1
Ngan N. Lam, Nagaraju Sarabu, Steven Habbous, and Amit X. Garg

2 Informed Consent and Framework of Living Donor Care 25
Anji E. Wall, Elisa J. Gordon, and Rebecca E. Hays

3 Evaluation of Glomerular Filtration Rate, Albuminuria and Hematuria in Living Donor Candidates 59
Andrew S. Levey, Nitender Goyal, and Lesley A. Inker

4 Evaluation of Renal Anatomy, Structure and Nephrolithiasis in Living Donor Candidates 93
Emilio D. Poggio, Nasir Khan, Christian Bolanos, Thomas Pham, and Jane C. Tan

5 Evaluation of Hypertension in Living Donor Candidates 119
Mona D. Doshi and Sandra J. Taler

6 Evaluation of Metabolic and Cardiovascular Risks in Living Donor Candidates 141
Margaux N. Mustian, Vineeta Kumar, and Jayme E. Locke

7 Infection and Cancer Screening in Living Donor Candidates 161
Mary Ann Lim, Eric Au, Blair Weikert, Germaine Wong, and Deirdre Sawinski

8 Evaluation of Genetic Kidney Disease in Living Donor Candidates . . . 189
Christie P. Thomas and Jasmin Divers

9 Perioperative Evaluation and Management of Living Donor Candidates 219
Gretchen Edwards, Beatrice P. Concepcion, and Rachel C. Forbes

10 Compatibility, Kidney Paired Donation, and Incompatible Living Donor Transplants 233
Neetika Garg, Jagbir Gill, and Didier A. Mandelbrot

**11 Psychosocial Evaluation, Care and Quality of Life
in Living Kidney Donation** 253
Mary Amanda Dew, Andrea F. DiMartini, Jennifer L. Steel,
and Sheila G. Jowsey-Gregoire

12 Risk Assessment Tools and Innovations in Living Kidney Donation . . . 283
Abimereki D. Muzaale, Allan B. Massie, and Dorry L. Segev

**13 Living Donor Nephrectomy: Approaches, Innovations,
and Outcomes** 291
Jonathan Merola, Matthew Cooper, and Sanjay Kulkarni

14 Follow-Up Care after Living Kidney Donation 303
Jane Long, Krista L. Lentine, and Macey L. Henderson

**15 Ethical and Policy Considerations in Living Kidney
Donor Evaluation and Care** 327
Jed Adam Gross and Marie-Chantal Fortin

**16 Living Donor Transplant Program Growth, Innovation
and Sustainability** 349
David A. Axelrod, David Serur, Matthew Abramson,
and Dianne LaPointe Rudow

Index 371

Contributors

Matthew Abramson, MD Transplant Nephrology, New York Presbyterian Hospital/Weill Cornell, New York, NY, USA

Eric Au, MBBS, MPH Sydney School of Public Health, University of Sydney, Sydney, NSW, Australia

David A. Axelrod, MD, MBA Department of Surgery, University of Iowa, Iowa City, IA, USA

Christian Bolanos, MD Division of Nephrology, Department of Medicine, Stanford University, Stanford, CA, USA

Beatrice P. Concepcion, MD Division of Nephrology and Hypertension, Department of Medicine, Vanderbilt University Medical Center, Nashville, TN, USA

Matthew Cooper, MD Medstar Georgetown Transplant Institute, Washington, DC, USA

Mary Amanda Dew, PhD Departments of Psychiatry, Psychology, Epidemiology, Biostatistics and the Clinical and Translational Science Institute, University of Pittsburgh, Pittsburgh, PA, USA

Andrea F. DiMartini, MD Departments of Psychiatry and Surgery and the Clinical and Translational Science Institute, University of Pittsburgh, Pittsburgh, PA, USA

Jasmin Divers, PhD Division of Health Services Research, Department of Foundations of Medicine, New York University Long Island School of Medicine, New York, NY, USA

Winthrop Research Institute, Mineola, NY, USA

Mona D. Doshi, MD Division of Nephrology, Department of Medicine, University of Michigan, Ann Arbor, MI, USA

Gretchen Edwards, MD Division of General Surgery, Department of Surgery, Vanderbilt University Medical Center, Nashville, TN, USA

Rachel C. Forbes, MD, MBA Division of Kidney and Pancreas Transplantation, Department of Surgery, Vanderbilt University Medical Center, Nashville, TN, USA

Marie-Chantal Fortin, MD, PhD Canadian Donation and Transplantation Research Program, Edmonton, AB, Canada

Centre de recherche du CHUM, Montreal, Canada

Department of Medicine, Université de Montréal, Montreal, Canada

Amit X. Garg, MD, PhD Division of Nephrology, Department of Medicine, Western University, London, ON, Canada

Neetika Garg, MD Division of Nephrology, Department of Medicine, University of Wisconsin-Madison, Madison, WI, USA

Jagbir Gill, MD, MPH Division of Nephrology, Department of Medicine, The University of British Columbia, Vancouver, BC, Canada

Elisa J. Gordon, PhD, MPH Department of Surgery, Northwestern University Feinberg School of Medicine, Chicago, IL, USA

Nitender Goyal, MD Division of Nephrology, Tufts Medical Center, Boston, MA, USA

Jed Adam Gross, J D, M Phil Bioethics Program, University Health Network, Toronto, ON, Canada

Canadian Donation and Transplantation Research Program, Edmonton, AB, Canada

Steven Habbous, PhD Ontario Health, Cancer Care Ontario, Toronto, ON, Canada

Rebecca E. Hays, MSW, APSW Department of Coordinated Care, University of Wisconsin Hospital and Clinics, Madison, WI, USA

Macey L. Henderson, PhD Department of Surgery, Division of Transplantation, Johns Hopkins School of Medicine, Baltimore, MD, USA

Lesley A. Inker, MD, MS Division of Nephrology, Tufts Medical Center, Boston, MA, USA

Sheila G. Jowsey-Gregoire, MD Department of Psychiatry, Mayo Clinic, Rochester, MN, USA

Nasir Khan, MD Department of Nephrology and Hypertension, Glickman Urological and Kidney Institute, Cleveland Clinic, Cleveland, OH, USA

Sanjay Kulkarni, MD Department of Surgery, Yale School of Medicine, New Haven, CT, USA

Vineeta Kumar, MD Department of Medicine, University of Alabama at Birmingham, Birmingham, AL, USA

Ngan N. Lam, MD, MSc Cumming School of Medicine and Department of Community Health Sciences, University of Calgary, Calgary, AB, Canada

Krista L. Lentine, MD, PhD Center for Abdominal Transplantation, Division of Nephrology, Saint Louis University School of Medicine, St. Louis, MO, USA

Andrew S. Levey, MD Division of Nephrology, Tufts Medical Center, Boston, MA, USA

Mary Ann Lim, MD Renal, Electrolyte and Hypertension Division, Department of Medicine, Perelman School of Medicine, Philadelphia, PA, USA

Jayme E. Locke, MD, MPH Department of Surgery, University of Alabama at Birmingham, Birmingham, AL, USA

Jane Long, MD, PhD Division of Transplantation, Department of Surgery, Johns Hopkins School of Medicine, Baltimore, MD, USA

Didier A. Mandelbrot, MD Division of Nephrology, Department of Medicine, University of Wisconsin-Madison, Madison, WI, USA

Allan B. Massie, PhD Johns Hopkins University, Baltimore, MD, USA

Jonathan Merola, MD, PhD Department of Surgery, Yale School of Medicine, New Haven, CT, USA

Margaux N. Mustian, MD, MSPH Department of Surgery, University of Alabama at Birmingham, Birmingham, AL, USA

Abimereki D. Muzaale, MD, MPH Johns Hopkins University, Baltimore, MD, USA

Thomas Pham, MD Division of Abdominal Transplantation, Department of Surgery, Stanford University, Stanford, CA, USA

Emilio D. Poggio, MD Department of Nephrology and Hypertension, Glickman Urological and Kidney Institute, Cleveland Clinic, Cleveland, OH, USA

Dianne La Pointe Rudow, ANP-BC, DNP Recanati Miller Transplantation Institute, Mount Sinai Hospital, New York, NY, USA

Nagaraju Sarabu, MD, MPH Division of Nephrology, Department of Medicine, University Hospitals Cleveland Medical Center, Cleveland, OH, USA

Deirdre Sawinski, MD Renal, Electrolyte and Hypertension Division, Department of Medicine, Perelman School of Medicine, Philadelphia, PA, USA

Dorry L. Segev, MD, PhD Johns Hopkins University, Baltimore, MD, USA

David Serur, MD Transplant Nephrology, New York Presbyterian Hospital/Weill Cornell, New York, NY, USA

Jennifer L. Steel, PhD Departments of Surgery, Psychiatry and Psychology, University of Pittsburgh, Pittsburgh, PA, USA

Sandra J. Taler, MD Division of Nephrology and Hypertension, College of Medicine, Mayo Clinic, Rochester, MN, USA

Jane C. Tan, MD, PhD Division of Nephrology, Department of Medicine, Stanford University, Stanford, CA, USA

Christie P. Thomas, MD Department of Internal Medicine and Pediatrics, Carver College of Medicine, University of Iowa and Veterans Affairs Medical Center, Iowa City, IA, USA

Anji E. Wall, MD, PhD Department of Abdominal Transplantation, Baylor University Medical Center, Dallas, TX, USA

Blair Weikert, MD Division of Infectious Diseases, Department of Medicine, Perelman School of Medicine, Philadelphia, PA, USA

Germaine Wong, MBBS, MMed, PhD Sydney School of Public Health, University of Sydney, Sydney, NSW, Australia

Rationale and Landscape of Living Kidney Donation in Contemporary Practice

1

Ngan N. Lam, Nagaraju Sarabu, Steven Habbous, and Amit X. Garg

Rationale for Living Donor Kidney Transplantation: The Organ Shortage

Chronic Kidney Disease and Kidney Failure

Chronic kidney disease (CKD) is defined as a sustained glomerular filtration rate (GFR) <60 mL/min per 1.73 m^2 [1]. The worldwide incidence and prevalence of CKD is growing, affecting 11% to 13% of the global population [2]. In some countries, these patterns are driven by noncommunicable risk factors, such as diabetes mellitus and hypertension, while in others, this is driven by premature births, low birth weight, malarial infection, and human immunodeficiency virus (HIV) infection [3–6]. Estimates from the World Health Organization (WHO) Global Burden of Disease show a 32% increase in death due to kidney failure between 2005 and 2015 [7].

N. N. Lam (✉)
Cumming School of Medicine and Department of Community Health Sciences,
University of Calgary, Calgary, AB, Canada
e-mail: ngan.lam@ucalgary.ca

N. Sarabu
Division of Nephrology, Department of Medicine,
University Hospitals Cleveland Medical Center, Cleveland, OH, USA
e-mail: Nagaraju.Sarabu@uhhospitals.org

S. Habbous
Ontario Health, Cancer Care Ontario, Toronto, ON, Canada
e-mail: steven.habbous@ontariohealth.ca

A. X. Garg
Division of Nephrology, Department of Medicine,
Western University, London, ON, Canada
e-mail: Amit.Garg@lhsc.on.ca

© Springer Nature Switzerland AG 2021
K. L. Lentine et al. (eds.), *Living Kidney Donation*,
https://doi.org/10.1007/978-3-030-53618-3_1

For most patients with CKD, disease progression can be slowed through medical, dietary, and lifestyle interventions [8]. Once a patient's kidney function declines to a GFR <20 mL/min per 1.73 m², renal replacement therapies including dialysis and kidney transplantation should be considered. The threshold for beginning a transplant candidate evaluation has been relaxed by some centers to enable more patients to receive a transplant before dialysis is required (preemptive transplantation).

Treatment options for kidney failure include dialysis, transplantation, or conservative care. Despite the high morbidity, mortality, and costs to the healthcare system, dialysis is the most common initial treatment modality provided to patients. In Canada, only 3% of patients with kidney failure receive a preemptive transplant, an estimate that has remained stable between 2006 and 2015 [6]. In the United States, 1% of adult kidney transplantations performed were preemptive [9]. This rate remains low, despite recognition from healthcare professionals that preemptive transplantation is the best treatment option for many patients with kidney failure [10].

Kidney Transplantation vs. Chronic Dialysis

For patients with end-stage kidney disease (ESKD), kidney transplantation is associated with improved patient and graft survival compared to chronic dialysis [11–14]. Among 228,552 patients who initiated dialysis between 1991 and 1996 in the United States, deceased donor kidney transplantation (DDKT) was associated with a 68% reduction in mortality compared to those who remained on the waitlist for transplant, after adjusting for age, sex, race, and cause of ESKD [11]. Among kidney transplants performed in the United States between 1996 and 2005, the median graft survival ranged from 10 to 27 years, depending on the type of donor [15]. Thus, kidney transplantation offers patients with ESKD the best chance for dialysis-free survival.

Compared to dialysis, kidney transplantation is also associated with a better patient quality of life and lower costs to the healthcare system [12, 16–20]. Two Canadian studies have shown that dialysis patients following successful kidney transplantation have improved quality of life and increased chance of employment [17, 18]. In 2016, annual transplant spending per patient was $34,780 US dollars (USD), which was lower than dialysis spending, irrespective of modality (peritoneal dialysis, $76,177 USD; hemodialysis, $90,971 USD) [21]. Despite the well-established benefits of kidney transplantation, the number of transplantable kidneys available from deceased donors does not meet the growing demand, and there is opportunity to reduce this gap through living donor kidney transplantation (LDKT).

Living vs. Deceased Donor Kidney Transplantation

Compared with DDKT, numerous studies have demonstrated superior medical and psychosocial outcomes with LDKT, which may reflect a variety of benefits [22, 23]. For patients who are approaching ESKD, LDKT offers the possibility of avoiding dialysis altogether (preemptive transplantation) [24, 25]. For patients on dialysis,

LDKT offers a shorter waiting time compared to DDKT, thereby reducing the duration and exposure of dialysis and its associated mortality, morbidity, and costs. In Canada, between 2013 and 2015, the median time spent on dialysis until transplant was 4.0 years for recipients of a DDKT and 1.6 years for recipients of a LDKT [6]. In addition to this, LDKT can be electively scheduled to allow for optimization of any donor or recipient comorbidities and thereby potentially reduce risks of perioperative complications. Recipients of LDKT may also benefit from improved genetic human leukocyte antigen (HLA) matching which may reduce short- and long-term risk of rejection. LDKT generally have a shorter cold ischemia time compared to DDKT with associated lower rates of delayed graft function [14, 22, 26]. All of these factors contribute to the superior patient and graft survival for recipients of LDKT vs. DDKT. In the United States, the probability of posttransplant patient survival at 1, 5, and 10 years for DDKT recipients in recent cohorts was 96%, 85%, and 64%, respectively, compared to 99%, 92%, and 79% for LDKT recipients (Fig. 1.1) [21, 27].

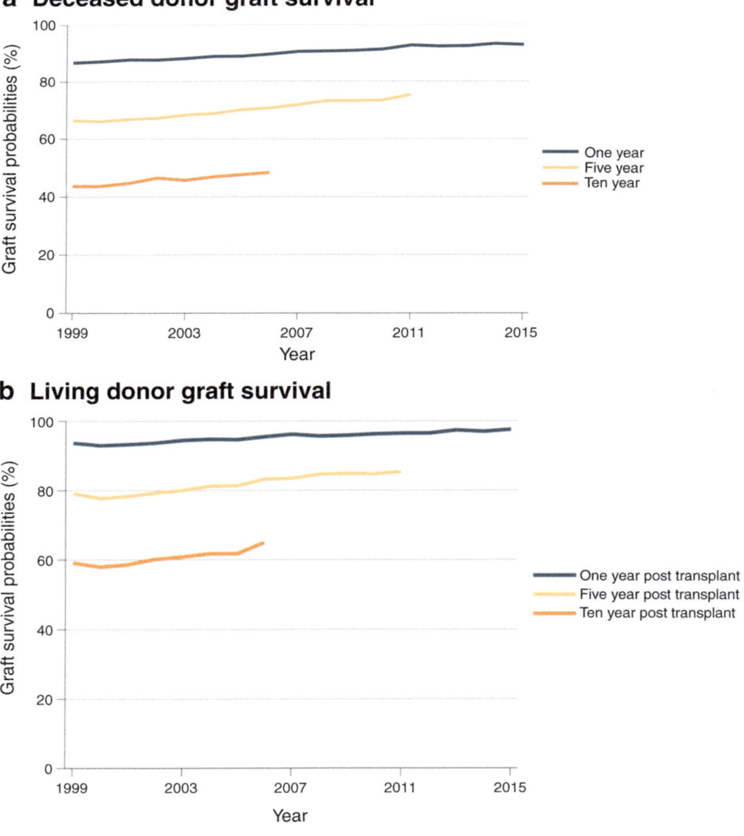

Fig. 1.1 Trends in 1-, 5-, and 10-year kidney transplant graft survival, 1999 to 2015, for (**a**) deceased donor and (**b**) living donor kidney transplants. (From the United States Renal Data System (USRDS) [21])

Similarly, the probability of graft survival at 1, 5, and 10 years for DDKT recipients was 93%, 75%, and 48%, respectively, compared to 98%, 85%, and 65% for LDKT recipients. Thus, from the perspective of best outcomes for the recipient, LDKT should be considered the preferred treatment for patients with ESKD.

Landscape of Living Kidney Donation

The successful first LDKT was performed in 1954 between identical twins, Ronald (donor) and Richard (recipient) Herrick [28]. The donor nephrectomy was performed by Dr. Hartwell Harrison, while the recipient transplant was performed by Dr. Joseph Murray at the Peter Bent Brigham Hospital in Boston, Massachusetts [28]. This landmark operation in the field of transplantation highlighted the culmination of multiple breakthroughs, including improved understanding of kidney disease, Dr. Alexis Carrel's technique of arterial anastomosis [29], and the success of skin allografts between identical twins [30, 31]. Since this transplant, the number of LDKT performed globally has risen to approximately 32,000 per year.

Geographic Variation and Trends in Living Donor Kidney Transplantation

The Global Observatory on Donation and Transplantation (GODT) is a collaborative effort between the WHO and Spanish Transplant Organization. In 2017, GODT reported that 32,990 LDKT were performed worldwide (representing 36.5% of the 90,306 total kidney transplants) [32]. Although this was a significant increase from the 27,000 LDKT performed in 2006, various WHO regions around the world have followed different patterns of growth during this era (Fig. 1.2). In America, which had the largest absolute number of registered LDKT performed per year, the incidence peaked in 2010 and had a slight decline in the subsequent years. In contrast, Europe had a steady increase in the total number of LDKT, while other WHO regions (Southeast Asia, Western Pacific, Eastern Mediterranean, and Africa) remained relatively stable. The greatest number of LDKT in 2016 were performed in India ($n = 5697$), the United States ($n = 5629$), and Turkey ($n = 2639$). The Netherlands had the highest rate of LDKT at 33.2 procedures per million population (pmp) followed by Turkey (33.1 pmp) and Israel (27.1 pmp) [32].

There are many factors that may have contributed to the rise in LDKT in the twenty-first century, such as advances in surgical techniques of donor nephrectomy and opportunities for paired donation [33]. In Hungary, the rise in LDKT may be due to support from the director of the Department of Transplantation and Surgery in Budapest in 2009 [34]. In Iran, the rise in LDKT may be the result of a controversial alternative funding model that remunerates unrelated donation [35, 36].

The reason for the recent stabilization or decline in LDKT rates in some countries remains unclear. In the United States, potential factors that may contribute to the decline in LDKT rates (from 2010 to 2017) include changes in the allocation of

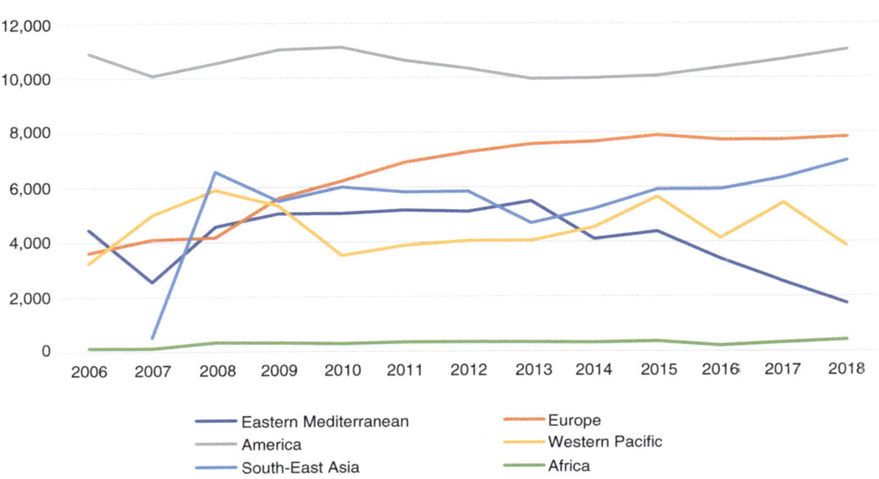

Fig. 1.2 Trends in living donor kidney transplants by World Health Organization (WHO) regions, 2006 to 2018 [32]. (Produced using 2017 data from the Global Observatory on Donation and Transplantation (GODT), compiled by the WHO-ONT collaboration)

high-quality deceased donor kidney with priority to pediatric recipients, increases in the prevalence of risk factors that may preclude donation in the general population (e.g., hypertension, diabetes mellitus, and obesity), inefficiencies in the living donor evaluation process, and disincentives for donors that hinder financial neutrality and insurability [37–42]. To better understand the national landscape of LDKT, the American Society of Transplantation (AST) held a consensus conference in 2014, which included members of its Live Donor Community of Practice [43]. The conference identified five main areas for improving practices to increase access to LDKT: 1) improving education outside of transplant centers about living donor transplantation [44]; 2) facilitating education about living kidney donation [45]; 3) improving efficiencies in living kidney donor evaluation [46]; 4) overcoming disparities in living kidney donation [47]; and 5) reducing financial barriers to living kidney donation [41]. The working groups identified the main barriers to LDKT and developed best practice recommendations to improve access, process, and utilization through partnerships and collaborations between healthcare providers, patients, and key stakeholders [43].

Temporal Trends in Living Kidney Donors

In addition to geographic variations, living donor nephrectomies also vary by age, sex, and other donor demographics. In the United States, over the last decade, there has been a decline in living kidney donation among those aged 18 to 34 years and an increase among those aged 50 to 64 years [9]. This may be due to concerns about lifetime risks of adverse events for younger donors, including kidney failure

[9, 48–50]. There is also a higher proportion of female donors compared to male donors (~60% vs. ~40%) [9]. In the United States, over 60% of donors are white and the reason for racial differences is likely multifactorial, including medical contraindications in nonwhite donor candidates, cultural and religious beliefs around organ transplantation, and socioeconomic barriers, as well as higher representation in the general population [9, 51, 52]. The proportion of obese living donors in the United States has also increased from 8% in 1963–1974 to 26% in 1997–2007, and the proportion of donors with glucose intolerance has also risen (9% to 25%) [53]. Between 2005 and 2015, living kidney donations declined among US men at all income household levels except the highest income quintile, suggesting financial barriers to donation in all but the highest income group [54, 55]. This suggests that particularly during times of economic instability, efforts should be made to develop policies that address financial barriers to donation [54]. Lastly, in part due to the success of the kidney paired exchange programs as well as recognition that HLA matching is not required for good LDKT outcomes in the era of modern immunosuppression, the number of unrelated and paired donations has increased over the last decade, while related donations have decreased [9].

Recipient Disparities in Access to Living Donor Kidney Transplantation

From the recipient perspective, certain demographic and clinical characteristics are associated with better access to LDKT. In Canada and the United States, older age, nonwhite race/ethnicity, lower education, and lower income level are associated with reduced rates of LDKT [9, 56, 57]. One study reported that these characteristics accounted for 14% of the variation in LDKT in the United States, more than recipient-, center-, or regional-level variation [56]. As shown in Fig. 1.3, LDKT was less common among nonwhite compared to white recipients. Further, racial disparities in LDKT in the United States have increased over time. After adjustment for baseline clinical factors, the relative likelihood of LDKT in Hispanic compared to white candidates declined from 17% lower access in 1995–1999 to 48% lower access in 2010–2014 [58]. Among Asian versus white candidates, LDKT was 44% less likely in 1995–1999 and 58% less likely in 2010–2014 [58]. As with donors, there are many factors contributing to these racial disparities, including educational barriers to pursuit of LDKT, and shared medical and economic risks within the patient's family and social network [47]. The AST consensus conference provided core recommendations to reduce disparities in access to LDKT [47]. This includes implementing diverse, culturally sensitive educational programs for patients and their social networks at every CKD stage and building partnerships between transplant centers, dialysis clinics, and community healthcare providers [47]. Overcoming educational and systemic barriers to living kidney donation and LDKT is vitally important for reducing disparities in access to LDKT.

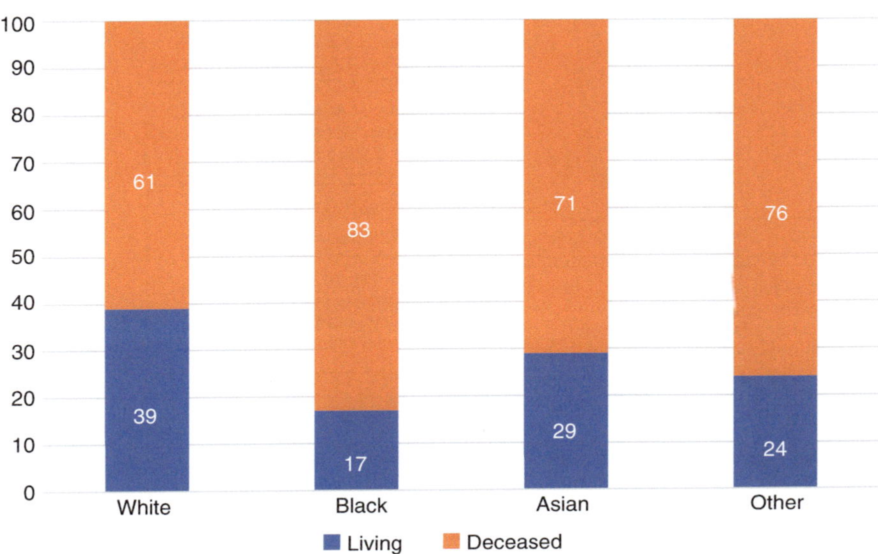

Fig. 1.3 Living vs. deceased donor kidney transplantation as a percentage of total transplants by race (United States, 2007–2016). (Produced using data from the 2018 USRDS Annual Data Report [21])

Primum Non Nocere: First, Do No Harm

Living organ donation seems to violate the Hippocratic Oath, an ethical standard that physicians abide by to do no harm to the patients that they care for. Living donors undergo a surgical procedure with no medical benefit for themselves. The practice of living organ donation is justified by the substantial benefit to the recipients and society, balanced by the minimal risks to the informed and consenting donor. Living donors may also derive personal benefit from donation, as the altruistic act provides psychological satisfaction in improving the life and well-being of their recipient who, in the majority of cases, are either genetically or emotionally related to the donor. In addition to this, the donor may be relieved of some burden of care if they were the recipient's primary caregiver prior to transplantation [59]. Posttransplant, recipients may be able to return to work which, in LDKT involving spouses, may alleviate financial burden for the donor as well.

There have been increasing efforts to better define and quantify donor risks in order to provide living donor candidates informed counseling to assist with patient-centered decision-making. Previous studies of living donor outcomes have been limited by single-center studies with small sample sizes and short observation periods, high proportion of donors lost to follow-up, insufficient power to estimate rare events, lack of appropriate control groups to define donation-attributable risk, and lack of donor diversity in race/ethnicity and comorbidities [60, 61]. Recent efforts

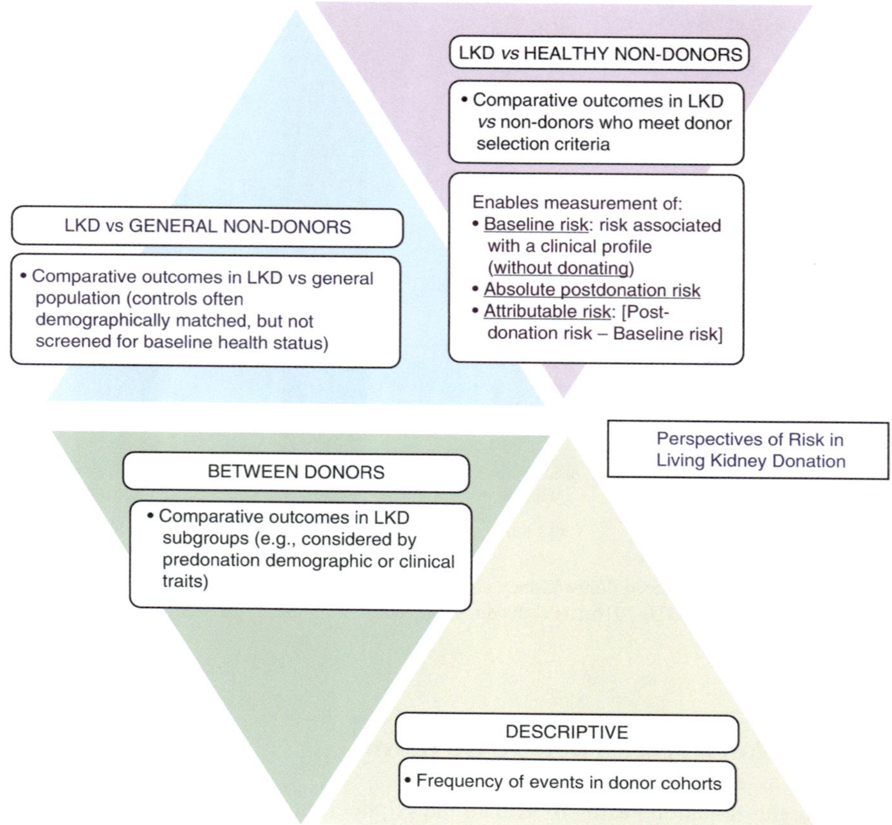

Fig. 1.4 Perspectives of risk in living kidney donation [74, 75]. (From Lentine et al. [74], S7–105)

have focused on developing better methodologies to improve understanding of risks associated with donation. These efforts include collaboration of multicentered cohorts [62, 63], novel linkages of national donor registries with other administrative healthcare databases to assess the incidence and outcomes of rare events [64–68], and the creation of healthy, non-donor control groups to estimate donation-attributable risks [61, 64, 69–73]. A clear understanding of the perspectives of risk in living kidney donation is needed to interpret observational studies assessing donor outcomes and provide a framework for donor candidates during the informed consent process (Fig. 1.4).

Risks to the Living Kidney Donor

Potential risks of living kidney donation to the donor include surgical, medical, psychological, and financial risks (Fig. 1.5) [61, 76]. These short- and long-term risks following living donor nephrectomy are discussed in further detail within their

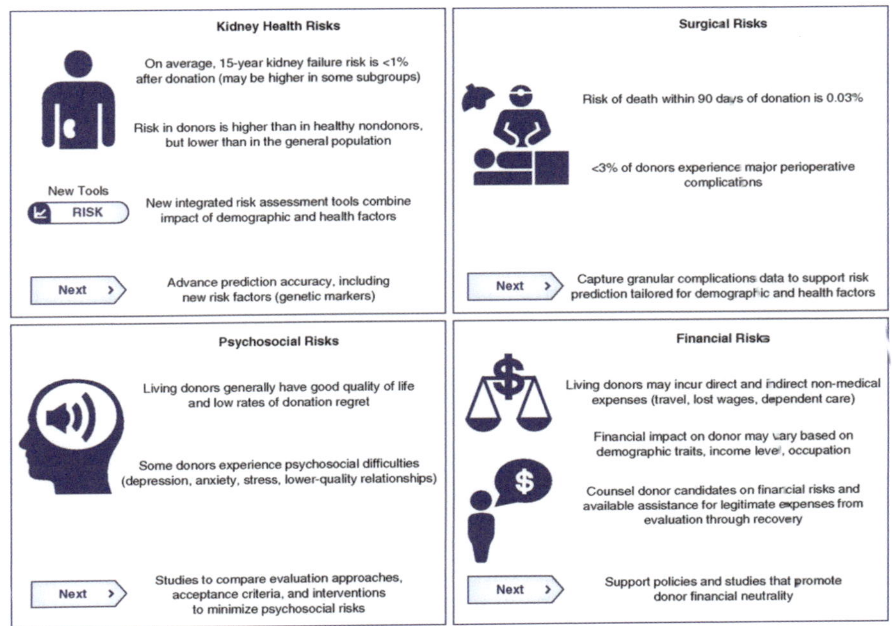

Fig. 1.5 Summary of medical, surgical, psychosocial, and financial risks to the living kidney donor with next steps for research and health policy. (From Lentine et al. [76])

respective sections. Briefly, the 90-day perioperative risk of mortality following living donor nephrectomy is estimated to be 3 per 10,000 (1 in 3000 or 0.03%) [77]. The risk of any perioperative complication ranges from 13% to 20% [67, 78, 79] and most commonly includes gastrointestinal (4%), bleeding (3%), respiratory (2%), and surgical/anesthesia-related injuries (2%) [67]. Major perioperative complications, defined by the Clavien grading system as level 4 or 5, are reported to affect <3% of donors [67, 78, 79]. A multicenter prospective cohort study of 1042 living kidney donors from 2004 to 2014 reported that 134 donors (13%) experienced 142 perioperative complications (55 intraoperative; 87 postoperative) [79]. Of these, 90% of all complications were considered minor; however, 1% of donors experienced at least one major complication. Perioperative complications did not seem to be influenced by donor characteristics, surgical experience, or center volume. There were no perioperative deaths in this study. A meta-analysis of 19 studies including 8098 living kidney donor reported that the pooled all-cause mortality was 3.8%, with ESKD-related deaths (0.3%) occurring at an average of 10 years following nephrectomy [80].

After living donor nephrectomy, there is compensatory hyperfiltration of the remaining kidney, such that the net reduction in GFR is between 25% and 40% [81–83]. The absolute 15-year risk of ESKD after live kidney nephrectomy is estimated to be <1% for most donors [76, 84–86]. This risk appears to be lower than the general population but may be higher compared to healthy, matched non-donors [85]. In certain subgroups of donors (e.g., older black men), this absolute 15-year risk may be higher [85, 87]. There are online risk assessment tools that integrate baseline characteristics to predict a donor candidate's risk of ESKD in the absence of donation and in the presence of donation (www.transplantmodels.com) [50, 88]. These tools can be used by healthcare professionals to provide living donor candidates information during the evaluation and informed consent process about their long-term risk of ESKD.

In addition to ESKD, compared to healthy, matched non-donor controls, there is evidence to suggest that living kidney donors are at higher risk of gestational hypertension or preeclampsia during pregnancy [71] and gout over their lifetime [64], whereas there appears to be no difference in the risk of acute kidney injury requiring dialysis [72], kidney stones requiring surgical intervention [70], gastrointestinal bleeding [73], or bone fractures [89].

From a psychosocial perspective, one systematic review found that the majority of donors scored high on health-related quality-of-life measurements, wherein psychosocial health was on average unchanged or even improved following donation [90]. As part of the donor evaluation process, candidates are assessed by various healthcare professionals, including social workers, psychologists, or psychiatrists. Donor candidates should be informed that a small number of donors may experience postdonation stress, anxiety, depression, or strained relationships with their recipient; however, even in rare circumstances when the recipient experiences a bad outcome, most donors do not regret their decision to donate [63].

As previously discussed, there are disparities in donation rates between low- and high-income populations [54]. The donation process may be associated with out-of-pocket expenses and loss of income for donor candidates as they proceed through the investigative laboratory and imaging tests; attend medical, surgical, and psychosocial appointments; and, if deemed acceptable, are admitted to hospital for the donor nephrectomy. Postdonation recovery requires time off from work or other responsibilities such as dependent care, the duration of which can vary with the type of occupation and associated physical demands. These out-of-pocket costs can include travel, parking, accommodations, child care, and lost productivity and may be significantly higher for donors who participate in national paired donation programs [91]. The costs of lost income or dependent care may not be remunerated. One Canadian study found that the median out-of-pocket costs for living kidney donors was $1254 Canadian dollars (CAD) and that for 25% of donors, the total cost (out-of-pocket and lost productivity) exceeded $5500 [92]. Policies should be implemented to aim for financial neutrality for living kidney donors, as for some, this may be a major barrier to proceeding with donation. Programs exist in many countries to reimburse donor candidates for their expenses, with the opportunity to further improve such programs [93]. In the United States, the Advancing American Kidney Health executive order recognized the importance of this issue by outlining plans to expand the scope of reimbursable expenses for living donors to include lost wages and childcare and eldercare expenses for those donors who lack other forms of financial support [94]. Living donor candidates should be counseled on the anticipated financial impact of the donation process and be made aware of any regional or national financial reimbursement programs [41].

In summary, while the medical, surgical, psychosocial, and financial risks following donor nephrectomy are low, donor care teams must have a comprehensive discussion of these risks with donor candidates. If the donor candidate's predicted risks are within the transplant program's boundaries of acceptable risk, then donor candidates who are appropriately informed of the potential risks and costs, along with any uncertainties, may make an autonomous decision whether (or not) to proceed with donation [95]. Living donor risk assessment and communication is discussed in detail in Chap. 12. Please also see Chap. 2 for detailed discussion of living donor informed consent.

Follow-Up Care of Living Kidney Donors

The favorable outcomes for donors are partly attributed to the rigorous screening and selection process. The 2017 Kidney Disease: Improving Global Outcomes (KDIGO) Clinical Practice Guideline on the Evaluation and Care of Living Kidney Donors also recommends that living kidney donors be followed at least annually after donation to monitor kidney health with blood pressure, serum creatinine, and albuminuria measurements, to promote healthy lifestyle choices, and to support psychosocial health and well-being [74]. The guideline highlights that the evaluation process should be regarded as the beginning of a long-term collaborative relationship between the donor and the transplant program. With better risk estimates, follow-up care has the added value of updating prior donors on emerging research and opportunities to mitigate complications based on individual risk assessments. The transplant community has an obligation to living donors to continue to seek and provide accurate risk estimates for donors and to support long-term health after donation by promoting healthy lifestyle, healthcare maintenance, and follow-up care.

Advances in the Field of Living Kidney Donation

In the last decade, there has been more research published in the field of living kidney donation than in the preceding 50 years. This highlights the growing body of work related to innovative strategies to increase rates of LDKT as well as a focus to better understand postdonation risks and benefits. The 2017 KDIGO Clinical Practice Guideline on the Evaluation and Care of Living Kidney Donors appointed working group members and an evidence review team to systematically review this literature to guide the development of evidence-based recommendations, whenever possible [74]. Unfortunately, the majority (>95%) of the recommendations were ungraded due to the lack of available evidence highlighting the ongoing need for high-quality research as well as the difficulty in subjecting some types of comparisons to highest-quality (e.g., randomized) study.

Surgical Approaches for Donor Nephrectomy

Overall, the chosen surgical approach to donor nephrectomy should be based on the donor's history (e.g., previous abdominal surgeries), physical examination (e.g., body mass index), renal anatomy (e.g., number of renal arteries and veins), surgical experience, and center availability.

Living donor nephrectomies were traditionally performed through an open flank incision, with or without a rib resection. The potential for perioperative or chronic pain, morbidity, and scarring or cosmetic deformation associated with open surgery may be a deterrent for some living donor candidates. In addition to this, the prolonged convalescent period with open surgery may lead to added financial burden to the donor with respect to lost wages and delayed return to dependent care responsibilities. One area that has advanced the field of living kidney donation is minimally invasive surgery. The first reported laparoscopic living donor nephrectomy was published by Ratner et al. in 1995, in which the donor experienced minimal discomfort and was discharged home on the first postoperative day [96]. Since then, laparoscopic donor nephrectomy has replaced the open technique as the standard of care for donor nephrectomy in the United States, accounting for more than 90% of all living donor nephrectomies performed [9].

A Cochrane review in 2011 of 6 studies that randomized 596 living donors to either laparoscopic or open donor nephrectomies found that the laparoscopic technique was associated with reduced analgesia use, shorter hospital stay, and faster return to normal physical functioning [97]. The conversion rate from laparoscopic to open nephrectomy ranged from 1% to 8% [97]. Kidneys extracted using the laparoscopic technique were exposed to longer warm ischemia time (mean difference range, -1.5 to -6.8 minutes) and longer overall surgery duration (range, 3 to 4 hours vs. 2 to 3 hours) compared to the open technique. There was no significant difference between laparoscopic and open techniques with respect to perioperative complications reoperations, early graft loss, delayed graft function, acute rejection, ureteric complications, or graft loss at 1 year [97].

An updated meta-analysis in 2013 found similar results between laparoscopic and open techniques and also compared outcomes between hand-assisted and standard laparoscopic donor nephrectomy techniques [98]. Hand-assisted laparoscopic nephrectomy involves the addition of port incision sites to allow surgeons to introduce their hands into the operative field. The authors found that hand-assisted laparoscopic donor nephrectomy was associated with a shorter warm ischemia time (mean difference, -1.02 minutes; 95% CI, -1.44 to -0.59) but a longer hospital stay (mean difference, 0.33 days; 95% CI, 0.10 to 0.56) than the standard laparoscopic donor nephrectomy approach [98]. Otherwise, operative duration (mean difference, -24.55 minutes; 95% CI, -50.8 to 1.71), intraoperative blood loss (mean difference, -20.65 mL; 95% CI, -43.88 to 2.57), and postoperative complications (odds ratio,

0.62; 95% CI, 0.27 to 1.39) were not significantly different between the two laparoscopic approaches [98].

In 2000, the da Vinci Surgical System (Intuitive Surgical, Inc.) was approved by the US Food and Drug Administration. Since then, advances in robotic systems for laparoscopic surgery have added three-dimensional vision to the traditional standard laparoscopic procedures by combining robotics and computer imaging [99]. In the non-donor population, the use of robotic-assisted laparoscopic radical nephrectomy for renal masses increased from 1.5% in 2003 to 27.0% in 2015 [100]. Compared to standard laparoscopic radical nephrectomies, there were no significant differences in the incidence of postoperative complications [100]. Robotic-assisted radical nephrectomies were associated with a higher incidence of prolonged (>4 hours) operative time (46.3% vs. 25.8%; risk difference, 20.5%; 95% CI, 14.2% to 26.8%) and a higher mean 90-day hospital cost ($19,530 USD vs. $16,851 USD; difference, $2678; 95% CI, $838 to $4519) [100].

In 2002, Horgan et al. were the first to describe a series of 12 living donors who had nephrectomies performed between 2000 and 2001 using the robotic-assisted approach [99]. Since then, robotic-assisted laparoscopic donor nephrectomies have been reported to be safe for living kidney donors and their recipients. The benefits of robotic-assisted nephrectomy include higher dissection facility, easier suturing and knotting, more accurate graft preservation, faster learning curve for surgeons, and higher surgeon comfort compared to standard laparoscopic approaches [101]. A systematic review of 18 studies involving 910 robotic-assisted laparoscopic donor nephrectomies from 2000 to 2018 found that the average operative time ranged from 139 to 306 minutes, the average warm ischemia time ranged from <1.5 to 5.8 minutes, and the average hospital stay ranged from 1.0 to 5.8 days [102]. Intraoperative complications ranged from 0% to 6.7%, early (<30 days) postoperative complications ranged from 0% to 15.7%, and the average estimated blood loss ranged from 30 to 146 mL [102]. The conversion rate to open nephrectomy ranged from 0% to 5% [102]. While potentially useful in some cases, the additional training required for use of the robotic system and associated costs, without established outcome advantages and possible risks, have limited its expansion.

Surgical advances in living donor nephrectomy aim to increase the number of LDKT by shortening donor recovery time and hospital stay, reducing perioperative pain, and improving the patient experience, including better cosmetic results [103]. Many living donors report that the availability of laparoscopic donor nephrectomy greatly influenced their decision to proceed with donation [103]. As a result, some transplant centers in the United States have seen upwards of an ~200% increase in the LDKT since the introduction of laparoscopic donor nephrectomy [103]. Please see Chap. 13 for detailed discussion of living donor nephrectomy approaches, outcomes, and innovations.

Kidney Paired Donation

Initially, LDKT were performed between genetically identical twins, confirmed through skin grafting since HLA typing did not exist at that time [104]. For non-identical/fraternal twins or other genetically related pairs, the recipient required whole-body irradiation and cytotoxic drugs to suppress the immune system to prevent rejection [104]. Advances in the field of transplantation immunology have led to the development of more potent and tolerable immunosuppression to allow LDKT from unrelated or emotionally related donors with essentially equivalent outcomes to genetically related donors [31, 105, 106].

Biologically incompatible pairs can be the result of either ABO blood type incompatibility or preformed donor-specific antibodies in the recipient. Approximately one-third of patients with a willing and healthy potential donor are unable to receive a transplant due to biologic incompatibility [107]. For highly sensitized patients who want to be transplanted, desensitization strategies can include removing or reducing the donor-specific antibodies through plasmapheresis, intravenous immunoglobulin, and anti-CD20 antibodies [108]. These strategies are associated with an increased risk of morbidity to the recipient and increased cost to the healthcare system when compared to compatible transplants but are still beneficial when compared to the cost and outcomes of long-term chronic dialysis treatments [107, 108].

Kidney paired donation programs allow recipients with an incompatible donor to have better access to LDKT, by exchanging donors to create acceptable compatible combinations. By increasing the donor pool, the likelihood of finding a successful match through kidney paired donation programs is increased. These programs are associated with better outcomes for the recipient and lower healthcare costs, as compatible LDKT may obviate the need for desensitization treatments [108]. In 2005, Segev et al. conducted a simulated model comparing a national kidney paired donation program to the local/regional first-accept matching scheme that was used at the time at participating centers. They reported that a national paired donation program would result in more transplants (47.7% vs. 42.0%), better HLA concordance (3.0 vs. 4.5 mismatched antigens), more grafts surviving at 5 years (34.9% vs. 28.7%), a reduction in the number of pairs required to travel (2.9% vs. 18.4%), and a savings of as much as $750 million USD for the healthcare system [109]. Other potential advantages of receiving a kidney through a paired donation program include finding a younger donor for a younger recipient or finding a better size match [107].

In its simplest form (two-way exchange), an incompatible pair can exchange kidneys with another incompatible pair so that both recipients receive compatible kidneys from an unrelated donor (Fig. 1.6) [110]. More complicated, longer chains can be formed using computer-based algorithms to help with matching compatible pairs from various geographical regions; however, these are more logistically complicated and require more resources to conduct. In a closed domino chain, an anonymous nondirected donor initiates a chain for incompatible pairs wherein the donor for the last recipient of the chain donates a kidney to a recipient on the deceased

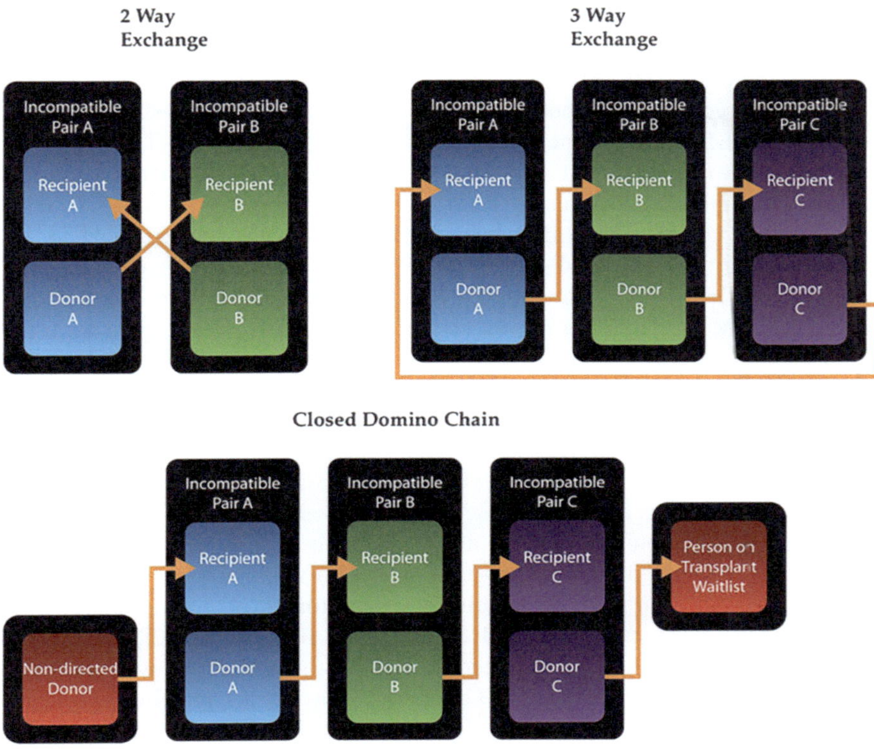

Fig. 1.6 Types of living donor exchange. (From Malik and Cole [110])

donor waiting list (Fig. 1.6) [110]. These types of domino exchanges are impactful strategies to increase the number of LDKT.

Although the concept of kidney paired donation was initially proposed in 1986 by Felix Rapaport [111], it was only in 2005 when the Netherlands became the first country to describe their national kidney paired donation registry [112]. Since then, many national kidney paired donation programs have been established worldwide, including the United States, Canada, France, the United Kingdom, Australia, Spain, and South Korea [110, 113]. In the United States, LDKT through kidney paired donation programs has been increasing over the last decade [9, 107]. In Canada, the kidney paired donation program was established in 2008 and expanded nationwide by 2010 [114]. By 2013, the program had facilitated 240 kidney transplants, including 10% of recipients who were considered highly sensitized (calculated panel-reactive antibody ≥97%) [114]. There have also been reports of international kidney paired donation transplants, including a ten-way domino transplant between the United States and Canada [113]. International cooperation and organ sharing can further increase the potential donor pool and can be logistically tenable between countries with shared border and language and short travel distances [113, 115].

There have been concerns raised about shipping living donor kidneys from paired donation programs and the association between prolonged cold ischemia time and increased risk of delayed graft function. One study from the United States compared outcomes between 1267 shipped and 205 non-shipped living donor kidneys from the kidney paired donation program [116]. They reported that there was no significant association between cold ischemia time and all-cause graft failure (adjusted hazard ratio, aHR, 1.01; 95% CI, 0.98–1.04; $p = 0.4$), death-censored graft failure (aHR, 1.02; 95% CI, 0.98–1.06; $p = 0.4$), or mortality (aHR, 1.00; 95% CI, 0.96–1.04; $p > 0.9$) [116]. This suggests that shipping living donor kidneys through the kidney paired donation program is not associated with an increased risk to patient or graft survival, despite an increase in the cold ischemia time. One major benefit of shipping living donor kidneys is eliminating the need for the donor (and their companion support) to travel to their matched recipient's transplant center, thus reducing donor-incurred costs and potentially eliminating a barrier to participating in paired donation programs [117].

Lastly, there has been interest in including ABO- and HLA-compatible pairs in kidney paired donation programs to further increase LDKT. Surveys of directed donors and recipients of compatible pairs suggest a willingness to participate in kidney paired donation programs if reimbursement for travel and lost wages were provided or if their recipient derived added benefit from the LDKT, such as the potential for a younger donor or better HLA match; however, this was not at the expense of delaying the LDKT [118]. One study estimated that allowing compatible pairs to participate in kidney paired donation programs could nearly double the match rate for incompatible pairs (e.g., 28.2% to 64.5% for single-center programs, 37.4% to 75.4% for national programs) [119].

Further strategies have been proposed to increase compatible pairs in kidney paired donation programs. An example is the creation of vouchers for future kidney transplant recipients. This would allow a donor to donate at a convenient time to a paired donation chain in exchange for a voucher for their intended recipient to redeem to receive a kidney, if and when needed, from another living donor at the end of a future paired donation chain [120]. This would be beneficial for pairs who are incompatible by time (i.e., "chronological incompatibility"), such as older donor candidates who have younger intended recipients, who may not be ready to receive a kidney at the time their loved one is ready to donate. The approach could also increase the opportunity for matches in that the voucher donors function similar to nondirected anonymous donors to trigger chains of transplants [117]. Another example is the reciprocity-based approach wherein the recipient of a compatible pair in a paired donation chain receives priority for a deceased donor transplant in the event that their primary LDKT fails [121]. Thus, kidney paired donation programs have increased access to LDKT for recipients who are incompatible with their willing, healthy potential donors, and there are innovative efforts to maximize LDKT through kidney paired donation programs. Please see Chap. 10 for detailed discussion of compatibility, paired donation, and incompatible living donor transplantation.

Conclusion

With the increasing burden of kidney failure worldwide, LDKT offers ESKD patients the optimal treatment to improve survival and quality of life at a reduced cost to the healthcare system. Living kidney donors and their recipients should be provided with clear information on the risks and benefits of living kidney donation and LDKT, reflective of the current state of evidence. Ongoing strategies are being developed and implemented to increase access to LDKT, particularly for those with racial/ethnic, socioeconomic, or geographic disparities in access to this optimal form of transplantation.

References

1. Kidney Disease: Improving Global Outcomes (KDIGO) CKD-MBD Work Group. KDIGO clinical practice guideline for the diagnosis, evaluation, prevention, and treatment of Chronic Kidney Disease-Mineral and Bone Disorder (CKD-MBD). Kidney Int Suppl. 2009;113:S1–130. https://doi.org/10.1038/ki.2009.188.
2. Hill N, Fatoba S, Oke J, Hirst J, O'Callaghan C, Lasserson D, et al. Global prevalence of chronic kidney disease – a systematic review and meta-analysis. PLoS One. 2016;11(7):e0158765. https://doi.org/10.1371/journal.pone.0158765.
3. Qaseem A, Hopkins RH, Sweet DE, Starkey M, Shekelle P, Clinical Guidelines Committee of the American College of Physicians. Screening, monitoring, and treatment of stage 1 to 3 chronic kidney disease: a clinical practice guideline from the American College of Physicians. Ann Intern Med. 2013;159(12):835–47. https://doi.org/10.7326/0003-4819-159-12-201312170-00726.
4. Luyckx VA, Tonelli M, Stanifer JW. The global burden of kidney disease and the sustainable development goals. Bull World Health Organ. 2018;96(6):414–422C. https://doi.org/10.2471/BLT.17.206441.
5. Ontario Renal Network. Ontario 2016 CKD System Atlas: Trends in kidney disease and care. Toronto: Ontario Renal Network; 2016. Available at: https://www.ccohealth.ca/en/access-data. Accessed: 7 Sept 2020.
6. Canadian Institute for Health Information. Treatment of End-Stage Organ Failure in Canada, Canadian Organ Replacement Register (CORR), 2009 to 2018: End-Stage Kidney Disease and Kidney Transplants – Data Tables. Available at: https://www.cihi.ca/en/access-data-and-reports. Accessed: 7 Sept 2020..
7. GBD 2015 Mortality and Causes of Death Collaborators. Global, regional, and national life expectancy, all-cause mortality, and cause-specific mortality for 249 causes of death, 1980–2015: a systematic analysis for the Global Burden of Disease Study 2015. Lancet. 2016;388(10053):1459–544. https://doi.org/10.1016/S0140-6736(16)31012-1
8. Stevens PE, Levin A. Evaluation and management of chronic kidney disease: synopsis of the kidney disease: improving global outcomes 2012 clinical practice guideline. Ann Intern Med. 2013;158(11):825–30. https://doi.org/10.7326/0003-4819-158-11-201306040-00007.
9. Hart A, Lentine KL, Smith JM, Miller JM, Skeans MA, Prentice M, et al. OPTN/SRTR 2019 Annual Data Report: Kidney. Am J Transplant. 2021;21(Suppl 2):21–137. https://doi.org/10.1111/ajt.16502.
10. Abramowicz D, Hazzan M, Maggiore U, Peruzzi L, Cochat P, Oberbauer R, et al. Does pre-emptive transplantation versus post start of dialysis transplantation with a kidney from a living donor improve outcomes after transplantation? A systematic literature review and position statement by the Descartes Working Group and ERBP. Nephrol Dial Transplant. 2016;31(5):691–7. https://doi.org/10.1093/ndt/gfv378.

11. Wolfe RA, Ashby VB, Milford EL, Ojo AO, Ettenger RE, Agodoa LY, et al. Comparison of mortality in all patients on dialysis, patients on dialysis awaiting transplantation, and recipients of a first cadaveric transplant. N Engl J Med. 1999;341(23):1725–30. https://doi. org/10.1056/NEJM199912023412303.

12. Tonelli M, Wiebe N, Knoll G, Bello A, Browne S, Jadhav D, et al. Systematic review: kidney transplantation compared with dialysis in clinically relevant outcomes. Am J Transplant. 2011;11(10):2093–109. https://doi.org/10.1111/j.1600-6143.2011.03686.x.

13. Rabbat CG, Thorpe KE, Russell JD, Churchill DN. Comparison of mortality risk for dialysis patients and cadaveric first renal transplant recipients in Ontario, Canada. J Am Soc Nephrol. 2000;11(5):917–22. http://www.ncbi.nlm.nih.gov/pubmed/10770970.

14. Medin C, Elinder CG, Hylander B, Blom B, Wilczek H. Survival of patients who have been on a waiting list for renal transplantation. Nephrol Dial Transplant. 2000;15(5):701–4. https:// doi.org/10.1093/ndt/15.5.701.

15. Cecka JM. Kidney transplantation in the United States. Clin Transpl. 2008:1–18. http://www. ncbi.nlm.nih.gov/pubmed/19711510.

16. Axelrod DA, Schnitzler MA, Xiao H, Irish W, Tuttle-Newhall E, Chang SH, et al. An economic assessment of contemporary kidney transplant practice. Am J Transplant. 2018;18(5):1168–76. https://doi.org/10.1111/ajt.14702.

17. Russell JD, Beecroft ML, Ludwin D, Churchill DN. The quality of life in renal transplantation - a prospective study. Transplantation. 1992;54(4):656–60. https://doi. org/10.1097/00007890-199210000-00018.

18. Laupacis A, Keown P, Pus N, Krueger H, Ferguson B, Wong C, et al. A study of the quality of life and cost-utility of renal transplantation. Kidney Int. 1996;50(1):235–42. https://doi. org/10.1038/ki.1996.307.

19. Ozcan H, Yucel A, Avşar UZ, Cankaya E, Yucel N, Gözübüyük H, et al. Kidney transplantation is superior to hemodialysis and peritoneal dialysis in terms of cognitive function, anxiety, and depression symptoms in chronic kidney disease. Transplant Proc. 2015;47(5):1348–51. https://doi.org/10.1016/j.transproceed.2015.04.032.

20. Whiting JF, Kiberd B, Kalo Z, Keown P, Roels L, Kjerulf M. Cost-effectiveness of organ donation: evaluating investment into donor action and other donor initiatives. Am J Transplant. 2004;4(4):569–73. https://doi.org/10.1111/j.1600-6143.2004.00373.x.

21. United States Renal Data System (USRDS). 2018 USRDS Annual Data Report: Epidemiology of kidney disease in the United States. End-stage Renal Disease (ESRD) in the United States. Chapter 6: Transplantation. National Institutes of Health, National Institute of Diabetes and Digestive and Kidney Diseases, Bethesda. Available at: https://www.usrds.org/annual-data-report/. Accessed: 7 Sept 2020.

22. Nemati E, Einollahi B, Lesan Pezeshki M, Porfarziani V, Fattahi MR. Does kidney transplantation with deceased or living donor affect graft survival? Nephrourol Mon. 2014;6(4):e12182. https://doi.org/10.5812/numonthly.12182.

23. Gozdowska J, Zatorski M, Torchalla P, Białek Ł, Bojanowska A, Tomaszek A, et al. Living-donor versus deceased-donor kidney transplantation: comparison of psychosocial consequences for recipients. Transplant Proc. 2016;48(5):1498–505. https://doi.org/10.1016/j. transproceed.2016.01.075.

24. Petrini C. Preemptive kidney transplantation: an ethical challenge for organ allocation policies. Clin Ter. 2017;168(3):e192–3. https://doi.org/10.7417/T.2017.2004.

25. Jay CL, Dean PG, Helmick RA, Stegall MD. Reassessing preemptive kidney transplantation in the United States: are we making progress? Transplantation. 2016;100(5):1120–7. https:// doi.org/10.1097/TP.0000000000000944.

26. Smith CR, Woodward RS, Cohen DS, Singer GG, Brennan DC, Lowell JA, et al. Cadaveric versus living donor kidney transplantation: a Medicare payment analysis. Transplantation. 2000;69(2):311–4. https://doi.org/10.1097/00007890-200001270-00020.

27. Saran R, Robinson B, Abbott KC, Agodoa LYC, Bragg-Gresham J, Balkrishnan R, et al. US renal data system 2018 annual data report: epidemiology of kidney disease in the United States. Am J Kidney Dis. 2019;73(3):A7–8. https://doi.org/10.1053/j.ajkd.2019.01.001.

28. Guild WR, Harrison JH, Merrill JP, Murray J. Successful homotransplantation of the kidney in an identical twin. Trans Am Clin Climatol Assoc. 1956;67:167–73. http://www.ncbi.nlm.nih.gov/pubmed/13360847.
29. Sade RM. Transplantation at 100 years: Alexis Carrel, Pioneer Surgeon. Ann Thorac Surg. 2005;80(6):2415–8. https://doi.org/10.1016/j.athoracsur.2005.08.074.
30. Murray JE. The first successful organ transplants in man. J Am Coll Surg. 2005;200(1):5–9. https://doi.org/10.1016/j.jamcollsurg.2004.09.033.
31. Starzl TE, Barker C. The origin of clinical organ transplantation revisited. JAMA. 2009;301(19):2041–3. https://doi.org/10.1001/jama.2009.644.
32. World Health Organization (WHO)- Organización Nacional de Trasplantes (ONT). Global Observatory on Donation and Transplantation (GODT). Available at: http://www.transplant-observatory.org/. Accessed: 7 Sept 2020.
33. Kuo PC, Johnson LB. Laparoscopic donor nephrectomy increases the supply of living donor kidneys: a center-specific microeconomic analysis. Transplantation. 2000;69(10):2211–3. https://doi.org/10.1097/00007890-200005270-00047.
34. Bäcker H, Piros L, Langer RM. Increasing living donor kidney transplantation numbers in Budapest. Transplant Proc. 2013;45(10):3678–81. https://doi.org/10.1016/j.transproceed.2013.10.001.
35. Ghods AJ, Savaj S. Iranian model of paid and regulated living-unrelated kidney donation. Clin J Am Soc Nephrol. 2006;1(6):1136–45. https://doi.org/10.2215/CJN.00700206.
36. Ghahramani N. Paid living donation and growth of deceased donor programs. Transplantation. 2016;100(6):1165–9. https://doi.org/10.1097/TP.0000000000001164.
37. Hanson CS, Chadban SJ, Chapman JR, Craig JC, Wong G, Tong A. Nephrologists' perspectives on recipient eligibility and access to living kidney donor transplantation. Transplantation. 2016;100(4):943–53. https://doi.org/10.1097/TP.0000000000000921.
38. Lam NN, Lentine KL, Garg AX. Renal and cardiac assessment of living kidney donor candidates. Nat Rev Nephrol. 2017;13(7):420–8. https://doi.org/10.1038/nrneph.2017.43.
39. Graham JM, Courtney AE. The adoption of a one-day donor assessment model in a living kidney donor transplant program: a quality improvement project. Am J Kidney Dis. 2018;71(2):209–15. https://doi.org/10.1053/j.ajkd.2017.07.013.
40. Habbous S, Woo J, Lam NN, Lentine KL, Cooper M, Reich M, et al. The efficiency of evaluating candidates for living kidney donation. Transplant Direct. 2018;4(10):e394. https://doi.org/10.1097/TXD.0000000000000833.
41. Tushla L, Rudow DL, Milton J, Rodrigue JR, Schold JD, Hays R, et al. Living-donor kidney transplantation: reducing financial barriers to live kidney donation–recommendations from a consensus conference. Clin J Am Soc Nephrol. 2015;10(9):1696–702. https://doi.org/10.1097/TXD.00000000000083310.2215/CJN.01000115.
42. Boyarsky BJ, Massie AB, Alejo JL, Van Arendonk KJ, Wildonger S, Garonzik-Wang JM, et al. Experiences obtaining insurance after live kidney donation. Am J Transplant. 2014;14(9):2168–72. https://doi.org/10.1111/ajt.12819.
43. Rodrigue JR, LaPointe Rudow D, Hays R, American Society of Transplantation. Living donor kidney transplantation: best practices in live kidney donation—recommendations from a consensus conference. Clin J Am Soc Nephrol. 2015;10(9):1656–7. https://doi.org/10.2215/CJN.00800115.
44. Waterman AD, Morgievich M, Cohen DJ, Butt Z, Chakkera HA, Lindower C, et al. Living donor kidney transplantation: improving education outside of transplant centers about live donor transplantation-recommendations from a consensus conference. Clin J Am Soc Nephrol. 2015;10(9):1659–69. https://doi.org/10.2215/CJN.00950115.
45. Tan JC, Gordon EJ, Dew MA, LaPointe Rudow D, Steiner RW, Woodle ES, et al. Living donor kidney transplantation: facilitating education about live kidney donation-recommendations from a consensus conference. Clin J Am Soc Nephrol. 2015;10(9):1670–7. https://doi.org/10.2215/CJN.01030115.
46. Moore DR, Serur D, Rudow DL, Rodrigue JR, Hays R, Cooper M, et al. Living donor kidney transplantation: improving efficiencies in live kidney donor evaluation – recommendations

from a consensus conference. Clin J Am Soc Nephrol. 2015;10(9):1678–86. https://doi.org/10.2215/CJN.01040115.

47. Rodrigue JR, Kazley AS, Mandelbrot DA, Hays R, LaPointe Rudow D, Baliga P. Living donor kidney transplantation: overcoming disparities in live kidney donation in the US – recommendations from a consensus conference. Clin J Am Soc Nephrol. 2015;10(9):1687–95. https://doi.org/10.2215/CJN.00700115.

48. Muzaale AD, Massie AB, Wang MC, Montgomery RA, McBride MA, Wainright JL, et al. Risk of end-stage renal disease following live kidney donation. JAMA. 2014;311(6):579–8. https://doi.org/10.1001/jama.2013.285141.

49. Steiner RW. "Normal for now" or "at future risk": a double standard for selecting young and older living kidney donors. Am J Transplant. 2010;10(4):737–41. https://doi.org/10.1111/j.1600-6143.2010.03023.x.

50. Delanaye P, Glassock RJ, Grams ME, Sang Y, Levey AS, Matsushita K, et al. Kidney-failure risk projection for the living kidney-donor candidate. N Engl J Med. 2016;374(5):411–21. https://doi.org/10.1056/NEJMoa1510491.

51. Purnell TS, Xu P, Leca N, Hall YN. Racial differences in determinants of live donor kidney transplantation in the United States. Am J Transplant. 2013;13(6):1557–65. https://doi.org/10.1111/ajt.12258.

52. Mostafazadeh-Bora M, Zarghami A. The crucial role of cultural and religious beliefs on organ transplantation. Int J organ Transplant Med. 2017;8(1):54. http://www.ncbi.nlm.nih.gov/pubmed/28299030.

53. Taler SJ, Messersmith EE, Leichtman AB, Gillespie BW, Kew CE, Stegall MD, et al. Demographic, metabolic, and blood pressure characteristics of living kidney donors spanning five decades. Am J Transplant. 2013;13(2):390–8. https://doi.org/10.1111/j.1600-6143.2012.04321.x.

54. Gill J, Dong J, Gill J. Population income and longitudinal trends in living kidney donation in the United States. J Am Soc Nephrol. 2015;26(1):201–7. https://doi.org/10.1681/ASN.2014010113.

55. Gill J, Joffres Y, Rose C, Lesage J, Landsberg D, Kadatz M, et al. The change in living kidney donation in women and men in the United States (2005-2015): a population-based analysis. J Am Soc Nephrol. 2018;29(4):1301–8. https://doi.org/10.1681/ASN.2017111160.

56. Gore JL, Danovitch GM, Litwin MS, Pham PTT, Singer JS. Disparities in the utilization of live donor renal transplantation. Am J Transplant. 2009;9(5):1124–33. https://doi.org/10.1111/j.1600-6143.2009.02620.x.

57. Mucsi I, Bansal A, Famure O, Li Y, Mitchell M, Waterman AD, et al. Ethnic background is a potential barrier to living donor kidney transplantation in Canada. Transplantation. 2017;101(4):e142–51. https://doi.org/10.1097/TP.0000000000001658.

58. Purnell TS, Luo X, Cooper LA, Massie AB, Kucirka LM, Henderson ML, et al. Association of race and ethnicity with live donor kidney transplantation in the United States from 1995 to 2014. JAMA. 2018;319(1):49. https://doi.org/10.1001/jama.2017.19152.

59. Van Pilsum Rasmussen SE, Henderson ML, Kahn J, Segev D. Considering tangible benefit for interdependent donors: extending a risk-benefit framework in donor selection. Am J Transplant. 2017;17(10):2567–71. https://doi.org/10.1111/ajt.14319.

60. Ommen ES, LaPointe Rudow D, Medapalli RK, Schröppel B, Murphy B. When good intentions are not enough: obtaining follow-up data in living kidney donors. Am J Transplant. 2011;11:2575–81. https://doi.org/10.1111/j.1600-6143.2011.03815.x.

61. Lam NN, Lentine KL, Levey AS, Kasiske BL, Garg AX. Long-term medical risks to the living kidney donor. Nat Rev Nephrol. 2015;11(7):411–9. https://doi.org/10.1038/nrneph.2015.58.

62. Jowsey SG, Jacobs C, Gross CR, Hong BA, Messersmith EE, Gillespie BW, et al. Emotional well-being of living kidney donors: findings from the RELIVE study. Am J Transplant. 2014;14(11):2535–44. https://doi.org/10.1111/ajt.12906.

63. Clemens K, Boudville N, Dew MA, Geddes C, Gill JS, Jassal V, et al. The long-term quality of life of living kidney donors: a multicenter cohort study. Am J Transplant. 2011;11(3):463–9. https://doi.org/10.1111/j.1600-6143.2010.03424.x.

64. Lam NN, McArthur E, Kim SJ, Prasad GVR, Lentine KL, Reese PP, et al. Gout after living kidney donation: a matched cohort study. Am J Kidney Dis. 2015;65(6):925–32. https://doi.org/10.1053/j.ajkd.2015.01.017.
65. Lentine KL, Koraishy FM, Sarabu N, Naik AS, Lam NN, Garg AX, et al. Associations of obesity with antidiabetic medication use after living kidney donation: an analysis of linked national registry and pharmacy fill records. Clin Transpl. 2019;33(10):e13696. https://doi.org/10.1111/ctr.13696.
66. Lam NN, Garg AX, Segev DL, Schnitzler MA, Xiao H, Axelrod D, et al. Gout after living kidney donation: correlations with demographic traits and renal complications. Am J Nephrol. 2015;41(3):231–40. https://doi.org/10.1159/000381291.
67. Lentine KL, Lam NN, Axelrod D, Schnitzler MA, Garg AX, Xiao H, et al. Perioperative complications after living kidney donation: a national study. Am J Transplant. 2016;16(6):1848–57. https://doi.org/10.1111/ajt.13687.
68. Lentine KL, Schnitzler MA, Xiao H, Axelrod D, Davis CL, McCabe M, et al. Depression diagnoses after living kidney donation: linking U.S. registry data and administrative claims. Transplantation. 2012;94(1):77–83. https://doi.org/10.1097/TP.0b013e318253f1bc.
69. Garg AX, Meirambayeva A, Huang A, Kim J, Prasad GVR, Knoll G, et al. Cardiovascular disease in kidney donors: matched cohort study. BMJ. 2012;344:e1203. https://doi.org/10.1136/bmj.e1203.
70. Thomas SM, Lam NN, Welk BK, Nguan C, Huang A, Nash DM, et al. Risk of kidney stones with surgical intervention in living kidney donors. Am J Transplant. 2013;13(11):2935–44. https://doi.org/10.1111/ajt.12446.
71. Garg AX, Nevis IF, McArthur E, Sontrop JM, Koval JJ, Lam NN, et al. Gestational hypertension and preeclampsia in living kidney donors. New Engl J Med. 2015;372(2):124–33. https://doi.org/10.1056/NEJMoa1408932.
72. Lam N, Huang A, Feldman LS, Gill JS, Karpinski M, Kim J, et al. Acute dialysis risk in living kidney donors. Nephrol Dial Transplant. 2012;27(8):3291–5. https://doi.org/10.1093/ndt/gfr802.
73. Thomas SM, Lam NN, Huang A, Nash DM, Prasad GV, Knoll GA, et al. Risk of serious gastrointestinal bleeding in living kidney donors. Clin Transpl. 2014;28(5):530–9. https://doi.org/10.1111/ctr.12344.
74. Lentine KL, Kasiske BL, Levey AS, Adams PL, Alberú J, Bakr MA, et al. KDIGO Clinical Practice Guideline on the Evaluation and Care of Living Kidney Donors. Transplantation. 2017;101(8):S1–109. https://doi.org/10.1097/TP.0000000000001769.
75. Lentine KL, Segev DL. Understanding and communicating medical risks for living kidney donors: a matter of perspective. J Am Soc Nephrol. 2017;28(1):12–24. https://doi.org/10.1681/ASN.2016050571.
76. Lentine KL, Lam NN, Segev DL. Risks of living kidney donation: current state of knowledge on outcomes important to donors. Clin J Am Soc Nephrol. 2019;14(4):597–608. https://doi.org/10.2215/CJN.11220918.
77. Segev DL, Muzaale AD, Caffo BS, Mehta SH, Singer AL, Taranto SE, et al. Perioperative mortality and long-term survival following live kidney donation. JAMA. 2010;303(10):959–66. https://doi.org/10.1001/jama.2010.237.
78. Mjøen G, Øyen O, Holdaas H, Midtvedt K, Line PD. Morbidity and mortality in 1022 consecutive living donor nephrectomies: benefits of a living donor registry. Transplantation. 2009;88(11):1273–9. https://doi.org/10.1097/TP.0b013e3181bb44fd.
79. Garcia-Ochoa C, Feldman LS, Nguan C, Monroy-Cuadros M, Arnold J, Boudville N, et al. Perioperative complications during living donor nephrectomy: results from a multicenter cohort study. Can J Kidney Heal Dis. 2019;6:1–14. https://doi.org/10.1177/2054358119857718.
80. Li SS, Huang YM, Wang M, Shen J, Lin BJ, Sui Y, et al. A meta-analysis of renal outcomes in living kidney donors. Medicine (Baltimore). 2016;95(24):e384. https://doi.org/10.1097/MD.0000000000003847.
81. Pabico RC, McKenna BA, Freeman RB. Renal function before and after unilateral nephrectomy in renal donors. Kidney Int. 1975;8(3):166–75. https://doi.org/10.1038/ki.1975.96.

82. Kasiske BL, Anderson-Haag T, Ibrahim HN, Pesavento TE, Weir MR, Nogueira JM, et al. A prospective controlled study of kidney donors: baseline and 6-month follow-up. Am J Kidney Dis. 2013;62(3):577–86. https://doi.org/10.1053/j.ajkd.2013.01.027.
83. Garg AX, Muirhead N, Knoll G, Yang RC, Prasad GVR, Thiessen-Philbrook H, et al. Proteinuria and reduced kidney function in living kidney donors: a systematic review, meta-analysis, and meta-regression. Kidney Int. 2006;70(10):1801–10. https://doi.org/10.1038/sj.ki.5001819.
84. Mjøen G, Hallan S, Hartmann A, Foss A, Midtvedt K, Øyen O, et al. Long-term risks for kidney donors. Kidney Int. 2014;86(1):162–7. https://doi.org/10.1038/ki.2013.460.
85. Massie AB, Muzaale AD, Segev DL. Outcomes after kidney donation. JAMA. 2014;312(1):94–5. https://doi.org/10.1001/jama.2014.6120.
86. Lam NN, Lentine KL, Garg AX. End-stage renal disease risk in live kidney donors: what have we learned from two recent studies? Curr Opin Nephrol Hypertens. 2014;23(6):592–6. https://doi.org/10.1097/MNH.0000000000000063.
87. Lentine KL, Segev DL. Health outcomes among non-Caucasian living kidney donors: knowns and unknowns. Transpl Int. 2013;26(9):853–64. https://doi.org/10.1111/tri.12088.
88. Massie AB, Muzaale AD, Luo X, Chow EKH, Locke JE, Nguyen AQ, et al. Quantifying postdonation risk of ESRD in living kidney donors. J Am Soc Nephrol. 2017;28(9):2749–55. https://doi.org/10.1681/ASN.2016101084.
89. Garg AX, Pouget J, Young A, Huang A, Boudville N, Hodsman A, et al. Fracture risk in living kidney donors: a matched cohort study. Am J Kidney Dis. 2012;59(6):770–6. https://doi.org/10.1053/j.ajkd.2012.01.013.
90. Wirken L, van Middendorp H, Hooghof CW, Sanders JS, Dam RE, van der Pant KAMI, et al. Pre-donation cognitions of potential living organ donors: the development of the donation cognition instrument in potential kidney donors. Nephrol Dial Transplant. 2017;32(3):573–80. https://doi.org/10.1093/ndt/gfw421.
91. Barnieh L, Klarenbach S, Arnold J, Cuerden M, Knoll G, Lok C, et al. Non-reimbursed costs incurred by living kidney donors: a case study from Ontario, Canada. Transplantation. 2019;103(6):e164–71. https://doi.org/10.1097/TP.0000000000002685.
92. Przech S, Garg AX, Arnold JB, Barnieh L, Cuerden MS, Dipchand C, et al. Financial costs incurred by living kidney donors: a prospective cohort study. J Am Soc Nephrol. 2018;29(12):2847–57. https://doi.org/10.1681/ASN.2018040398.
93. Sickand M, Cuerden MS, Klarenbach SW, Ojo AO, Parikh CR, Boudville N, et al. Reimbursing live organ donors for incurred non-medical expenses: a global perspective on policies and programs. Am J Transplant. 2009;9(12):2825–36. https://doi.org/10.1111/j.1600-6143.2009.02829.x.
94. Lentine KL, Mannon RB. The Advancing American Kidney Health (AAKH) Executive Order: Promise and Caveats for Expanding Access to Kidney Transplantation. Kidney360. 2020;1(6):557–60. https://doi.org/10.34067/KID.0001172020.
95. Glannon W, Cronin AJ. Is it unethical for doctors to encourage healthy adults to donate a kidney to a stranger? No. BMJ. 2011;343:d7140. https://doi.org/10.1136/bmj.d7140.
96. Ratner LE, Ciseck LJ, Moore RG, Cigarroa FG, Kaufman HS, Kavoussi LR. Laparoscopic live donor nephrectomy. Transplantation. 1995;60(9):1047–9. http://www.ncbi.nlm.nih.gov/pubmed/7491680.
97. Wilson CH, Sanni A, Rix DA, Soomro NA. Laparoscopic versus open nephrectomy for live kidney donors. In: Wilson CH, editor. Cochrane database of systematic reviews. Chichester: Wiley; 2011. p. CD006124. https://doi.org/10.1002/14651858.CD006124.pub2.
98. Yuan H, Liu L, Zheng S, Yang L, Pu C, Wei Q, et al. The safety and efficacy of laparoscopic donor nephrectomy for renal transplantation: an updated meta-analysis. Transplant Proc. 2013;45(1):65–76. https://doi.org/10.1016/j.transproceed.2012.07.152.
99. Horgan S, Vanuno D, Sileri P, Cicalese L, Benedetti E. Robotic-assisted laparoscopic donor nephrectomy for kidney transplantation. Transplantation. 2002;73(9):1474–9. https://doi.org/10.1097/00007890-200205150-00018.

100. Jeong IG, Khandwala YS, Kim JH, Han DH, Li S, Wang Y, et al. Association of robotic-assisted vs laparoscopic radical nephrectomy with perioperative outcomes and health care costs, 2003 to 2015. JAMA. 2017;318(16):1561. https://doi.org/10.1001/jama.2017.14586.
101. Giacomoni A, Di Sandro S, Lauterio A, Concone G, Buscemi V, Rossetti O, et al. Robotic nephrectomy for living donation: surgical technique and literature systematic review. Am J Surg. 2016;211(6):1135–42. https://doi.org/10.1016/j.amjsurg.2015.08.019.
102. Creta M, Calogero A, Sagnelli C, Peluso G, Incollingo P, Candida M, et al. Donor and recipient outcomes following robotic-assisted laparoscopic living donor nephrectomy: a systematic review. Biomed Res Int. 2019;2019:1–10. https://doi.org/10.1155/2019/1729138.
103. Ratner LE, Buell JF, Kuo PC. Laparoscopic donor nephrectomy: pro. Transplantation. 2000;70(10):1544–6. https://doi.org/10.1097/00007890-200011270-00029.
104. Starzl T, Brittain R, Stonnington O, Coppinger W, Waddell W. Renal transplantation in identical twins. Arch Surg. 1963;86(4):600–7. https://doi.org/10.1001/archsurg.1963.01310100084013.
105. Terasaki PI, Cecka JM, Gjertson DW, Takemoto S. High survival rates of kidney transplants from spousal and living unrelated donors. N Engl J Med. 1995;333(6):333–6. https://doi.org/10.1056/NEJM199508103330601.
106. Halloran PF. Immunosuppressive drugs for kidney transplantation. N Engl J Med. 2004;351(26):2715–29. https://doi.org/10.1056/NEJMra033540.
107. Gentry SE, Montgomery RA, Segev DL. Kidney paired donation: fundamentals, limitations, and expansions. Am J Kidney Dis. 2011;57(1):144–51. https://doi.org/10.1053/j.ajkd.2010.10.005.
108. Kuppachi S, Axelrod DA. Desensitization strategies: is it worth it? Transpl Int. 2019;tri.13532. https://doi.org/10.1111/tri.13532.
109. Segev DL, Gentry SE, Warren DS, Reeb B, Montgomery RA. Kidney paired donation and optimizing the use of live donor organs. JAMA. 2005;293(15):1883. https://doi.org/10.1001/jama.293.15.1883.
110. Malik S, Cole E. State of the art practices and policies in kidney paired donation. Curr Transplant Rep. 2014;1(1):10–7. https://doi.org/10.1007/s40472-013-0002-5.
111. Rapaport FT. The case for a living emotionally related international kidney donor exchange registry. Transplant Proc. 1986;18(3 Suppl. 2):5–9. http://www.ncbi.nlm.nih.gov/pubmed/11649919.
112. de Klerk M, Keizer KM, Claas FHJ, Witvliet M, Haase-Kromwijk BJJM, Weimar W. The Dutch National Living Donor Kidney Exchange Program. Am J Transplant. 2005;5(9):2302–5. https://doi.org/10.1111/j.1600-6143.2005.01024.x.
113. Garonzik-Wang JM, Sullivan B, Hiller JM, Cass V, Tchervenkow J, Feldman L, et al. International Kidney Paired Donation. Transplant J. 2013;96(7):e55–e56. https://doi.org/10.1097/TP.0b013e3182a68879.
114. Cole EH, Nickerson P, Campbell P, Yetzer K, Lahaie N, Zaltzman J, et al. The Canadian kidney paired donation program: a National Program to increase living donor transplantation. Transplantation. 2015;99(5):985–90. https://doi.org/10.1097/TP.0000000000000455.
115. Shukhman E, Hunt J, LaPointe-Rudow D, Mandelbrot D, Hays RE, Kumar V, et al. Evaluation and care of international living kidney donor candidates: strategies for addressing common considerations and challenges. Clin Transpl. 2020;34(3):e13792. https://doi.org/10.1111/ctr.13792.
116. Treat E, Chow EKH, Peipert JD, Waterman A, Kwan L, Massie AB, et al. Shipping living donor kidneys and transplant recipient outcomes. Am J Transplant. 2018;18(3):632–41. https://doi.org/10.1111/ajt.14597.
117. D'Alessandro T, Veale JL. Innovations in kidney paired donation transplantation. Curr Opin Organ Transplant. 2019;24(4):429–33. https://doi.org/10.1097/MOT.0000000000000669.
118. Hendren E, Gill J, Landsberg D, Dong J, Rose C, Gill JS. Willingness of directed living donors and their recipients to participate in kidney paired donation programs. Transplantation. 2015;99(9):1894–9. https://doi.org/10.1097/TP.0000000000000533.

119. Gentry SE, Segev DL, Simmerling M, Montgomery RA. Expanding kidney paired donation through participation by compatible pairs. Am J Transplant. 2007;7(10):2361–70. https://doi.org/10.1111/j.1600-6143.2007.01935.x.
120. Veale JL, Capron AM, Nassiri N, Danovitch G, Gritsch HA, Waterman A, et al. Vouchers for future kidney transplants to overcome "chronological incompatibility" between living donors and recipients. Transplantation. 2017;101(9):2115–9. https://doi.org/10.1097/TP.0000000000001744.
121. Gill JS, Tinckam K, Fortin MC, Rose C, Shick-Makaroff K, Young K, et al. Reciprocity to increase participation of compatible living donor and recipient pairs in kidney paired donation. Am J Transplant. 2017;17(7):1723–8. https://doi.org/10.1111/ajt.14275.

Informed Consent and Framework of Living Donor Care

2

Anji E. Wall, Elisa J. Gordon, and Rebecca E. Hays

Background and History of Living Donation

In 1954, Joseph Murray performed the first living donor kidney transplant, in which one identical twin donated to the other at the Peter Bent Brigham Hospital in Boston. The donor, Ronald Herrick, lived for 54 years after his donation [1]. The decision to operate on a healthy person and to remove a normal kidney was a challenging one. Murray assembled a separate team to evaluate and care for the donor to reduce conflict of interest (perceived or real) on the part of the transplant team [2].

Living donor kidney transplantation (LDKT) now accounts for over 30% of the kidney transplants performed in the United States and 40% of kidney transplants performed worldwide and is the preferred treatment for people with end-stage kidney disease (ESKD). LDKT confers improved survival and quality of life compared to deceased donor transplantation or dialysis, at lower costs to the healthcare system [3–6]. Improved understanding of immunology, and the development of immunosuppressive agents to overcome immunologic barriers, led to improved LDKT recipient outcomes and allowed both biologically related and unrelated individuals to be living donors. In turn, the advent of laparoscopic donor surgery in the late 1990s increased public acceptance of the procedure (through shorter recovery times and improved cosmesis) and encouraged the growth of both kidney paired donation

A. E. Wall (✉)
Department of Abdominal Transplantation, Baylor University Medical Center, Dallas, TX, USA
e-mail: anji.wall@bswhealth.org

E. J. Gordon
Department of Surgery, Northwestern University Feinberg School of Medicine, Chicago, IL, USA

R. E. Hays
Department of Coordinated Care, University of Wisconsin Hospital and Clinics, Madison, WI, USA

© Springer Nature Switzerland AG 2021
K. L. Lentine et al. (eds.), *Living Kidney Donation*,
https://doi.org/10.1007/978-3-030-53618-3_2

(KPD) and nondirected donation in the mid-2000s, leading to expanded opportunities for living donation [7].

With thorough evaluation and stringent candidacy criteria in place, living donor nephrectomy is considered a low-risk surgical procedure, with a 90-day mortality rate of 3.1 in 10,000 donors [8]. There is a low incidence rate of ESKD after donation, although recent evidence suggests a higher rate of ESKD among donors than in healthy nondonor controls. Kidney donors also have higher rates of preeclampsia, but data remain inconclusive as to whether donors have increased cardiovascular risk compared to healthy controls [9, 10]. Most donors have stable quality of life after donation and a low rate of regret. However, a small percentage describes postoperative depression, and many describe associated financial burdens [11–14]. Donors have also described diverse other challenges in their clinical interactions and postdonation experiences [15].

Living Donor Evaluation and Care Overview for Donors

Given the extraordinary nature of living donation as a surgical procedure comprising no medical benefit to the donor, oversight agencies have developed minimum standards for donor candidate evaluation, informed consent, care, and follow-up [16–19]. Regulatory guidance and consensus recommendations have been built across many healthcare systems to safeguard donor interests and safety [20–22]. Internationally, the World Health Organization (WHO) issued guiding principles on living donation, and the Kidney Disease: Improving Global Outcomes (KDIGO) consensus group issued a clinical practice guideline [17, 23]. In the United States, Centers for Medicare and Medicaid Services (CMS) and the Organ Procurement and Transplantation Network (OPTN) promulgated regulatory guidelines and policies on care practices and documentation requirements [16, 24].

As is the case in all aspects of transplantation, living donor candidates and actual living donors are provided care by members of a multidisciplinary team who conduct evaluation, provide education and counseling, offer candidacy recommendations and determinations, and deliver care. The specific membership of the donor care team varies to some degree across healthcare systems, but there are some common themes. The clinicians caring for donors and donor candidates typically include physicians (surgeons, nephrologists, and/or primary care physicians depending on the setting), nurse coordinators, psychosocial providers (psychologist, clinical social worker, and/or psychiatrist), and often additional consults, including dieticians and histocompatibility specialists. In terms of the informed consent process, each clinician provides education, counseling, and risk assessment relevant to their field of expertise [16, 17].

Between healthcare systems and regions, there may be wide variation in the makeup of donor teams [17]. We offer the following summary to illustrate the ways that a donor team functions together to support the informed consent process for living donor candidates. The donor candidate's physicians provide education about the procedure's risks and benefits, assess the candidate's medical risk profile, and offer input about anticipated outcomes and aftercare. The nurse coordinator provides preparatory guidance about the process and medical education; the dietitian provides guidance on nutrition status, including modifiable risks as appropriate. The social worker, psychologist, and psychiatrist assesses psychosocial risk profile and provides education about potential quality of life impacts.

Benefits of living donor-specific care teams have been described. Specifically, clinicians on a donor-specific care team focus on the needs of the donor candidate, reducing risks of conflict of interest associated with caring for transplant candidates and affording the opportunity to build expertise in the needs of a donor population [22, 25]. However, an independent donor care team may not be economically or practically feasible in all settings and has not been regulatorily mandated [16, 17].

Prior to participating in an evaluation in the United States, living donor candidates must receive psychoeducation about their rights and the risks of the evaluation process. In fact, they must sign a separate consent document to undergo donor evaluation. Donor candidates should be advised that donor evaluation is voluntary and confidential and that they can choose to withdraw from donation confidentially at any time. They should be informed that members of the multidisciplinary donor team will conduct evidence-informed assessment of health status and risk profile and that living donor candidacy is determined in a multidisciplinary selection meeting. They should be advised that some contraindications to living donation are defined in regulation; individual transplant programs may further define candidacy criteria. More details about donor rights and process, particularly regarding confidentiality, are discussed in detail later in this chapter. The role of an independent living donor advocate (ILDA) is described below and in Table 2.1.

The Role of an Independent Living Donor Advocate

An emerging role in the care of living donors is that of an "independent living donor advocate," a team member uninvolved in recipient care and whose role is to act as a safeguard to living donor rights, care process, and informed consent. In the United States, as required by CMS and the OPTN, all living donor candidates and actual living donors must be provided an ILDA or ILDA team. The KDIGO guidelines also recognize the role of the ILDA as part of the evaluation and care team [17]. Individual member states of the European Union (EU) have also

Table 2.1 Roles of the independent living donor advocate. (From Rudow et al. [30])

Independence	Not part of the recipient care team, separation from the program pressures to increase volume
Advocacy	Assess donor ability to give consent and facilitate donor understanding
Transparency	Openness and honesty with the donor regarding process and information
Partnership	Promote education and guidance
Confidentiality	Maintain separation of donor information from recipient team

developed varying practices in implementing the role [20, 26]. In the United States, the ILDA as a designated role was first recommended in 2002 by the Federal Advisory Committee on Organ Transplantation to the Secretary of Health and Human Services (HHS) following the death of a living liver donor [27]. In 2007, the CMS Conditions for Transplant Center Participation mandated the integration of an ILDA or ILDA team into the care of all US living donor candidates, which, in turn, was further codified by the OPTN [16, 24, 25]. Some aspects of the ILDA role are defined in US regulatory guidance; others remain open to interpretation by transplant centers (Table 2.1). A guidance document produced by the American Society of Transplantation (AST) under the auspices of its Live Donor Community of Practice, and reviewed by representatives from both CMS and the OPTN, specified that the US ILDA role requires completion of particular assessment components with the donor candidate, a clinical skill set to do so appropriately, and independence from recipient care and concerns related to transplant center volume pressures [28]. Individual transplant centers can determine the ILDA's professional discipline, assessment timing, and role at donor candidate selection meetings [28]. The ILDA provides navigation support and voice to promote the donor candidate's autonomy and understanding during all stages of the donation process. Ideally, the ILDA strives to align the donor candidate's expectations with likely outcomes and risks and serves as a bridge between the donor candidate and the rest of the care team, by helping the donor candidate process the benefits and risks of donation and communicating these wishes to the donor team [29, 30]. The ILDA plays a central role in ensuring that donor evaluation and care meets ethical standards. The following section outlines the ethical framework for living kidney donation.

Ethical Framework for Living Kidney Donation

Living kidney donation is an ethically unique surgical procedure because it involves operating on one healthy person and removing a healthy kidney for no personal medical benefit, in order to achieve a medical benefit in another person [21, 22, 31]. The risks and benefits of the donor and recipient operations must be considered both separately and collectively [22]. The application of general bioethical principles is different with living donation as compared to other medical interventions because of the unique characteristics of this practice: non-maleficence is understood to encompass more than physical harm even in the absence of a medically beneficial procedure; beneficence must take into account the risks and benefits for both the donor and recipient; and "respect for persons" or autonomy is held to a high standard because donor candidates must understand that donation confers medical risk without direct medical benefit [23, 32]. This section describes how the bioethical principles of non-maleficence, beneficence, and respect for persons (autonomy) are balanced to achieve ethical soundness of living kidney donation. Please see the Ethical Principles chapter for more information.

Non-maleficence

The first principle to consider in the analysis of living kidney donation is non-maleficence, which follows the Hippocratic maxim to do-no-harm. This principle states that healthcare providers should not perform interventions that are exclusively harmful to patients [32]. The living donation context challenges this principle because living donor nephrectomy is not in the donor's medical best interest. The primary question with respect to non-maleficence is whether donor nephrectomy is an exclusively harmful practice. If living donation is of absolute harm without any benefit to the donor, then this procedure would be construed as unacceptable, stopping any further need to evaluate the ethics of this procedure. However, living donation can be identified as part of a shared transaction, in which harms to the donor (e.g., nephrectomy) can be balanced with expected benefits to the recipient (e.g., receiving a transplant) and with psychosocial gains to the donor associated with the act of donation [33]. Because donation is performed with the intent of directly helping another, the donor chooses to do so, and may derive psychosocial benefit from the act of donation, the procedure becomes ethically justified. Moreover, there is precedent for permitting clinical tests or procedures that harm one person for the benefit of another, such as blood and bone marrow donation.

Beneficence

The second principle, beneficence, requires that healthcare providers maximize the benefits and minimize the harms of medical interventions [32]. Beneficence in the living kidney donation context requires an acceptable balance between the risks and expected benefits of the operative interventions to both the donor and the recipient. The multifaceted considerations of recipient need, donor risk, and the chance of a good recipient outcome have been termed triangular equipoise [34] The general calculation must show that the risks to the donor are acceptable, the donor will achieve psychological benefit, the recipient's risks are acceptable, and the recipient is likely to benefit from the kidney transplant. At issue, of course, in the clinical context is that each of these qualifiers – "acceptable" and "likely" – is subjective and must be assessed in light of the individual donor candidate's goals and values [35].

Respect for Persons or Autonomy

If the conditions of non-maleficence and beneficence are met, the final principle to consider is respect for persons, or autonomy. This principle states that individuals have the right to make choices regarding their own health and medical care to align with their values and life goals; respect for autonomy is expressed through the process of informed consent [32]. In living donation, the donor candidate must have adequate knowledge about risks to themselves and risks, benefits, and alternatives available to the recipient candidate, as well as adequate understanding of the donor evaluation process and understanding of living donor transplantation as a shared transaction involving three "deciders" (recipient, donor, and transplant team) [17, 31, 36]. Donor teams can create a climate of care in which donor candidates are encouraged to articulate their values, goals, and wishes about donation; discuss any undue influences affecting their donation decision-making; and are informed and reminded of the right to stop the donation process at any time [31]. The following section details the general informed consent process for medical interventions as well as special considerations for the living donor candidate.

General Requirements for Informed Consent

The requirements for informed consent are decisional capacity, disclosure, comprehension, voluntariness, and agreement [32]. Every member of the donor team is responsible for ensuring that these general requirements are met, although each team member may be evaluating different components of the potential donor's readiness or understanding [17]. Moreover, in the US context, and in a growing number of other countries, donor evaluation teams include an ILDA, who ensures that the donor candidate proceeds voluntarily and with adequate understanding. The role of an ILDA in the donor informed consent process is further described throughout this section.

Decisional Capacity

The first requirement for informed consent is that patients must have decisional capacity, which means that they have the ability to make decisions about their medical care. The term competence is commonly used interchangeably with capacity. Competence is a legal term that means a person is able to make decisions as determined by a judge, while capacity is the ability to make decisions as determined by a physician. While competence and capacity can be used to describe the same characteristics, the term capacity is more suited for a discussion of the healthcare team members' determination of the ability of living donor candidates to make decisions about donation. The essential requirements of capacity include the ability to understand and appreciate the proposed intervention; deliberate about the risks, benefits, and alternatives; and be able to make a reasoned decision based on this deliberation [37]. A patient's decisional capacity can be determined by any physician, but if there is a question about the donor's capacity, psychiatrists or psychologists can assist using capacity assessment tools.

In living kidney donation, additional steps to assess capacity are advised if the donor candidate has a diagnosis associated with cognitive impairment (i.e., developmental delay, dementia, history of traumatic brain injury, Huntington's disease, etc.) or if care team members notice the donor candidate exhibiting problems retaining information or processing choices. Additional assessment might include psychiatric evaluation, neurocognitive assessment, or review of legal competency determinations (i.e., social security disability determinations in the United States, guardian ad litem assignment, etc.).

Disclosure

The second requirement for informed consent is that the treating provider discloses information including the details of the proposed procedure as well as the risks, benefits, and alternatives. There are two general legal standards in the United States for disclosure of information about medical procedures: the reasonable patient standard and the professional practice standard [37]. The reasonable patient standard requires disclosing information to the patient that a reasonable patient in the same situation would want to know. The professional practice standard requires disclosure of the same information that another physician in the same situation would disclose. Failure to disclose information in accordance with these standards can result in legal action against the physician for negligence. Outside of the United States, disclosure standards and guidelines vary [18, 38–40].

Informed consent does not end with the physician's disclosure and recommendation; it involves communication over time, in which provider and patient share a reciprocal process of disclosure and information-sharing, with the goal of comprehension. As such, the clinician provides patient-centered psychoeducation, the patient shares knowledge of personal history and concerns, and the clinician in turn offers follow-up education and risk assessment based on what the patient has shared [40, 41].

Specific Disclosure Requirements for Living Donors

For living donation, professional practice guidelines and policies have been established regarding information that should be disclosed to donor candidates [24, 42, 43]. Specifics of required content elements vary by country and healthcare system. In 2017, the KDIGO consensus group developed a guideline from a broad international perspective, describing essential elements that should be disclosed regardless of healthcare setting. Recommendations include disclosing processes of donor evaluation, risks and expected outcomes of donation, confidentiality guidelines, alternative treatments available to recipients, and transplant recipient selection processes [17].

In the United States, OPTN policy identifies aspects of living donor rights, care, and evaluation process; evaluation components, candidacy requirements, and confidentiality aspects for transplant candidates; and risks to be disclosed as part of living donor informed consent [16]. The OPTN also specified information for disclosure to living donor candidates participating in KPD and nondirected donors [16, 44]. OPTN policy has changed several times between 2012 and 2018 to incorporate emerging evidence and the expansion of paired exchange. Tables 2.2, 2.3, and 2.4 list the living donor disclosure requirements in the United States per OPTN

Table 2.2 Elements of OPTN requirements for living donor informed consent. Part 1 of 3, (From [16])

1. It is a federal crime for any person to knowingly acquire, obtain, or otherwise transfer any human organ for anything of value including, but not limited, to cash, property, and vacations
2. The recovery hospital must provide an ILDA
3. Alternate procedures or courses of treatment for the recipient, including deceased donor transplantation
4. A deceased donor organ may become available for the candidate before the recovery hospital completes the living donor's evaluation or the living donor transplant occurs
5. Transplant hospitals determine candidacy for transplantation based on existing hospital-specific guidelines or practices and clinical judgment
6. The recovery hospital will take all reasonable precautions to provide confidentiality for the living donor and recipient
7. Any transplant candidate may have an increased likelihood of adverse outcomes (including but not limited to graft failure, complications, and mortality) that: • Exceed local or national averages   • Do not necessarily prohibit transplantation   • Are not disclosed to the living donor
8. The recovery hospital can disclose to the living donor certain information about candidates only with permission of the candidate, including: • The reasons for a transplant candidate's increased likelihood of adverse outcomes   • Personal health information collected during the transplant candidate's evaluation, which is confidential and protected under privacy law
9. Health information obtained during the living donor evaluation is subject to the same regulations as all medical records and could reveal conditions that must be reported to local, state, or federal public health authorities
10. The recovery hospital is required to: • Report living donor follow-up information, at the time intervals specified in Policy 18.5: Living Donor Data Submission Requirements   • Have the donor commit to postdonation follow-up testing coordinated by the recovery hospital
11. Any infectious disease or malignancy that is pertinent to acute recipient care discovered during the donor's first 2 years of follow-up care: • May need to be reported to local, state, or federal public health authorities   • Will be disclosed to their recipient's transplant hospital   • Will be reported through the OPTN Improving Patient Safety portal
12. A living donor must undergo a medical evaluation according to Policy 14.4: Medical Evaluation Requirements for Living Donors and a psychosocial evaluation as required by Policy 14.1: Psychosocial Evaluation Requirements for Living Donors
13. The hospital may refuse the living donor. In such cases, the recovery hospital must inform the living donor that a different recovery hospital may evaluate him/her using different selection criteria
14. The following are inherent risks associated with evaluation for living donation: • Allergic reactions to contrast   • Discovery of reportable infections   • Discovery of serious medical conditions   • Discovery of adverse genetic findings unknown to the living donor   • Discovery of certain abnormalities that will require more testing at the living donor's expense or create the need for unexpected decisions on the part of the transplant team

Table 2.3 Elements of OPTN requirements for living donor informed consent. Part 2 of 3, (From [16])

Potential medical or surgical risks to donor candidates:
• Death
• Scars, hernia, wound infection, blood clots, pneumonia, nerve injury, pain, fatigue, and other consequences typical of any surgical procedure
• Abdominal symptoms such as bloating, nausea, and developing bowel obstruction
• The morbidity and mortality of the living donor may be impacted by age, obesity, hypertension, or other donor-specific preexisting conditions
Potential psychosocial risks to donor candidates:
• Problems with body image
• Postsurgery depression or anxiety
• Feelings of emotional distress or grief if the transplant recipient experiences any recurrent disease or if the transplant recipient dies
• Changes to the living donor's lifestyle from donation
Potential financial impacts on donor candidates:
• Personal expenses of travel, housing, childcare costs, and lost wages related to donation might not be reimbursed; however, resources might be available to defray some donation-related costs
• Need for lifelong follow-up at the living donor's expense
• Loss of employment or income
• Negative impact on the ability to obtain future employment
• Negative impact on the ability to obtain, maintain, or afford health insurance, disability insurance, and life insurance
• Future health problems experienced by living donors following donation may not be covered by the recipient's insurance

Table 2.4 Elements of OPTN requirements for living donor informed consent. Part 3 of 3, (From [16])

Education about expected postdonation kidney function and how - CKD - and - ESKD - might potentially impact the living donor in the future, to include:
• On average, living donors will have a 25–35% permanent loss of kidney function after donation
– Although risk of ESKD for living kidney donors does not exceed that of the general population with the same demographic profile, risk of ESKD for living kidney donors may exceed that of healthy nondonors with medical characteristics similar to living kidney donors
• Living donor risks must be interpreted in light of the known epidemiology of both CKD and ESKD.
– When CKD or ESKD occurs, CKD generally develops in midlife (40–50 years old) and ESKD generally develops after age 60
– The medical evaluation of a young living donor cannot predict lifetime risk of CKD or ESKD
• Living donors may be at a higher risk for CKD if they sustain damage to the remaining kidney.
– The development of CKD and subsequent progression to ESKD may be faster with only one kidney
• Dialysis is required if the living donor develops ESKD
• Current practice is to prioritize prior living kidney donors who become kidney transplant candidates according to Policy 8.3: Kidney Allocation Points

(continued)

Table 2.4 (continued)

Surgical risks may be transient or permanent and include but are not limited to: • Decreased kidney function   • Acute kidney failure and the need for dialysis or kidney transplant for the living donor in the immediate postoperative period
Disclose to all female living kidney donors: risks of preeclampsia or gestational hypertension are increased in pregnancies after donation
As part of the informed consent process, recovery hospitals must also provide transplant recipient outcome and transplanted organ survival data to living donors

Abbreviations: *CKD* chronic kidney disease; *ESKD* end-stage kidney disease

policy. Disclosure guidelines have also been defined within other healthcare systems, including the United Kingdom and Spain, with concepts affirmed by the Working Group on Living Donation under the European Union [18, 20, 45]. The following sections address different disclosure elements organized thematically.

Living Donor Rights and Care Processes

OPTN policy mandates and the KDIGO guideline recommends that transplant centers describe donor confidentiality, limits to confidentiality, and the donor candidate's right to withdraw at any time. Donor confidentiality in the United States is protected under the Health Insurance Portability and Accountability Act (HIPAA); methods to protect donor confidentiality should be discussed and clarified with donor candidates [46]. Limits to confidentiality should also be disclosed. For example, donor candidates in the United States should be informed about components of the donor evaluation that assess US Public Health Service (US PHS) increased risk status and that findings of increased risk status must be disclosed to the recipient if the donation is to be approved [47]. Similarly, donor candidates should be informed of any mandated reporting of specific disease test results to local departments of public health (i.e., Lyme disease, syphilis, HIV). Donor candidates should be advised of their rights to confidentially withdraw from donation at any time. Transplant center practices to facilitate donor withdrawal should be explicitly described (i.e., some centers provide a general statement of "unsuitability to donate") [48, 49]. Donor candidates considering KPD should be advised they do not get to choose their actual recipient and be informed of policies regarding meetings between pairs. Nondirected donors should be informed of all donation options, including participation in KPD or donation to someone on the deceased donor waitlist.

Transplant centers should describe and disclose composition of the donor team, including the requirement to designate an ILDA (if applicable); an overview of the donation process, including candidacy process and the transplant center's right to decline a transplant or donation candidate; and any recommendations for follow-up after living donation (i.e., 2 years of follow-up in the United States). Donor candidates considering KPD should be informed about unpredictable aspects of paired exchange, including potential delays in finding a match for their intended recipient, complicated timing and logistics, potential for additional testing burden, potential differences in outcomes between pairs, and remedies for a failed exchange.

Moreover, timing differences of "bridge donation," in which the originally intended donor's surgery occurs days, weeks, or months after the intended recipient has received a transplant, should be disclosed.

Recipient Care, Rights, and Processes

Living donor candidates should also receive fundamental information about transplant recipient care and general expected outcomes, rights, and evaluation process; this is codified by OPTN and offered in the KDIGO guideline [16, 17]. This includes an overview of ESKD treatment options, average expected recipient graft and patient survival, and disclosure that some transplant candidates may be at higher risk for poor outcomes than national averages. Living donor candidates should be informed of recipient confidentiality protections: in most settings including the United States and the European Union, specifics of the recipient risk profile are only disclosed with recipient written consent. Some scholars have proposed disclosure of increased recipient risk for meaningful living donor informed consent (i.e., when recipients have a poor prognosis), but this is not a policy requirement in the United States or internationally [50–52]. Nondirected donor candidate or donor candidates considering KPD must also be informed of recipients' rights to anonymity.

Donation Risks

The OPTN policy requires and KDIGO recommends disclosures regarding surgical, medical, psychosocial, and insurability risks of donation [16, 17] (Tables 2.3 and 2.4). Even with these prescribed content elements, many authors and consensus groups have called for increased standardization to ensure key elements are described and understood [3, 22, 53, 54]. Beyond disclosing the known risks, providers must disclose that there are potentially unknown outcomes including the relative and absolute risks of mortality and long-term morbidity among donors as compared to healthy nondonor populations [3, 54, 55].

Methods of Disclosure

Although information points have been minutely prescribed, there is limited procedural guidance about how disclosure should occur. The OPTN specifies that education should be conducted in a language the potential donor understands [16]. KDIGO recommends information be disclosed in a sympathetic environment with simple language, allowing time for questions with appropriate information and pace [17]. The ILDA is tasked by the OPTN to confirm the donor candidate has received required information and by CMS to ensure the donor candidate understands the information received [16, 24]. The method of education is left to the discretion of the transplant program: some provide one-on-one education with members of the clinical team; others offer group sessions; still others rely on videos. Studies have documented much variation in the disclosure process nationally and internationally [36].

Benefits to standardized approaches for the disclosure process and the overall consent process include improved consistency and thoroughness of education for donor candidates [3, 53, 56]. Standardization also ensures that donor candidates have access to adequate information. Disclosure approaches that aim to target infor-mation to specific groups (e.g., culturally targeted by ethnic group) or to tailor infor-mation to individuals' personal needs can potentially complement a standardized approach. Disclosure can be targeted in terms of presenting unique information desired by the targeted group in addition to standardized approaches and presenting that information in ways that are optimally comprehended by the targeted group. Disclosure can be tailored through layering information according to each person's desire for additional information. Challenges may arise in developing a single approach that accommodates all learning needs. However, decision aids that com-bine standardized and personalized approaches illustrate how to target or tailor dis-closure [57, 58].

The Dilemma of the "Recommendation" and Shared Decision-Making

In addition to disclosing required information to patients, physicians typically have a duty to provide a recommendation [37]. Unlike other informed consent scenarios, in which the physician offers a recommendation about what is in the patient's best interest based on available evidence, the donor candidates must weigh pros and cons themselves [35]. Transplant physicians strongly encourage patients with ESKD to seek living donors because LDKT is the best treatment option. However, while donor candidates may be informed that living donation is the best treatment for the transplant recipient, donor teams must also avoid unduly influencing donor candi-dates to undergo an operation that is not medically indicated. The goal should be to allow the donor candidate to express their autonomous desire to proceed without influence by the transplant team. Such caution about preventing undue influence underscores the value of a separate donor evaluation team that can prioritize the needs and best interests of the potential donor.

Shared decision-making models can be applied to living donation, without requiring physician recommendation [59]. For living donor candidates, a shared decision-making model involves formal consideration of the donor candidate's risk tolerance, expectations, and strength of motivation, in conjunction with living donor candidacy criteria and risk thresholds set by healthcare systems and transplant cen-ters. Incorporation of shared decision-making principles strengthens donor candi-date autonomy and allows transplant centers to employ different risk thresholds for donor candidates with relative contraindications (e.g., hypertension, obesity, and glucose intolerance) [60, 61].

Comprehension

Comprehension is the next requirement for informed consent, which can be assessed in multiple ways including teach-back, quizzes, and peer mentoring. Not only does comprehension involve an assessment of understanding, but it also requires delivery of information in a way that fosters understanding. A 2014 Best Practices in Live Donation Consensus Conference, convened by the AST and supported by 11 profes-sional societies, affirmed best practices for donor candidate education should meet health literacy guidelines, incorporate education in the donor candidate's first language, and be culturally targeted, in order to foster comprehension [3]. Ideally, education should be provided at multiple time points, and donor candidates should have the opportunity to ask questions and to reflect back their comprehension over time and certainly prior to donation [3, 17, 62].

Living donor psychosocial assessment should document specific learning needs, and the donor team should adapt teaching as needed [11]. In addition, a growing body of evidence describes benefits of culturally relevant education in improving engagement and understanding of LDKT and living donation [63, 64]. Unfortunately, most online donor education websites have been shown to be lacking in readability, content quality, and racial/ ethnic diversity, with few exceptions [58, 65, 66]. Moreover, most transplant centers do not formally assess candidate comprehension of the information that is disclosed [31].

In the United States, one of the key roles of the ILDA is to assess the understanding of the donor candidate and to help donor candidates access additional education as needed [16, 24]. Hays recommends that the ILDA utilize a structured interview that incorporates a teach-back of the disclosure elements required by OPTN [28]. This approach enables donor candidates to demonstrate their comprehension, recognize deficits in their knowledge, and offer an opportunity for donor clinicians to repeat teaching when appropriate.

Voluntariness

The fourth requirement for informed consent is voluntariness, in which a person decides without undue influence or coercion. Living donor candidates must make an affirmative, voluntary decision to proceed, without undue influence or what the OPTN has termed "undue pressure" [16, 67]. In the following section, we offer strategies for the assessment of voluntariness, risk, and the donor candidate's desire to proceed.

Protections Against Undue Influence or "Undue Pressure"

Influence on the donor candidate is common during the evaluation process, whether internally felt or externally imposed. In one single-center study, Valapour et al. found that 40% of donors felt pressure in their decision-making [68]. Donors must make an autonomous decision to proceed, without undue influence/undue pressure (including coercion). Psychosocial assessment and the ILDA evaluation explore donor candidate motivation and illuminate the presence of coercion and pressure influence (Section "Case Scenario 1"). Coercion and undue influence can be difficult to assess, particularly because of their subjective character. A nuanced clinical interview, integrating a process of gradual shared disclosure, psychoeducation, and assessment of risk factors, is recommended. KDIGO recommends the donor candidate psychosocial evaluation be done at least partially in the absence of the recipient candidate in order to ensure voluntariness [17]. In the United Kingdom, living donor candidate voluntariness is evaluated by an independent assessor; Spain has instituted a review by an independent judge prior to donor candidacy approval [20, 26].

Many donor candidates are motivated to donate by an internally experienced drive to help or part of a moral obligation associated with their family role (Section "Case Scenario 2") [68]. For others, the family relationship between donor and recipient may entail an explicitly described role obligation – "this is what sisters do" – but one in which the donor candidate can articulate her right (and ability) to make an autonomous decision about donation [69]. As such, influence in and of itself is not a contraindication to donation. In our view, external influences meet the standard of "undue" when they are strong enough to limit or steer the donor candidate's decision about whether or not to donate.

Undue influence goes hand in hand with power differentials. Therefore, assessment of donor motivation and autonomy should include discussion of the power imbalance between the donor candidate and intended recipient (i.e., status, age, potential donor dependence on the recipient, cognitive or emotional vulnerability of the donor) and the impact of power imbalance on decisions related to donation. Power imbalance alone is not a contraindication to donation, but options should be explored to mitigate its impact. Assessment of influence should include discussion of what the donor candidate believes would happen, should he or she decide not to donate (i.e., will he/she be penalized in some way?) [28, 49].

Protections Against Coercion

Coercion is a plausible threat of force or harm toward an individual aimed at influencing that individual to make a particular decision to act in a way that goes against the individual's preferences. Outright coercion to donate is thankfully rare, though it does occur, and must be assessed as part of the donor candidate evaluation (Section "Case Scenario 3"). Unfortunately, data on the rate of coercion experienced by donor candidates are lacking. In the authors' clinical experience, coercion might include an undocumented donor candidate being threatened with a call to US Immigration and Customs Enforcement if he does not agree to donate; a work site in which the supervisor advises employees to get tested for donation or face layoff; and a battered woman ordered to donate by her abuser. Clearly, donation is contraindicated in each of these scenarios, and a confidential means to withdrawal is indicated, which might include donor team coaching on a general statement of unsuitability to donate.

Absence of "Valuable Consideration"

In the United States and in most countries around the world, living donation must occur without expectations of pay or valuable consideration [17, 67]. In the United States, the National Organ Transplant Act (NOTA) has been amended to clarify that neither KPD nor reimbursement of donor expenses constitutes valuable consideration. OPTN policy mandates that donor candidates confirm understanding of NOTA provisions and agreement to abide by them [16]. At minimum, US transplant centers must document that living donors understand NOTA provisions, agree to comply with them, and are proceeding with donation voluntarily. Clearly, if a donor candidate discloses expectations of financial compensation in a country in which compensation is illegal, donation is contraindicated. If there are multiple risk factors for financial compensation or promise of valuable consideration disclosed, this should be considered carefully during donor candidacy selection meeting.

Agreement

The final step in the informed consent process is providing agreement, which typically occurs when the patient and physician sign a written consent form for the surgery. Although the donor candidate may sign the consent form to donate days or weeks before the actual operation, this form is not a binding agreement to donate. Donor candidates have the option to withdraw at any time up to the point when they undergo administration of anesthesia.

In the United States and across the world, there are no nationally or internationally standardized consent forms for living donor workup or surgery, though there is a UK project underway to develop them [70, 71]. A 2013 survey showed that the majority of US transplant programs used consent forms that did not have all of the CMS- or OPTN-mandated elements [72]. Additionally, consent forms are typically written at a college reading grade level [73]. Given that the disclosure requirements are well defined and mandated in regulatory guidance, some have called for standardizing consent forms and informed consent processes for both donor evaluation and living kidney donation, as discussed below [53, 72, 73].

Presence of an Affirmative Decision

For many donor candidates, decision-making happens smoothly, quickly, and from the "gut." Studies show that decision-making is mostly emotionally driven [74]. However, some donor candidates experience ambivalence about whether to donate. Many donor candidates simultaneously wish to donate but are afraid of the surgical risks; others may feel responsibility to help a family member but are worried about the recipient's ability to engage in self-care to effectively maintain the kidney; still others may be exploring donation in spite of objections by a significant other. In the context of living donation, the absence of a "no" is not equivalent to a definitive "yes": the donor candidate must voice an affirmative decision to proceed. The donor candidate's desire to proceed is a necessary element of living donor candidacy: surgery scheduling should not occur until a donor candidate states they do, in fact, want to donate.

Data suggest that donors who proceed despite ambivalence are at higher risk for poor psychosocial outcomes [75, 76]. In a single-center study, Dew et al. showed that an intervention to reduce donor candidates' ambivalence effectively reduced poor outcomes after donation including somatic symptoms, family problems, anxiety, and recovery time [77]. Others have proposed additional approaches to assist ambivalent donor candidates, including provision of a waiting or "cooling off" period to support reflection about the donation decision, psychoeducation, and counseling, reiterating that the donor candidate has the right to withdraw from donation and providing a description of confidential withdrawal options [49, 78].

Special Considerations in Informed Consent

In this section, we discuss special circumstances in living donation that may increase vulnerability for populations of potential living donors and may warrant specialized care practices by donor teams. Regarding aspects of donor evaluation that may warrant clarification for informed consent, we explore misattributed paternity and apolipoproteinL1 (*APOL1*) genetic variants. We discuss potentially vulnerable donor populations warranting additional protections, including incarcerated people and minors. We discuss specific scenarios that may warrant specialized informed consent processes, including nondirected donation, publicly solicited donation, and advanced donation.

Dilemmas About Disclosure of Misattributed Paternity

Misattributed relationship (typically paternity) can be an incidental finding in the donor evaluation process; transplant center practices vary regarding disclosure of this finding. Ross made compelling arguments not to disclose, as paternity is outside of the scope or expertise of living donor teams [79]. Whatever the transplant center policy, Hays recommends care practices regarding paternity be communicated with donor candidates up front as part of the donor evaluation consent process [49].

Dilemmas About Testing for Genetic Risk Factors

The *APOL1* has garnered much attention in the living kidney donation literature as certain genotypes are a genetic marker of risk of ESKD for both donors and recipients [80]. Living donors with two *APOL1* renal risk variants may have a steeper decline in kidney function after donation compared to those with one or no gene variant [81]. *APOL1* risk variants appear predominantly in populations with Western African genetic ancestry and may provide part of the explanation for why black living kidney donors have a greater risk of kidney failure postdonation as compared to European American donors [9, 82]. The transplant community has debated whether all living kidney donor candidates of recent African ancestry should undergo *APOL1* genetic testing and, if so, if the results of testing should be used for counseling about donor candidates' potentially increased risk versus as a strict contraindication to donation [83, 84]. Comprehensive genetic testing of living donor candidates has also been described [85].

To date, no standards of informed consent have been established for *APOL1* or other genetic marker testing. Research among African American living kidney donors reports their desire to have undergone such testing to foster greater informed consent, their information needs about *APOL1* for decision-making, and their concerns about psychosocial risks of undergoing testing [84, 86]. The 2017 KDIGO guideline recommends that *APOL1* genotyping be offered to donor candidates with sub-Saharan African ancestors and that donor candidates should be informed that having two *APOL1* risk alleles increases the lifetime risk of kidney failure but that the precise kidney failure risk for an affected individual after donation cannot currently be quantified [17]. However, qualitative interviews with African American living kidney donors point out that many people do not know their ancestry, particularly in the United States, which has a history of genetic admixture across "racial" groups. Thus, exploratory community studies of African American living kidney donors have recommended that all donor candidates, not just African American donors, be offered *APOL1* genetic testing [86]. The KDIGO guideline also recommends continued research to define the role of *APOL1* genotyping in the evaluation of donor candidates of African ancestry. In the United States, the "*APOL1* Long-Term Outcomes" (APOLLO) and "Living Donor Extended Time" (LETO) studies are being launched as national studies to strengthen the evidence base for use of *APOL1* genotyping in living and deceased donor transplantation [87].

Vulnerable Populations: Incarcerated Donors

Prisoners are considered a vulnerable population with respect to biomedical research; this view of vulnerability has been extended to living donors [88]. Incarcerated living donor candidates have limited access to information and support; with limited online and library access, they may be unable to independently research aspects of living donation and may have limited opportunity to weigh risks and benefits with loved ones (Section "Case Scenario 4"). Prison sentences may be lengthened or shortened by a parole board's evaluation of "good behavior," which may serve as a pressure to donate (Section "Case Scenario 5"). Security needs may entail additional costs and logistics burdens for the incarcerated donor and recipient. Ross and Thistlethwaite suggest that psychosocial evaluation of an incarcerated living donor candidate include feedback from a provider who works specifically with prisoners to facilitate adequate assessment and protections [88].

Other Vulnerable Populations

There are other donor candidate populations with characteristics that can contribute to vulnerability. For example, in the Unites States and in other countries lacking universal healthcare, some donors may lack access to follow-up care. For example, people with undocumented immigration status may be allowed to donate but may have difficulty accessing their own kidney treatment in the future. Likewise, uninsured donors in the United States have the donation medical costs covered by the recipient's insurance but may not have access to healthcare in the future if they develop a complication such as hypertension or chronic kidney disease [12, 89]. Jehovah's Witnesses who refuse blood products are at higher risk than other donors because of risks associated with bleeding complications that would usually be treated with blood product administration [90]. This is not an exhaustive list of vulnerable populations but serves to illustrate some potential vulnerabilities. All providers who evaluate donor candidates must be aware that any donor candidate may be vulnerable and may need further evaluation to ensure this vulnerability is adequately protected.

Nondirected Donors and Directed Donors with Limited Relationship

Nondirected donors must have a realistic understanding of expected process and outcomes of their donation. Nondirected donors proceed without knowledge about their actual transplant recipient, and they agree to abide by transplant center policies regarding anonymity and confidentiality, as previously described in the disclosure section of this chapter. They should demonstrate realistic expectations, which may include the generalized psychological benefits associated with acts of altruism, but should not be dependent on witnessing their kidney recipient thrive the way that directed donors may [91, 92].

Potential Donors Solicited via Social Media or Public Pleas

Potential living donors who respond to social media pleas or public solicitations should have clear and realistic expectations confirmed prior to proceeding with donation. The nature of the relationship between donor and recipient may not be entirely clear to any of the parties, and it is not unusual for publicly solicited living donors to have high hopes for a long-term connection. During the informed consent process, the transplant center team should clarify confidentiality regulations and offer education about the range of relationships that can occur after donation and transplantation and ascertain the presence of realistic expectations on the part of the donor candidate [93].

Donors in "Advanced Donation"

Advanced donation, in which an individual donates a kidney in exchange for a voucher for a specific individual to receive a kidney transplant in the future, is an emerging practice incorporated in some KPD systems [94]. These programs raise multiple ethical issues including uncertainty over whether the intended recipient will need a kidney in the future, uncertainty regarding whether the exchange program will have the authority to honor the voucher by the time the intended recipient is in need, and uncertainty about how the intended recipient will be prioritized when they do meet criteria for kidney transplantation [95, 96]. Informed consent for "advance" donors, then, must include recognition of these unknowns and desire to proceed in any case.

Donors with "Increased Risk Status" per the US Public Health Service Criteria

The OPTN requires that transplant centers obtain "specific informed consent" from transplant candidates in order to accept organs considered at "increased risk" for transmitting HIV, hepatitis B virus (HBV), or hepatitis C virus (HCV) to the recipient. Given that this disclosure may cause psychological harm to the donor, Gordon et al. recommend that potential donors be informed early in the evaluation process the requirement for assessment of increased risk and disclosure of such status (as indicated) to the intended recipient prior to donation [97]. The potential donor should be advised of the individual transplant center's disclosure policy, whether this entails describing the specific increased risk behavior or providing a general statement of increased risk status to the recipient (Section "Case Scenario 6"). The donor candidate should be given the option to withdraw from the donation process to avoid disclosure or, in some risk categories, to delay donation until the time period of "increased risk status" has passed.

Future Research

While most living kidney donors report satisfaction with the decision to donate, there is a significant minority who incur complications and/or have negative outcomes associated with donation [98–100]. In a questionnaire study of 167 donors, Schover found that one of the strongest correlates with donor dissatisfaction was a belief that information given preoperatively was inadequate [100]. Another questionnaire study of over 2000 donors found that recipient graft failure was the only predictor of negative psychosocial outcomes [99]. An interview study of kidney donors who developed ESKD found that many lacked appreciation for the need for postdonation self-care and recommended that living donors are informed that they should consider themselves healthy, but at risk [101]. Moreover, studies of living kidney donors have found that some donors do not believe information is well explained, sufficient, or understandable [102, 103]. Given that donors have expressed dissatisfaction with the informed consent process, and this translated for some into dissatisfaction with the donation experience as a whole, more research is needed to understand and improve the donor candidate informed consent process. Research should focus on both substantive and processual aspects of each informed consent element as each uniquely applies to living donors. Table 2.5 provides an outline of future research questions.

Disclosure

Studies should assess what information needs living donor candidates have. Few studies have investigated this [56, 104, 105]. For example, Traino and colleagues conducted semi-structured interviews with living kidney donors about which

Table 2.5 Questions for future research on informed consent for living kidney donation

Disclosure
- What are the current disclosure practices of transplant centers?
- What are the disclosure needs of donor candidates?
- Do disclosure needs vary among different donor candidate populations?
- What disclosure methods are most effective for fostering comprehension?
- What are the disclosure needs of donor candidates regarding recipient outcomes?
- What are the best practice methods for shared disclosure of increased USPHS risk status?

Comprehension
- How should comprehension assessment be used in the evaluation process?
- How can teaching be adapted to meet different learning needs, priorities, and comfort in the medical environment, to best foster comprehension?
- What are the pros and cons of using mechanisms to measure effectiveness of patient education and ultimately measuring patient comprehension?
- Should a transplant program proceed to surgery with a donor candidate who has not yet demonstrated comprehension on a comprehension assessment test?
- For how long after disclosure should donor candidates be required to retain and recall information?
- When should comprehension assessment occur during the donor evaluation process?
- What are the benefits of peer mentoring for information retention?
- Which methods of teaching and comprehension assessment are most effective in achieving the goal of informing donor candidates about the essentially needed information?
- Which methods of teaching and comprehension assessment do donors like the most?
- Which methods of teaching and comprehension assessment best retain cultural relevance among different ethnic and cultural groups?

Voluntariness
- What is the spectrum of undue influence experienced among donor candidates?
- Do donor candidates feel protected from undue influence and coercion when making their decisions?
- How do donor candidates perceive their level of certainty for donation?
- What are best practice standards for assessment of undue influence?
- What are best practice standards for assessment of valuable consideration?

Standardization
- What processes work the best for minimizing variation in the consent process?
- Can standardization in the consent process also meet specific donor information needs?

Satisfaction
- How do donor candidates use the informed consent process in their decision-making process about donating?
- Which aspects of the informed consent process do donor candidates perceive as satisfactory or in need of revision?

Priority setting
- How can donor candidates be engaged in priority setting for research on informed consent on donation?
- How can researchers be encouraged to align research on informed consent with the priorities of candidate and actual donors?

Development and evaluation of interventions
- How can the informed consent process for living donation become culturally targeted?
- What donor candidate populations benefit from culturally targeted informed consent?
- How should culturally targeted interventions be evaluated?

CMS-required information for disclosure helped donors with decision-making [56]. However, more ethnographic qualitative research is needed to understand, from the donor's perspective, what information needs about living donation they have overall. Some research has shown that donors with different ethnic/racial backgrounds have different information needs about donation, such as in the Latinx population, but little is known about the needs of other ethnic/racial or cultural groups [106]. This raises the question of whether donor candidates' information needs vary by gender, age, or other demographic traits. Observational studies should assess actual disclosure practices in order to determine what information gets disclosed and not disclosed [73].

At the heart of the matter about disclosure is the question about how much knowledge and which specific knowledge items are essential to ensuring the donor candidates' informed consent [107]. This issue is not unique to donors but applies to all clinical contexts. What clinicians believe to be essential information is not always the same as what patients (or donors) believe to be critical for decision-making. Variability in disclosure practices – in terms of content – can result in under-disclosure or overwhelming donor candidates with too much information. It is unclear how much information living donor candidates desire. Either of these scenarios can undermine the informed consent process. Thus, identifying the right content and amount of information is critically needed.

Moreover, further research should identify donor candidates' preferred method of information disclosure. Current approaches used include group education, one-on-one education, video presentation, and written information. Information is often communicated in one sitting, but little is known about which method of disclosure donors experience as most effective in conveying information, and in fostering retention, and whether some information should be spaced out over more than one session. Disclosure method preferences may differ by individual learning styles in terms of written or verbal communication and/or may vary by sociodemographic factors, all of which remain to be empirically examined [108].

Comprehension

Studies should assess whether donor candidates comprehend information disclosed to them. As new data emerge over time about donor risks, long-term donor outcomes, and gender, age, and ethnic/racial differences in donor outcomes, potential living donors need to be apprised of such information. Accordingly, ongoing evaluation of potential donors' understanding is crucial to identify gaps and undertake quality improvement efforts to ensure that donor candidates understand implications of their choices.

Approaches for evaluating donor candidates' comprehension are needed. Currently, no standard approach exists across transplant programs, despite CMS requirements that assessment be performed [109]. Transplant programs use a variety of ways to ascertain donor candidates' comprehension including teach-back, brief quizzes, peer mentoring, or no approach at all. No vetted, validated, standardized knowledge assessment tool has been developed for potential living kidney donors, as has been developed for potential living liver donors [73, 110]. The use of comprehension assessment deserves greater reflection and further deliberation.

Voluntariness

Studies are needed to understand the spectrum of undue influence in the donation context. Research should assess perceptions of factors that contribute to undue influence and then identify ways to enhance voluntariness and reduce undue influence to donate. As recommended, research should assess how effective ILDAs and policies are in protecting potential donors' perceptions of voluntariness [73]. Little research has investigated donor candidates' level of certainty about undergoing donation [111]. Future research should investigate the source of uncertainty and ways to overcome it.

Standardization

Given the variation in living donor consent processes, several transplant scholars have called for standardizing the informed consent process for living donors so that all donors receive the same content [31, 53, 111]. Research is needed to minimize variability in the consent process, evaluate what processes work most optimally, and determine the best methods to meet a range of donor information needs.

Value, Use of, and Satisfaction with Informed Consent

Research is also needed to assess what donor candidates believe is the value of informed consent for living donation. Interviews with living liver donor candidates found that information was valued for preparation rather than decision-making [111]. Prospective studies should assess potential living donors' expectations to see if they match their postdonation experiences in the short and longer term [31]. Research should ascertain the source of discrepancies and identify how to revise the information disclosure process accordingly.

Priority Setting and Donor Engagement

Research is needed to ascertain potential and actual living kidney donors' perspectives on the kinds of research that should be conducted on living donors and donor candidates and how they would prioritize such research. In a meta-analysis of research and stakeholder priorities in solid organ transplantation, Tong and colleagues found that seven (25%) studies focused on priorities for living donation. Of these seven, a subset prioritized research on informed consent that focuses on "improve[ing] consistency in the information provided to donors by physicians and transplant programs" (two studies) and "improving awareness about nondirected donor programs" (one study) [112]. They recommended patient involvement in establishing priorities.

Develop and Evaluate Interventions

Although a number of decision aids have been developed to increase recipient understanding of the benefits of LDKT, future research is needed to develop and evaluate interventions to focus on specifically enhancing informed consent [31, 113]. Informed consent interventions have been developed; but still fewer have targeted specific sociodemographic groups of donors and/or used novel delivery modes. Developing and evaluating culturally targeted interventions to address shared culturally based concerns among ethnic/racial and religious donor groups are needed to increase comprehension of donation information and reduce disparities in donation. For example, Gordon and colleagues developed and evaluated a bilingual website targeted to Hispanics that effectively increased knowledge about living donation and transplantation among Hispanic potential donors, patients, and family members beyond current education alone [58]. Others have followed suit among African American donors [63, 114]. However, interventions should also be designed for other ethnic minority donors. Other donor candidate groups with unique information needs might include First Nations donors. As educational materials are typically written at a high reading grade level, education materials are also needed that are written in plain language (i.e., fifth- to eighth-grade reading level). Additionally, informed consent interventions developed for other clinical contexts may be adapted to the donation context.

In sum, we recommend that living donor candidates and actual living kidney donors, as key stakeholders, be engaged as partners in research activities so that their perspectives inform the study design, data collection, and interpretation of study results in future research.

Case Scenario #1: Undue Pressure

A 30-year-old female undergoes evaluation for living kidney donation to her uncle. The recipient is the daycare provider for the donor candidate's two children. The donor candidate's mother (not the recipient) has participated in all initial calls. The donor candidate's affect is quiet and withdrawn when she meets with the independent living donor advocate.

Case Evaluation

- **Motivation:** the donor candidate discloses that multiple family members have said she *owes* donation to her uncle, after the kindness the uncle has shown. Family members have said that to have doubts about donation is to be "ungrateful."
- **Status of decision-making:** the donor candidate says she is *expected to*.
- **Consequences if she opted not to donate:** she believes that if she withdraws, she will be *shunned by her family*. She reports that family describes her as a "leech" for utilizing her uncle for childcare; her brother told her "it's the least you can do." The donor candidate believes family relationships will be broken if she does not proceed.

Recommendations

- Help the donor candidate differentiate between internally felt and externally imposed pressure. Define "undue pressure," and explain that donating solely out of fear of reprisal is doing so under "undue pressure."
- Advise the donor candidate of her rights, including the right to withdraw confidentially from the donation process at any time, and information about the center's policy for confidential withdrawal from the donor workup should she so choose.
- For donor candidates describing confusing family pressures, support the donor candidate's decision-making process. This may include a waiting period to consider options and sort out complex emotions or counseling to resolve family role conflicts.
- Support donor candidate autonomy in decision-making and right to make a decision about donation independent of family pressures.

Case Scenario #2: Internally Felt Pressure

A 32-year-old female is evaluated as a living donor candidate for her mother. The donor candidate expresses gratitude and appreciation for the care provided her by the recipient; she attributes her adult career path to the sacrifices the recipient made while raising her. The donor candidate is intermittently tearful when describing this history.

Case Evaluation

- **Motivation:** the donor candidate describes feeling love and gratitude for her mother. She identifies reciprocal roles of love, support, and assistance in her family and with the intended recipient in particular. She reports, "how could I let her suffer? Helping her is only right, and I'm glad to do it."
- **Status of decision-making:** the donor candidate says she *has to*.

- **Consequences if she opted not to donate:** the potential donor says, "I could never live with myself if she died on dialysis."

Recommendations

- Explore past helping acts and helping roles in the family and in the community. This helps identify consistency between donation decision-making and way of life and/or self-schema.
- Discuss the differences between internal and external pressure with the donor candidate, and ensure that the pressure is not an undue external pressure that she has internalized.
- Make sure the donor candidate understand the alternative option for the recipient, especially deceased donation, and the projected waiting time for that option.

Case Scenario #3: Coercion

A 23-year-old female starts evaluation to donate to her grandmother. She is healthy and there are no medical contraindications to donation. She is unemployed and lives rent-free in her grandmother's basement. The intended recipient first leaves messages for the donor coordinator herself about the donor candidate's evaluation and later can be heard in the background of intake calls between the donor candidate and donor coordinator. The intended recipient becomes irate when she is asked to leave the exam room for the donor evaluation. The evaluating nephrologist notes that the donor candidate's affect is intermittently flat and irritated.

Case Evaluation

- **Motivation:** the donor candidate says she "guesses [she] owes it" to the recipient.
- **Status of decision-making:** the donor candidate says she *has to*.
- **Consequences if she opted not to donate:** the donor candidate reports she has been told that if she doesn't donate, she can "find a different place to live." The donor candidate believes that if she doesn't donate, she will be *evicted*.

Recommendations

- This donor candidate is facing coercive pressures. Provide the donor candidate education about the definition of coercion. Affirm that donating in order to avoid eviction is doing so under duress, is ethically contraindicated, and does not meet donor candidacy standards.
- Inform the donor candidate of the ability to confidentially withdraw with a general statement of unsuitability.

Case Scenario #4: An Incarcerated Donor Candidate

A 55-year-old man hopes to donate to his brother. He is incarcerated. His initial donor screening appears to be within normal limits, and there are no identified medical contraindications.

Case Evaluation

- **Motivation:** he states that his brother has been a consistent source of support during a long incarceration, and he wants to give back.
- **Status of decision-making:** the donor candidate says he wants to donate to keep his brother around as long as possible.
- **Consequences of donating (or not donating):** "None, other than feeling bad about myself if I cannot donate." He has been convicted and his sentence has been determined. No parole hearings are scheduled. In this case, donating should have no effect on his status in the criminal justice system.

Recommendations

- Explore patient's current status in the criminal justice system to identify any secondary pressures that may influence donation decision-making. This may include upcoming trials, sentencing, or parole hearings, in which there would be pressures and potential gains associated with appearing civic-minded.
- With the donor candidate's permission, confirm with the Department of Corrections that the donor will receive appropriate accommodations for donation recovery and follow-up.
- The donor candidate should be advised of costs associated with donating while incarcerated, which may include significant security costs during the hospitalization.

Case Scenario #5: An Incarcerated Donor Candidate

A 38-year-old man hopes to donate to his neighbor. He is in jail pending trial. Initial medical evaluation appears to be within normal limits, and there are no medical contraindications.

Case Evaluation

- **Motivation:** he wants to help his neighbor. He also acknowledges donation may improve his profile during the trial.
- **Status of decision-making:** clear and determined. The donor candidate *wants to donate* and also hopes donation will decrease the severity of his sentence.

- **Consequences of donating or not donating:** he reports that the judge expressed enthusiasm for his donation during an early hearing. Donation may affect the outcome of the trial.

Recommendations

- The transplant program should consider pending the donor evaluation process until this candidate's case has been decided and sentencing has occurred. In this way, his decision about donation is separate from external pressures to "do good."
- Given that his psychosocial situation and access to care may significantly change based on whether or not he is incarcerated (and in what facility), pending his donor evaluation also ensures he receives adequate assessment and education.
- If possible, the donor team should collaborate with a social worker or psychologist familiar with prison/jail systems, so as to better understand potential systemic influences on the individual donor candidate's decision-making or access to care.

Case Scenario #6: Clinical Care for Donor Candidates Who Meet US Public Health Service "Increased Risk" Criteria

A 19-year-old woman wants to donate to her uncle. She is healthy. There are no medical contraindications to donation. HIV, hepatitis B, and hepatitis C nucleic acid testing is negative. She has had one sexual partner, contracted chlamydia 6 months ago, and completed treatment. She is not currently sexually active. However, because of the recent diagnosis of chlamydia, she meets US Public Health Service definition of being a donor at increased risk of transmitting infectious diseases, specifically hepatitis B, hepatitis C, and HIV, to the transplant recipient. The donor candidate is advised of US policy requirements for disclosure of this status to her intended recipient, should she choose to proceed with donation.

Case Evaluation

- **Motivation:** she wants to donate to help her uncle.
- **Status of decision-making:** clear, decided.
- **Complicating factor affecting her donation decision-making and process:** upon hearing about mandated disclosure of increased risk status, she is distressed. She feels torn between her desire to help her uncle and her desire for privacy.

Recommendations

- Provide information. The donor candidate should be informed of what information will be disclosed and how it will be disclosed to the recipient, should she choose to donate. The transplant center may provide a general statement of increased risk but keep the specific reason confidential versus disclosing the specific reason.

- Describe options to preserve donor confidentiality. For example, donor candidates are no longer considered increased risk once 12 months have elapsed following sexually transmitted infection diagnosis/treatment. She could elect to delay donation until she no longer meets the "increased risk" criteria.
- Alternatively, she could also elect to participate in a paired exchange program so an unknown recipient receives the disclosure of her increased risk status.
- Provide education about donor rights, including her right to withdraw from donation so as to avoid disclosure.

References

1. Kasiske BL. Outcomes after living kidney donation: what we still need to know and why. Am J Kidney Dis. 2014;64(3):335–7. https://doi.org/10.1053/j.ajkd.2014.04.013.
2. Murray JE. Surgery of the soul: reflections on a curious career. Science History Publications. Sagamore Beach, MA, USA; 2004.
3. Tan JC, Gordon EJ, Dew MA, LaPointe RD, Steiner RW, Woodle ES, Hays R, Rodrigue JR, Segev DL, American Society of Transplantation. Living donor kidney transplantation: facilitating education about live kidney donation–recommendations from a consensus conference. Clin J Am Soc Nephrol. 2015;10(9):1670–7. https://doi.org/10.2215/CJN.01030115.
4. Hart A, Lentine KL, Smith JM, Miller JM, Skeans MA, Prentice M, et al. OPTN/SRTR 2019 Annual Data Report: Kidney. Am J Transplant. 2021;21(Suppl 2):21–137. https://doi.org/10.1111/ajt.16502.
5. Axelrod DA, Schnitzler MA, Xiao H, Irish W, Tuttle-Newhall E, Chang S-H, Kasiske BL, Alhamad T, Lentine KL. An economic assessment of contemporary kidney transplant practice. Am J Transplant. 2018;18(5):1168–76. https://doi.org/10.1111/ajt.14702.
6. World Health Organization (WHO)- Organización Nacional de Trasplantes (ONT). Global Observatory on Donation and Transplantation (GODT). Available at: http://www.transplant-observatory.org/. Accessed: 7 Sept 2020.
7. United States Renal Data System (USRDS). 2018 USRDS Annual Data Report: Epidemiology of kidney disease in the United States. Bethesda: National Institutes of Health, National Institute of Diabetes and Digestive and Kidney Diseases. Available at: https://www.usrds.org/annual-data-report/. Accessed: 7 Sept 2020.
8. Segev DL, Muzaale AD, Caffo BS, Mehta SH, Singer AL, Taranto SE, et al. Perioperative mortality and long-term survival following live kidney donation. JAMA. 2010;303(10):959–66. https://doi.org/10.1001/jama.2010.237.
9. McKay DB, Josephson MA. Reproduction and Transplantation: Report on the AST Consensus Conference on Reproductive Issues and Transplantation. Am J Transplant. 2005;5(7):1592–99. https://doi.org/10.1111/j.1600-6143.2005.00969.x.
10. Matas AJ, Hays RE, Ibrahim HN. Long-term non–end-stage renal disease risks after living kidney donation. Am J Transplant. 2017;17(4):893–900. https://doi.org/10.1111/ajt.14011.
11. Dew MA, Myaskovsky L, Steel JL, DiMartini AF. Managing the psychosocial and financial consequences of living donation. Curr Transplant Rep. 2013;1(1):24–34. https://doi.org/10.1007/s40472-013-0003-4.
12. Tushla L, Rudow DL, Milton J, Rodrigue JR, Schold JD, Hays R. Living-donor kidney transplantation: reducing financial barriers to live kidney donation--recommendations

from a consensus conference. Clin J Am Soc Nephrol. 2015;10(9):1696–702. https://doi.org/10.2215/CJN.01000115.

13. Lentine KL, Schnitzler MA, Xiao H, Axelrod D, Davis CL, McCabe M, et al. Depression diagnoses after living kidney donation: linking U.S. registry data and administrative claims. Transplantation. 2012;94(1):77–83. https://doi.org/10.1097/TP.0b013e318253f1bc.

14. Wirken L, van Middendorp H, Hooghof CW, Rovers MM, Hoitsma AJ, Hilbrands LB, et al. The course and predictors of health-related quality of life in living kidney donors: a systematic review and meta-analysis. Am J Transplant. 2015;15(12):3041–54. https://doi.org/10.1111/ajt.13453.

15. Gordon EJ. Living organ donors' stories: (unmet) expectations about informed consent, outcomes, and care. Narrat Inq Bioeth. 2012;2(1):1–6. https://doi.org/10.1353/nib.2012.0001.

16. Organ Procurement and Transplantation Network (OPTN)/United Network for Organ Sharing (UNOS). Policy 14: Living Donation. Available at: https://optn.transplant.hrsa.gov/governance/policies/. Accessed: 7 Sept 2020.

17. Lentine KL, Kasiske BL, Levey AS, Adams PL, Alberú J, Bakr MA, et al. KDIGO clinical practice guideline on the evaluation and care of living kidney donors. Transplantation. 2017;101(8S Suppl 1):S1–S109. https://doi.org/10.1097/TP.0000000000001769.

18. British Transplantation Society (BTS). Guidelines for living donor kidney transplantation. Available at: https://bts.org.uk/wp-content/uploads/2018/07/FINAL_LDKT-guidelines_June-2018.pdf. Accessed: 7 Sept 2020.

19. Abramowicz D, Cochat P, Claas FHJ, Heemann U, Pascual J, Dudley C, et al. European renal best practice guideline on kidney donor and recipient evaluation and perioperative care. Nephrol Dial Transplant. 2015;30:1790–7. https://doi.org/10.1093/ndt/gfu216.

20. Working Group on Living Donation under the European Union. Action plan on organ donation and transplantation (2009–2015): strengthened cooperation between member states. Available at: https://ec.europa.eu/health//sites/health/files/blood_tissues_organs/docs/eutoolbox_living_kidney_donation_en.pdf. Accessed: 7 Sept 2020.

21. Delmonico F, Council of the Transplantation Society. A report of the Amsterdam forum on the Care of the Live Kidney Donor: data and medical guidelines. Transplantation. 2005;79(6 Suppl):S53–66. https://pubmed.ncbi.nlm.nih.gov/15785361/.

22. Ethics Committee of the Transplantation Society. The consensus statement of the Amsterdam forum on the Care of the Live Kidney Donor. Transplantation. 2004;78(4):491–2. https://doi.org/10.1097/01.TP.0000136654.85459.1E.

23. World Health Organization (WHO). World Health Organization guiding principles on human cell, tissue, and organ transplantation. Available at: www.who.inttransplantationGuidingPrinciplesTransplantationWHA.en.pdf. Accessed: 7 Sept 2020.

24. U.S. Department of Health and Human Services (HHS), Centers for Medicare and Medicaid Services (CMS). CFR parts 405, 482, 488, and 498 Medicare program; Hospital Conditions of Participation: Requirements for Approval and Reapproval of Transplant Centers; Final Rule. Available at: https://www.cms.gov/Medicare/Provider-Enrollment-and-Certification/GuidanceforLawsAndRegulations/Downloads/TransplantFinalLawandReg.pdf. Accessed: 7 Sept 2020.

25. Rudow DL. The living donor advocate: a team approach to educate, evaluate, and manage donors across the continuum. Prog Transplant. 2009;19(1):64–70. https://doi.org/10.7182/prtr.19.1.53n8ju8520238465.

26. Lennerling A, Lovén C, Dor FJMF, Ambagtsheer F, Duerinckx N, Frunza M, et al. Living organ donation practices in Europe – results from an online survey. Transplant Int. 2013;26(2):145–53. https://doi.org/10.1111/tri.12012.

27. Advisory Committee on Organ Transplantation, U.S. Department of Health and Human Services Recommendations 1-18, issued November 18–19, 2002. Available at: organdonor.gov/about-dot/acot/acotrecs118.html. Accessed: 7 Sept 2020.

28. Hays RE, Rudow DL, Dew MA, Taler SJ, Spicer H, Mandelbrot DA. The independent living donor advocate: a guidance document from the American Society of Transplantation's Living Donor Community of Practice (AST LDCOP). Am J Transplant. 2015;15(2):518–25. https://doi.org/10.1111/ajt.13001.

29. Hays R, Matas AJ. Ethical review of the responsibilities of the patient advocate in living donor liver transplant. Clin Liver Dis. 2016;7(3):57–9. https://doi.org/10.1002/cld.533.

30. Rudow DL, Swartz K, Phillips C, Hollenberger J, Smith T, Steel JL. The psychosocial and independent living donor advocate evaluation and post-surgery care of living donors. J Clin Psychol Med Settings. 2015;22(2–3):136–49. https://doi.org/10.1007/s10880-015-9426-7.

31. Gordon EJ. Informed consent for living donation: a review of key empirical studies, ethical challenges and future research. Am J Transplant. 2012;12(9):2273–80. https://doi.org/10.1111/j.1600-6143.2012.04102.x.

32. Beauchamp TL, Childress JF. Principles of biomedical ethics. New York: Oxford University Press, USA; 2001.

33. Jowsey SG, Jacobs C, Gross CR, et al. Emotional well-being of living kidney donors: findings from the RELIVE study. Am J Transplant. 2014;14(11):2535–44. https://doi.org/10.1111/ajt.12906.

34. Miller CM. Ethical dimensions of living donation: experience with living liver donation. Transplant Rev. 2008;22(3):206–9. https://doi.org/10.1016/j.trre.2008.02.001.

35. Ross LF, Thistlethwaite JR. Developing an ethics framework for living donor transplantation. J Med Ethics. 2018;44(12):843–50. https://doi.org/10.1136/medethics-2018-104762.

36. Henderson ML, Gross JA. Living organ donation and informed consent in the United States: strategies to improve the process. J Law Med Ethics. 2017;45(1):66–76. https://doi.org/10.1177/1073110517703101.

37. Ferreres AR, Angelos P, Singer EA, editors. Ethical issues in surgical care. Chicago: American College of Surgeons; 2017.

38. Parekh AM, Gordon EJ, Garg AX, Waterman AD, Kulkarni S, Parikh CR. Living kidney donor informed consent practices vary between US and non-US centers. Nephrol Dial Transplant. 2008;23(10):3316–24. https://doi.org/10.1093/ndt/gfn295.

39. Housawi AA, Young A, Boudville N, Thiessen-Philbrook H, Muirhead N, Rehman F, et al. Transplant professionals vary in the long-term medical risks they communicate to potential living kidney donors: an international survey. Nephrol Dial Transplant. 2007;22(10):3040–5. https://doi.org/10.1093/ndt/gfm305.

40. General Medical Council UK. Consent: patients and doctors making decisions together, proposed document under review 2019. Available at: www.gmc-uk.orgethical-guidanceethical-guidance-for-doctorsconsent.pdf. Accessed: 7 Sept 2020.

41. Faden RR, Beauchamp TL. A history and theory of informed consent. New York: Oxford University Press; 1986.

42. Organ Procurement and Transplantation Network (OPTN)/United Network for Organ Sharing (UNOS). Living donor informed consent checklist. 2017. Available at: optn.transplant.hrsa.gov/media/2162/living_donor_consent_checklist.pdf. Accessed: 7 Sept 2020.

43. Abecassis M, Adams M, Adams P, et al. Consensus statement on the live organ donor. JAMA. 2000;284(22):2919–26. https://doi.org/10.1001/jama.284.22.2919.

44. Organ Procurement and Transplantation Network (OPTN)/United Network for Organ Sharing (UNOS). Policy 13: Kidney Paired Donation. Available at: https://optn.transplant.hrsa.gov/media/1200/optn_policies.pdf. Accessed: 7 Sept 2020.

45. Ministerior de Sanidad. Disposiciones generales. Available at: https://www.finanzas.gob.ec/disposiciones-generales/. Accessed: September 7, 2020.

46. U.S. Department of Health and Human Services Health Information Privacy. Available at: www.hhs.gov/hipaa/for-professionals/privacy/laws-regulations/index.html. Accessed: 7 Sept 2020.

47. Organ Procurement and Transplantation Network (OPTN)/United Network for Organ Sharing (UNOS). Understanding the risk of transmission of HIV, Hepatitis B and Hepatitis C from U.S. PHS increased risk donors. Available at: https://optn.transplant.hrsa.gov/media/2116/guidance_increased_risk_organ_offers_20170327.pdf. Accessed: 7 Sept 2020.

48. Thiessen C, Kim YA, Formica R, Bia M, Kulkarni S. Opting out: confidentiality and availability of an "alibi" for potential living kidney donors in the USA. J Med Ethics. 2015;41(7):506–10. https://doi.org/10.1136/medethics-2014-102184.

49. Hays RE. Informed consent of living kidney donors: pitfalls and best practice. Curr Transplant Rep. 2015;2(1):29–34. https://doi.org/10.1007/s40472-014-0044-3.
50. Meadow J, Thistlethwaite JR, Rodrigue JR, Mandelbrot DA, Ross LF. To tell or not to tell: attitudes of transplant surgeons and transplant nephrologists regarding the disclosure of recipient information to living kidney donors. Clin Transpl. 2015;29(12):1203–12. https://doi.org/10.1111/ctr.12651.
51. Mataya L, Meadow J, Thistlethwaite JR, Mandelbrot DA, Rodrigue JR, Ross LF. Disclosing health and health behavior information between living donors and their recipients. Clin J Am Soc Nephrol. 2015;10(9):1609–16. https://doi.org/10.2215/CJN.02280215.
52. Rodrigue JR, Ladin K, Pavlakis M, Mandelbrot DA. Disclosing recipient information to potential living donors: preferences of donors and recipients, before and after surgery. Am J Transplant. 2011;11(6):1270–8. https://doi.org/10.1111/j.1600-6143.2011.03580.x.
53. Kortram K, Lafranca JA, Ijzermans JNM, Dor FJMF. The need for a standardized informed consent procedure in live donor nephrectomy: a systematic review. Transplantation. 2014;98(11):1134–43. https://doi.org/10.1097/TP.0000000000000518.
54. Lentine KL, Segev DL. Understanding and communicating medical risks for living kidney donors: a matter of perspective. J Am Soc Nephrol. 2017;28(1):12–24. https://doi.org/10.1681/ASN.2016050571.
55. Serur D, Gordon EJ. Kidney donors at risk: how to inform the donor. Prog Transplant. 2015;25(4):284–6. https://doi.org/10.7182/pit2015682.
56. Traino HM, Nonterah CW, Gupta G, Mincemoyer J. Living kidney donors' information needs and preferences. Prog Transplant. 2016;26(1):47–54. https://doi.org/10.1177/1526924816633943.
57. Gordon EJ, Sohn M-W, Chang C-H, McNatt G, Vera K, Beauvais N, Warren E, Mannon RB, Ison MG. Effect of a mobile web app on kidney transplant candidates' knowledge about increased risk donor kidneys: a randomized controlled trial. Transplantation. 2017;101(6):1167–76. https://doi.org/10.1097/TP.0000000000001273.
58. Gordon EJ, Feinglass J, Carney P, et al. A culturally targeted website for Hispanics/Latinos about living kidney donation and transplantation: a randomized controlled trial of increased knowledge. Transplantation. 2016;100(5):1149–60. https://doi.org/10.1097/TP.0000000000000932.
59. Gordon EJ, Butt Z, Jensen SE, et al. Opportunities for shared decision making in kidney transplantation. Am J Transplant. 2013;13(5):1149–58. https://doi.org/10.1111/ajt.12195.
60. Thiessen C, Gordon EJ, Reese PP, Kulkarni S. Development of a donor-centered approach to risk assessment: rebalancing nonmaleficence and autonomy. Am J Transplant. 2015;15(9):2314–23. https://doi.org/10.1111/ajt.13272.
61. Reese PP, Allen MB, Carney C, et al. Outcomes for individuals turned down for living kidney donation. Clin Transpl. 2018;10(9):e13408. https://doi.org/10.1111/ctr.13408.
62. LaPointe Rudow D, Hays R, Baliga P, et al. Consensus conference on best practices in live kidney donation: recommendations to optimize education, access, and care. Am J Transplant. 2015;15(4):914–22. https://doi.org/10.1111/ajt.13173.
63. Strigo TS, Ephraim PL, Pounds I, et al. The TALKS study to improve communication, logistical, and financial barriers to live donor kidney transplantation in African Americans: protocol of a randomized clinical trial. BMC Nephrol. 2015;16(1):160. https://doi.org/10.1186/s12882-015-0153-y.
64. Gordon EJ, Lee J, Kang R, Ladner DP, Skaro AI, Holl JL, French DD, Abecassis MM, Caicedo JC. Hispanic/Latino disparities in living donor kidney transplantation: role of a culturally competent transplant program. Transplant Direct. 2015;1(8):e29. https://doi.org/10.1097/TXD.0000000000000540.
65. Gordon EJ, Rodde J, Gil S, Caicedo JC. Quality of internet education about living kidney donation for Hispanics. Prog Transplant. 2012;22(3):294–303. https://doi.org/10.7182/pit2012802.
66. Rodrigue JR, Feranil M, Lang J, Fleishman A. Readability, content analysis, and racial/ethnic diversity of online living kidney donation information. Clin Transpl. 2017;31(9):e13039. https://doi.org/10.1111/ctr.13039.

67. U.S. Department of Health and Human Services. National Organ Transplant Act. 1984. Available at: www.congress.gov/bill/98th-congress/senate-bill/2048. Accessed: 7 Sept 2020.

68. Valapour M, Kahn JP, Bailey RF, Matas AJ. Assessing elements of informed consent among living donors. Clin Transpl. 2011;25(2):185–90. https://doi.org/10.1111/j.1399-0012.2010.01374.x.

69. Halverson CME, Crowley-Matoka M, Ross LF. Unspoken ambivalence in kinship obligation in living donation. Prog Transplant. 2018;28(3):250–5. https://doi.org/10.1177/1526924818781562.

70. Kortram K, Spoon EQW, Ismail SY, d'Ancona FCH, Christiaans MHL, van Heurn LWE, et al. Towards a standardised informed consent procedure for live donor nephrectomy: the PRINCE (Process of Informed Consent Evaluation) project-study protocol for a nationwide prospective cohort study. BMJ Open. 2016;6(4):e010594. https://doi.org/10.1136/bmjopen-2015-010594.

71. Kortram K, IJzermans JNM, Dor FJMF. Towards a standardized informed consent procedure for live donor nephrectomy: what do surgeons tell their donors? Int J Surg. 2016;32:83–8. https://doi.org/10.1016/j.ijsu.2016.05.063.

72. Thiessen C, Kim YA, Formica R, Bia M, Kulkarni S. Written informed consent for living kidney donors: practices and compliance with CMS and OPTN requirements. Am J Transplant. 2013;13(10):2713–21. https://doi.org/10.1111/ajt.12406.

73. Gordon EJ, Bergeron A, McNatt G, Friedewald J, Abecassis MM, Wolf MS. Are informed consent forms for organ transplantation and donation too difficult to read? Clin Transpl. 2012;26(2):275–83. https://doi.org/10.1111/j.1399-0012.2011.01480.x.

74. Tong A, Chapman JR, Wong G, Kanellis J, McCarthy G, Craig JC. The motivations and experiences of living kidney donors: a thematic synthesis. Am J Kidney Dis. 2012;60(1):15–26. https://doi.org/10.1053/j.ajkd.2011.11.043.

75. Switzer GE, Dew MA, Simmons RG. Donor ambivalence and postdonation outcomes: implications for living donation. Transplant Proc. 1997;29(1–2):1476. https://doi.org/10.1016/s0041-1345(96)00590-8.

76. Dew MA, Zuckoff A, DiMartini AF, DeVito Dabbs AJ, McNulty ML, Fox KR, Switzer GE, Humar A, Tan HP. Prevention of poor psychosocial outcomes in living organ donors: from description to theory-driven intervention development and initial feasibility testing. Prog Transplant. 2012;22(3):280–92. https://doi.org/10.1002/14651858.CD002098.

77. Dew MA, DiMartini AF, DeVito Dabbs AJ, Zuckoff A, Tan HP, McNulty ML, Switzer GE, Fox KR, Greenhouse JB, Humar A. Preventive intervention for living donor psychosocial outcomes: feasibility and efficacy in a randomized controlled trial. Am J Transplant. 2013;13(10):2672–84. https://doi.org/10.1111/ajt.12393.

78. Guerin RM, O'Toole E, Daly B. The will reconsidered: hard choices in living organ donation. Narrat Inq Bioeth. 2018;8(2):179–86. https://doi.org/10.1353/nib.2018.0055.

79. Ross LF. Good ethics requires good science: why transplant programs should not disclose misattributed parentage. Am J Transplant. 2010;10(4):742–6. https://doi.org/10.1111/j.1600-6143.2009.03011.x.

80. Lentine KL, Mannon RB. Apolipoprotein L1: role in the evaluation of kidney transplant donors. Curr Opin Nephrol Hypertens. 2020;29(6):645–55. https://pubmed.ncbi.nlm.nih.gov/33009133/; https://doi.org/10.1097/MNH.0000000000000653.

81. Doshi MD, Ortigosa-Goggins M, Garg AX, Li L, Poggio ED, Winkler CA, Kopp JB. APOL1 genotype and renal function of black living donors. J Am Soc Nephrol. 2018;29(4):1309–16. https://doi.org/10.1681/ASN.2017060658.

82. Nadkarni GN, Gignoux CR, Sorokin EP, Daya M, Rahman R, Barnes KC, Wassel CL, Kenny EE. Worldwide frequencies of APOL1 renal risk variants. N Engl J Med. 2018;379(26):2571–2. https://doi.org/10.1056/NEJMc1800748.

83. Newell KA, Formica RN, Gill JS, Schold JD, Allan JS, Covington SH, Wiseman AC, Chandraker A. Integrating APOL1 gene variants into renal transplantation: considerations arising from the American Society of Transplantation Expert Conference. Am J Transplant. 2017;17(4):901–11. https://doi.org/10.1111/ajt.14173.

84. Gordon EJ, Amórtegui D, Blancas I, Wicklund C, Friedewald J, Sharp RR. African American living donors' attitudes about APOL1 genetic testing: a mixed methods study. Am J Kidney Dis. 2018;72(6):819–33. https://doi.org/10.1053/j.ajkd.2018.07.017.

85. Thomas CP, Mansilla MA, Sompallae R, et al. Screening of living kidney donors for genetic diseases using a comprehensive genetic testing strategy. Am J Transplant. 2017;17(2):401–10. https://doi.org/10.1111/ajt.13970.

86. Gordon EJ, Amortegui D, Blancas I, Wicklund C, Friedewald J, Sharp RR. African American living donors' treatment preferences, sociocultural factors, and health beliefs about Apolipoprotein L1 genetic testing. Prog Transplant. 2019. In Press. https://doi.org/10.1177/1526924819854485.

87. Freedman BI, Moxey-Mims MM, Alexander AA, Astor BC, Birdwell KA, Bowden DW, et al. APOL1 Long-term Kidney Transplantation Outcomes Network (APOLLO): design and rationale. Kidney Int Rep. 2020;5(3):278–88. https://doi.org/10.1016/j.ekir.2019.11.022.

88. Ross LF, Thistlethwaite JR. Prisoners as living donors: a vulnerabilities analysis. Camb Q Healthc Ethics. 2018;27(1):93–108. https://doi.org/10.1017/S0963180117000433.

89. Rodrigue JR, Fleishman A. Health insurance trends in United States living kidney donors (2004 to 2015). Am J Transplant. 2016;16(12):3504–11. https://doi.org/10.1111/ajt.13827.

90. Lawson T, Ralph C. Perioperative Jehovah's witnesses: a review. Br J Anaesth. 2015;115(5):676–87. https://doi.org/10.1093/bja/aev161.

91. Dew MA, Jacobs CL, Jowsey SG, Hanto R, Miller C, Delmonico FL. Guidelines for the psychosocial evaluation of living unrelated kidney donors in the United States. Am J Transplant. 2007;7:1047–54. https://doi.org/10.1111/j.1600-6143.2007.01751.x.

92. Jacobs C, Berglund DM, Wiseman JF, Garvey C, Larson DB, Voges M, Radecki Breitkopf C, Ibrahim HN, Matas AJ. Long-term psychosocial outcomes after nondirected donation: a single-center experience. Am J Transplant. 2018;343(6):433. https://doi.org/10.1111/ajt.15179.

93. Henderson ML, Adler JT, Van Pilsum Rasmussen SE, et al. How should social media be used in transplantation? A survey of the American Society of Transplant Surgeons. Transplantation. 2018. April 21: Publish Ahead of Print. https://doi.org/10.1097/TP.0000000000002243.

94. Veale JL, Capron AM, Nassiri N, et al. Vouchers for future kidney transplants to overcome "chronological incompatibility" between living donors and recipients. Transplantation. 2017;101(9):2115–9. https://doi.org/10.1097/TP.0000000000001744.

95. Ross LF, Rodrigue JR, Veatch RM. Ethical and logistical issues raised by the advanced donation program "pay it forward" scheme. J Med Philos. 2017;42(5):518–36. https://doi.org/10.1093/jmp/jhx018.

96. Wall AE, Veale JL, Melcher ML. Advanced donation programs and deceased donor-initiated chains-2 innovations in kidney paired donation. Transplantation. 2017;101(12):2818–24. https://doi.org/10.1097/TP.0000000000001838.

97. Gordon EJ, Beauvais N, Theodoropoulos N, Hanneman J, McNatt G, Penrod D, Jensen S, Franklin J, Sherman L, Ison MG. The challenge of informed consent for increased risk living donation and transplantation. Am J Transplant. 2011;11(12):2569–74. https://doi.org/10.1111/j.1600-6143.2011.03814.x.

98. Rodrigue JR, Vishnevsky T, Fleishman A, Brann T, Evenson AR, Pavlakis M, Mandelbrot DA. Patient-reported outcomes following living kidney donation: a single center experience. J Clin Psychol Med Settings. 2015;22(2–3):160–8. https://doi.org/10.1007/s10880-015-9424-9.

99. Jacobs CL, Gross CR, Messersmith EE, et al. Emotional and financial experiences of kidney donors over the past 50 years: the RELIVE study. Clin J Am Soc Nephrol. 2015;10(12):2221–31. https://doi.org/10.2215/CJN.07120714.

100. Schover LR, Streem SB, Boparai N, Duriak K, Novick AC. The psychosocial impact of donating a kidney: long-term follow-up from a urology based center. J Urol. 1997;157(5):1596–601. https://doi.org/10.1016/s0022-5347(01)64803-1.

101. Halverson CME, Wang JY, Poulson M, Karlin J, Crowley-Matoka M, Ross LF. Living kidney donors who develop kidney failure: excerpts of their thoughts. Am J Nephrol. 2016;43(6):389–96. https://doi.org/10.1159/000446161.

102. Haljamäe U, Nyberg G, Sjöström B. Remaining experiences of living kidney donors more than 3 yr after early recipient graft loss. Clin Transpl. 2003;17(6):503–10. https://doi.org/10.1046/j.1399-0012.2003.00078.x.
103. Cabrer C, Oppenhaimer F, Manyalich M, et al. The living kidney donation process: the donor perspective. Transplant Proc. 2003;35(5):1631–2. https://doi.org/10.1016/s0041-1345(03)00697-3.
104. Ruck JM, Van Pilsum Rasmussen SE, Henderson ML, Massie AB, Segev DL. Interviews of living kidney donors to assess donation-related concerns and information-gathering practices. BMC Nephrol. 2018;19(1):130. https://doi.org/10.1186/s12882-018-0935-0.
105. Hanson CS, Ralph AF, Manera KE, Gill JS, Kanellis J, Wong G, Craig JC, Chapman JR, Tong A. The lived experience of "being evaluated" for organ donation: focus groups with living kidney donors. Clin J Am Soc Nephrol. 2017;12(11):1852–61. https://doi.org/10.2215/CJN.03550417.
106. Gordon EJ, Mullee JO, Ramirez DI, MacLean J, Olivero M, Feinglass J, Carney P, O'Connor K, Caicedo JC. Hispanic/Latino concerns about living kidney donation: a focus group study. Prog Transplant. 2014;24(2):152–62. https://doi.org/10.7182/pit2014946.
107. Tong A, Chapman JR, Wong G, Craig JC. Living kidney donor assessment: challenges, uncertainties and controversies among transplant nephrologists and surgeons. Am J Transplant. 2013;13(11):2912–23. https://doi.org/10.1111/ajt.12411.
108. Grady C. Enduring and emerging challenges of informed consent. N Engl J Med. 2015;372(9):855–62. https://doi.org/10.1056/NEJMra1411250.
109. U.S. Department of Health and Human Services (HHS), Centers for Medicare and Medicaid Services (CMS). Organ Transplant Interpretive Guidelines. Available at: https://www.cms.gov/Regulations-and-Guidance/Guidance/Transmittals/2019Downloads/R189SOMA.pdf. Accessed: 7 Sept 2020.
110. Freeman J, Emond J, Gillespie BW, et al. Computerized assessment of competence-related abilities in living liver donors: the adult-to-adult living donor liver transplantation cohort study. Clin Transpl. 2013;27(4):633–45. https://doi.org/10.1111/ctr.12184.
111. Gordon EJ, Rodde J, Skaro A, Baker T. Informed consent for live liver donors: a qualitative, prospective study. J Hepatol. 2015;63(4):838–47. https://doi.org/10.1016/j.jhep.2015.05.003.
112. Tong A, Sautenet B, Chapman JR, et al. Research priority setting in organ transplantation: a systematic review. Transplant Int. 2017;30(4):327–43. https://doi.org/10.1111/tri.12924.
113. Gander JC, Gordon EJ, Patzer RE. Decision aids to increase living donor kidney transplantation. Curr Transplant Rep. 2017;4(1):1–12. https://doi.org/10.1007/s40472-017-0133-1.
114. Rodrigue JR, Paek MJ, Egbuna O, Waterman AD, Schold JD, Pavlakis M, Mandelbrot DA. Making house calls increases living donor inquiries and evaluations for blacks on the kidney transplant waiting list. Transplantation. 2014;98(9):979–86. https://doi.org/10.1097/TP.0000000000000165.

Evaluation of Glomerular Filtration Rate, Albuminuria and Hematuria in Living Donor Candidates

3

Andrew S. Levey, Nitender Goyal, and Lesley A. Inker

Introduction

The 2017 guideline on the evaluation of kidney donor candidates from the international organization KDIGO adopts a framework for shared decision-making for kidney donor candidates based on benefits and risks to the donor [1]. Unlike prior guidelines, the KDIGO donor evaluation guideline proposes a comprehensive and integrated evaluation of all risk factors for adverse outcomes, rather than an evaluation of single risk factors in isolation. Recent data suggest that kidney donors have an increased risk for subsequent development of kidney failure and other conditions associated with CKD, compared to nondonors with equivalent risk profiles. Reasons for increased risk are not defined, but may relate to increased susceptibility to CKD from the impact of a second "hit" in the context of donation-related alterations in kidney function or structure [2], particularly in the presence of predonation alterations which do not meet the criteria for CKD. Evaluations of GFR, albuminuria, and hematuria are the main methods for the detection of predonation CKD in kidney donor candidates, and alterations in these measures have been related to increased risk of kidney failure in the general population. Imaging of the kidney (as reviewed elsewhere) is obtained principally for the evaluation of vessels, collecting system, and ureters to guide surgery, but may also disclose evidence of kidney disease that informs risk for the donor or appropriateness of the kidney for the recipient. This chapter reviews the pathophysiology and measurement methods for GFR, albuminuria, and hematuria and risk of kidney failure related to these measures, including recommendations from the recent KDIGO donor evaluation guideline and how they compare with previous guidelines.

A. S. Levey (✉) · N. Goyal · L. A. Inker
Division of Nephrology, Tufts Medical Center, Boston, MA, USA
e-mail: alevey@tuftsmedicalcenter.org

© Springer Nature Switzerland AG 2021
K. L. Lentine et al. (eds.), *Living Kidney Donation*,
https://doi.org/10.1007/978-3-030-53618-3_3

Recommendations in the KDIGO donor evaluation guideline related to measurement are based on physiological principles and recommendations for general clinical practice from the 2012 KDIGO Clinical Practice Guideline for the Evaluation and Management of Chronic Kidney Disease for GFR and albuminuria [3] and from the AUA 2012 guidelines for hematuria [4]. There is no evidence to suggest that living kidney donor candidates or kidney donors differ from other populations in a way that is relevant to recommendations for measurements.

Glomerular Filtration Rate

Pathophysiology and Measurement

The level of GFR is widely accepted as the best overall index of kidney function in healthy people and those with diseases. The rationale is that GFR is a property of the kidney, has a wide range, and is affected by physiologic, pharmacologic, and pathologic conditions. Furthermore, GFR decline is associated with many physiologic and clinical consequences and is correlated with decline in other kidney functions. Decreased GFR is one criterion in the definition and staging of acute and chronic kidney diseases [3].

Normal range and variability. GFR is proportional to kidney size, which is proportional to body size; hence, normative levels of GFR are expressed per 1.73 m^2 body surface area (BSA), thereby reducing the variability in GFR in healthy individuals. Similarly, for assessment of kidney donor candidates, adjusting GFR to BSA allows communication of GFR thresholds for decision-making that can be applied across the usual distribution of body size.

Mean GFR in healthy young white adults is approximately 125 mL/min per 1.73 m^2, but with a wide range around this normal value [5]. GFR is affected by numerous physiologic and pathologic conditions and varies with time of day, dietary protein intake, exercise, age, pregnancy, obesity, hyperglycemia, use of antihypertensive drugs, surfeit or deficit of extracellular fluid, and acute and chronic kidney disease. Some but not all evidence suggests that the normal level of GFR varies among ethnic groups [6, 7]. The average kidney length and volume in healthy adults are approximately 12 cm and 300 mL, respectively, and correlate with GFR, but vary based on age, sex, and body size [8–10]. On average the normal right kidney is approximately 5% smaller than the normal left kidney.

GFR is lower at older age. Most studies have been cross-sectional (Fig. 3.1) [5]; the few longitudinal studies show a wide variability in rates of decline among individuals. The cause of decline is often not known. Other kidney functions are also lower in older populations (e.g., renal plasma flow, maximal urinary concentration), and kidney structure is altered in older populations (e.g., cortical atrophy, global glomerulosclerosis, nephrosclerosis). As such, there is debate about whether abnormalities in kidney function and structure in older people represent normal aging or disease.

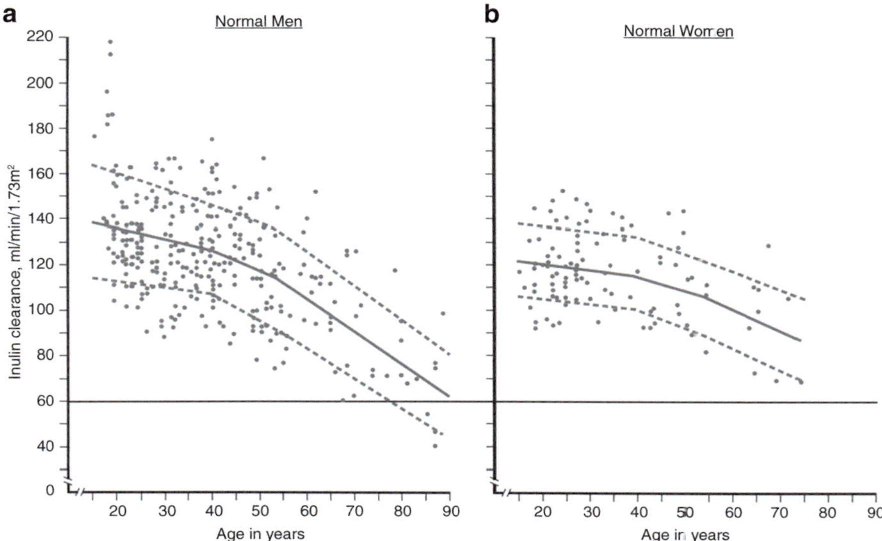

Fig. 3.1 Normal values for GFR in men and women. Normal values for GFR (inulin clearance) are shown for men and women of various ages. Solid lines represent the mean value of GFR per decade of age, and dashed lines represent the value 1 standard deviation from the mean value of GFR per decade of age. (From Wesson [5])

The 2012 KDIGO CKD guideline defines GFR < 60 mL/min per 1.73 m² for 3 months or more as satisfying the criteria for CKD [3]. GFR in young men and women >90 mL/min per 1.73 m² is considered normal, and GFR between 60 and 89 mL/min per 1.73 m² is considered decreased compared to the usual level for young adults. GFR < 30 mL/min per 1.73 m² is defined as severely reduced, and GFR < 15 mL/min per 1.73 m² is defined as kidney failure. *2012 KDIGO CKD recommendations for evaluation.* It is not possible to directly measure GFR in humans; thus, the "true" GFR cannot be known with certainty. GFR can be measured indirectly as the clearance of exogenous filtration markers or estimated from serum levels of endogenous filtration markers, but both measured GFR (mGFR) and estimated GFR (eGFR) are associated with error in their determination. The accuracy of various methods for measuring and estimating GFR is not known with sufficient certainty to define specific thresholds for each method.

The 2012 KDIGO CKD guideline recommends expressing kidney function as GFR, not as serum concentrations of endogenous filtration markers, and recommends expressing GFR in mL/min per 1.73 m² rather than mL/min [3]. The guideline recommends two-stage testing (initial testing followed by confirmatory testing as necessary). eGFR based on serum creatinine (eGFR$_{cr}$) is the recommended initial test. Confirmatory tests are indicated in specific circumstances when eGFR$_{cr}$ is less accurate.

The 2012 KDIGO CKD guideline recommends that serum creatinine assays should be traceable to the international reference standard. Assay traceability is important for all endogenous filtration markers and is especially important for GFR estimation at higher GFR ranges, corresponding to low values for serum concentrations.

The 2012 KDIGO CKD guideline recommends use of the 2009 CKD-EPI creatinine equation in North America, Europe, and Australia, where it has been extensively validated. The equation has minimal bias at normal GFR; however, it is imprecise (Fig. 3.2), and thus it is useful for an initial evaluation [11]. In regions other than North America, Europe, and Australia, the 2009 CKD-EPI creatinine equation is less accurate, and other equations are recommended if they are more accurate in the given region. A variety of confirmatory tests for GFR are available. The 2012 KDIGO CKD guideline suggests confirmation of GFR with either GFR estimation using serum cystatin C ($eGFR_{cys}$) or the combination of serum creatinine and cystatin C ($eGFR_{cr-cys}$) or a clearance measurement. The guideline further suggests measuring GFR with an exogenous filtration marker under circumstances where more accurate ascertainment of GFR will impact treatment decisions and gives the specific example of evaluating kidney donors.

GFR estimating equations are developed using regression to relate the mGFR to steady-state serum creatinine (S_{cr}) or serum cystatin C (S_{cys}) concentration and a combination of demographic and clinical variables as surrogates of the non-GFR determinants of S_{cr} or S_{cys}. GFR estimates using S_{cr} or S_{cys} concentrations are more accurate in estimating mGFR than the serum concentrations alone in the study population in which they were developed. Sources of error in GFR estimation from S_{cr}

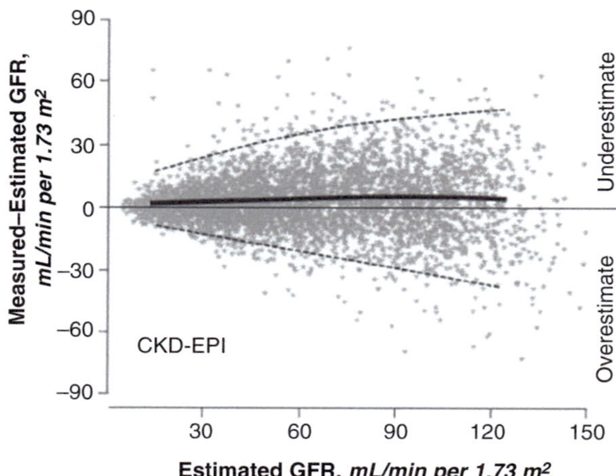

Fig. 3.2 Performance of the CKD-EPI equation to estimate measured GFR. The figure shows the difference between measured and estimated GFR (bias) vs estimated GFR in the CKD-EPI external validation dataset ($N = 3896$). A smoothed regression line is shown with the 95% CI. *Abbreviation: CKD-EPI* Chronic Kidney Disease Epidemiology Collaboration. (From Levey et al. [11])

Table 3.1 Sources of error in using estimated GFR

Sources of Error	Examples using eGFR$_{cr}$	Examples using eGFR$_{cys}$
Nonsteady state Non-GFR determinants[a]	Acute kidney injury	Acute kidney injury
Generation	• Race/ethnicity other than US and European black and white • Extremes of body size • Diet and nutritional status (high-protein diet, creatine supplements)	• Race/ethnicity other than US and European black and white • Disorder of thyroid function • Administration of corticosteroids • Other hypothesized factors (diabetes, adiposity)
Tubular reabsorption or secretion	• Inhibition of tubular secretion (trimethoprim, cimetidine, fenofibrate)	None identified
Extra-renal elimination	• Dialysis • Inhibition of gut creatininase by antibiotics • Large extracellular fluid losses	Severe decreased GFR
Interferences with assay	• Spectral interferences (bilirubin, some drugs) • Chemical interferences (glucose, ketones, bilirubin, some drugs)	Heterophilic antibodies
Higher GFR	• Higher biological variability in non-GFR determinants relative to GFR • Higher measurement error in GFR • Higher measurement error in S$_{cr}$	• Higher biological variability in non-GFR determinants relative to GFR • Higher measurement error in GFR • Higher measurement error in S$_{cys}$

Abbreviations: eGFR estimated GFR, *S$_{cr}$* serum creatinine, *S$_{cys}$* serum cystatin C
[a]Non-GFR determinants that differ from the study populations in which GFR estimating equations were developed
(From KDIGO 2012 [3])

or S$_{cys}$ concentrations include nonsteady-state conditions, non-GFR determinants of S$_{cr}$ or S$_{cys}$, measurement error at higher GFR, and interferences with S$_{cr}$ or S$_{cys}$ assays (Table 3.1) [3]. GFR estimates are less precise at higher GFR levels than at lower levels. Interpretation of GFR estimates in donor candidates requires appreciation of these sources of error.

In general eGFR$_{cys}$ is not more accurate then eGFR$_{cr}$; however using two filtration markers improves precision of GFR estimates compared to using either marker alone; thus eGFR$_{cr-cys}$ is generally recommended over eGFR$_{cr}$ or eGFR$_{cys}$ [12, 13]. Advantages of cystatin C compared to creatinine are that S$_{cys}$ is not affected by muscle mass and current equations do not require specification of race. Therefore, eGFR$_{cys}$ may be more accurate than eGFR$_{cr-cys}$ in people with very large or very small muscle mass, very high or very low meat intake, or race ethnicity other than black (African American or African European) or white. If S$_{cys}$ is measured, assays should be traceable to an international reference standard (which is in the early stages of implementation), and the 2012 CKD-EPI eGFR$_{cys}$ or eGFR$_{cr-cys}$ equation should be used unless other equations have been shown to be more accurate.

Many methods for mGFR determination using exogenous filtration markers and clearance calculations are available, with variable accuracy [14]. mGFR is not available in all centers, so other alternatives are acceptable. Measured creatinine clearance (mCl$_{cr}$) is less accurate than mGFR [14], but is acceptable if mGFR is not available. mCl$_{cr}$ overestimates mGFR due to creatinine secretion [15]. The magnitude of overestimation is 15% or more at normal GFR, based on older data using nonstandardized S$_{cr}$ assays. The magnitude of overestimation may be higher using standardized assays. At lower levels of GFR, averaging the clearances of creatinine and urea nitrogen can provide an accurate estimate of mGFR, but this is less accurate at the higher levels of GFR encountered in the evaluation of donor candidates.

One study suggests that eGFR may be sufficiently accurate for decision-making in kidney donor candidates [16]. Posttest probabilities were computed from pretest probabilities for mGFR and test performance for eGFR$_{cr}$ or eGFR$_{cr-cys}$. Very high posttest probabilities provide reassurance that mGFR is above the threshold level for decision-making, while very low posttest probabilities provide reassurance that mGFR is below the threshold levels for decision-making. A web-based calculator is available to compute posttest probabilities for mGFR above or below threshold probabilities for decision-making: *http://ckdepi.org/equations/donor-candidate-gfr-calculator/*. Transplant centers can determine what posttest probabilities are sufficient for clinical decision-making in the absence of mGFR and mCl$_{cr}$. Another study validating these computations in donor candidates has been reported [17], but validations have not yet been performed to determine accuracy among racial and ethnic groups for whom the accuracy of eGFR is less certain (e.g., nonblack, nonwhite persons).

In the United States, performance of mGFR or mCl$_{cr}$ is required by Organ Procurement and Transplantation Network (OPTN) policy for donor evaluation [18]. In countries where clearances are required for assessment of GFR, an efficient strategy could be to omit timed urine collections and to rely on mGFR using clearance of an exogenous filtration marker along with urine albumin-to-creatinine ratio (ACR) (discussed below). In countries where clearance measures are not required for assessment of GFR, transplant programs could take the approach of obtaining eGFR$_{cr}$, eGFR$_{cr-cys}$, and urine ACR prior to a candidate donor's visit to the center [19].

All kidney donor candidates undergo kidney imaging to detect parenchymal, vascular, or urologic abnormalities. Asymmetry in kidney size suggests asymmetry in kidney function. In these cases, single-kidney ("divided" or "split") GFR can be assessed by radionuclide imaging.

Risk of Kidney Failure Related to Decreased GFR

Risk in the general population. Decreased GFR in the general population is associated with a higher risk of complications of CKD, including end-stage renal disease

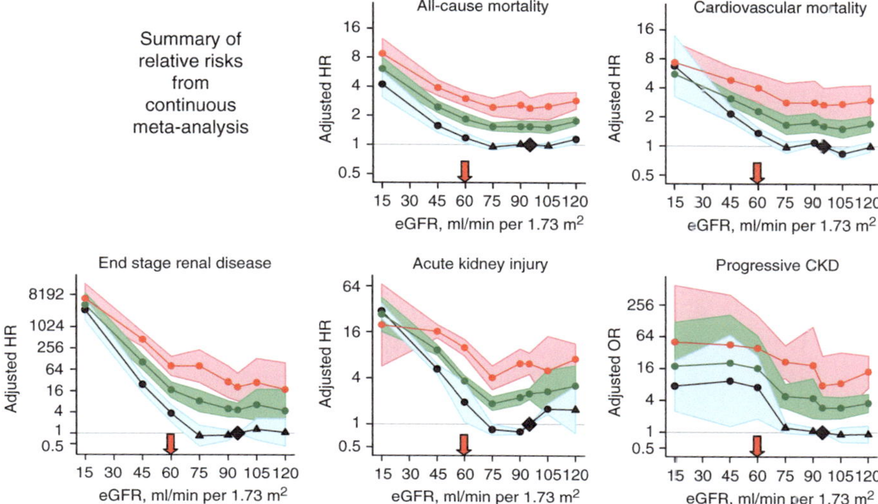

Fig. 3.3 Summary of relative risks for mortality and kidney disease outcomes based on eGFR and albuminuria. The data above are based on $eGFR_{cr}$ using the MDRD study equation. Comparable data are not available for mGFR. However, studies using the CKD-EPI 2009 creatinine equation and the CKD-EPI 2012 cystatin C and creatinine-cystatin C equations confirm these results. Color shading represents ACR categories: blue <30 mg/g; green 30–300 mg/g; red (>300 mg/g). *Abbreviations*: *eGFR* estimated GFR, $eGFR_{cr}$ eGFR based on creatinine, *MDRD* Modification of Diet in Renal Disease, *CKD-EPI* Chronic Kidney Disease Epidemiology Collaboration, *ACR* albumin-creatinine ratio. (From Levey et al. [20])

(ESRD), defined by initiation of kidney replacement therapy, cardiovascular disease, and death. In general populations, compared to a reference eGFR of 95 mL/min per 1.73 m², the relative risk (RR) for complications related to decreased eGFR is apparent between 60 and 75 mL/min per 1.73 m² and is exponentially higher at lower eGFR (Fig. 3.3) [20–22]. However, the association of lower eGFR with a higher risk of adverse outcomes is also strongly associated with the presence of other conditions that co-occur with low GFR, such as hypertension, diabetes, and cardiovascular disease. Lower GFR in older people is associated with increased risk for CKD outcomes, including ESRD, cardiovascular disease, and death. The relative risk for these outcomes in older people with lower eGFR compared to the reference eGFR is less than the RR in younger people; however, the increment in absolute risk is higher in older people than in younger people [23]. However, the applicability of these studies to donor candidates may be limited because donors are usually selected for the absence of these conditions and sometimes for younger age.

A recent meta-analysis based on data from nearly 5 million healthy persons identified from seven US general population cohorts with health characteristics similar to kidney donor candidates found that lower GFR (in the absence of donation) is associated with an increased risk for ESRD over a median cohort follow-up of 4–16 years [24]. A web-based calculator is available to compute 15-year and lifetime

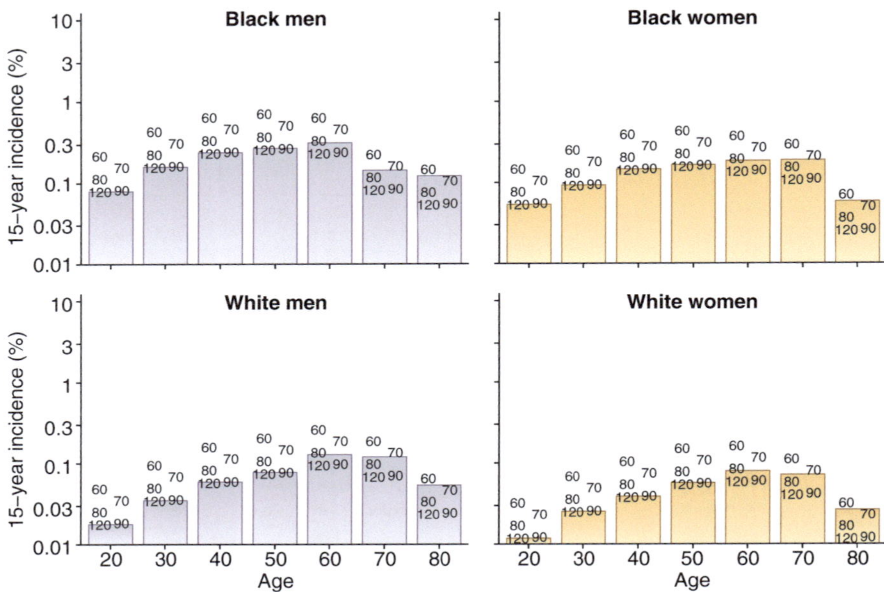

Fig. 3.4 Estimated 15-year incidence (%) of ESKD in the United States according to baseline eGFR and demographic profile. The base-case scenario is the following: age-specific eGFR (114, 106, 98, 90, 82, 74, and 66 mL/min per 1.73 m² for ages 20, 30, 40, 50, 60, 70, and 80 years, respectively), systolic blood pressure 120 mmHg, urine ACR 4 mg/g [0.4 mg/mmol], BMI 26 kg/m², and no diabetes mellitus or antihypertensive medication use. These were selected as being representative of recent US living kidney donors where, with the exception of eGFR, there was little variation in health characteristics by age. *Abbreviations*: *eGFR* estimated GFR, *ACR* albumin-creatinine ratio, *BMI* body mass index. (From Grams et al. [24])

risks for ESRD (in the absence of donation) based on baseline demographic and health characteristics: *http://www.ckdpcrisk.org/esrdrisk/*. Variations in the projected risks according to level of eGFR from this analysis are displayed graphically in Figs. 3.4 and 3.5 [24] according to age, sex, and race for healthy persons [1]. This analysis demonstrates that lower eGFR is associated with increased lifetime risk for ESRD in all demographic subgroups. For eGFR ≥90 mL/min per 1.73 m², lifetime risk for white men and white women was less than 1% at all ages, but exceeded 2% for black men and women younger than 30 and 20 years, respectively (Fig. 3.5). Lifetime risk for eGFR 60–89 was less than 1% at ages older than 60 years.

Risk after kidney donation. Following the approximate reduction of renal mass by 50% with donor nephrectomy, there is rapid compensatory hyperfiltration leading to a net reduction in GFR of only 30% (25–40%) after donation (decrement in GFR of 25–40 mL/min per 1.73 m²) [25–28]. There is theoretical justification for concern about development of kidney disease after nephrectomy. In experimental animals, hemodynamic alterations associated with hyperfiltration after reduction in renal

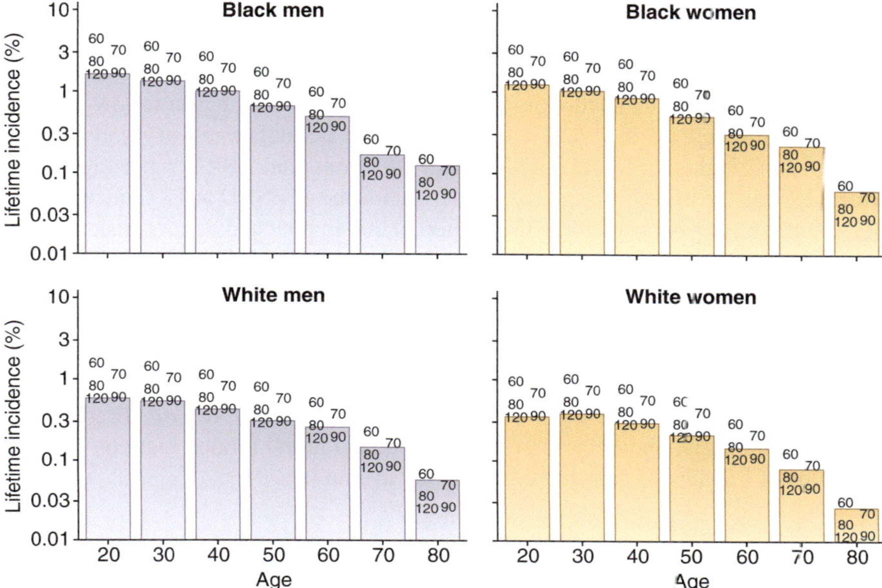

Fig. 3.5 Estimated lifetime incidence (%) of ESKD in the United States according to baseline eGFR and demographic profile. The base-case scenario is the following: age-specific eGFR (114, 106, 98, 90, 82, 74, and 66 mL/min per 1.73 m² for ages 20, 30, 40, 50, 60, 70, and 80 years, respectively), systolic blood pressure 120 mmHg, urine ACR 4 mg/g [0.4 mg/mmol], BMI 26 kg/m², and no diabetes mellitus or antihypertensive medication use. These were selected as being representative of recent US living kidney donors where, with the exception of eGFR, there was little variation in health characteristics by age. Lifetime risk projections are based on 15 years of follow-up data and calibrated to the incidence of ESRD in the low-risk population and thus are likely imprecise. *Abbreviations*: *eGFR* estimated GFR, *ACR* albumin-creatinine ratio, *BMI* body mass index. (From Grams et al. [24])

mass are followed by development of structural and functional abnormalities associated with kidney disease. In general, the severity of reduction in renal mass is directly associated with the rate of development of subsequent kidney disease. Recent studies in humans document similar hemodynamic alterations associated with hyperfiltration following kidney donation [28, 29]. Limited data show a higher risk for lower GFR among kidney donors with lower predonation GFR.The risk of ESRD after kidney donation does not exceed ESRD rates in the general population [26, 30, 31]. An analysis of living kidney donors in the United States between 1994 and 2003 quantified a postdonation ESRD rate of 0.134 per 1000 person-years over an average follow-up of 9.8 years, which was not higher than the ESRD rate in the general population, even though GFR was lower [32]. However, the general population is a limited comparison group given that donors undergo careful medical evaluation and selection [33]. Two recent studies comparing kidney donors to individuals selected for baseline good health suggest that donation is associated with an increase in the risk of ESRD, although the risk increase is small and the absolute postdonation risk remains low. In comparing 1901 kidney donors with 32,621 healthy, demographically matched controls, Mjøen et al. reported that nine donors (0.47%) developed ESRD versus 22 healthy nondonors (0.07%) over a median 15.2-year follow-up [34]. Based on linking data for 96,217 donors from the US donor registry and data for healthy participants drawn from NHANES III to national ESRD reporting forms, Muzzale et al. estimated that the cumulative incidence of ESRD at 15 years was 30.8 per 10,000 in donors compared with 3.9 per 10,000 in matched donors (risk attributable to donation of 26.9 per 10,000) [35]. In this study, the incidence of ESRD was higher in individuals who are older vs younger at the time of donation, in men vs women, in blacks vs whites, and in biologically related vs unrelated donors. The authors of this report subsequently developed a model to predict postdonation ESRD risk over 20 years, based on age, sex, race, BMI, and family history of ESRD [36], and a web-based calculator: *http://www.transplantmodels.com/donesrd/*. Predonation eGFR, albuminuria, and hematuria are not included in the model. Data on lifetime estimates of ESRD in donors are currently not available.

Box 3.1: 2017 KDIGO Living Donor Guideline Recommendations related to Predonation GFR

Measurement

- 5.1: Donor kidney function should be expressed as glomerular filtration rate and not as serum creatinine concentration.
- 5.2: Donor GFR should be expressed in mL/min per 1.73 m^2 rather than mL/min.
- 5.3: Donor GFR should be estimated from serum creatinine (eGFRcr) for initial assessment, following recommendations from the KDIGO 2012 CKD guideline.
- 5.4: Donor GFR should be confirmed using one or more of the following measurements depending on their availability:
  - Measured GFR using an exogenous filtration marker, preferably urinary or plasma clearance of inulin, urinary or plasma clearance of iothalamate, urinary or plasma clearance of 51Cr-EDTA, urinary or plasma clearance of iohexol, and urinary clearance of 99mTc-DTPA
  - Measured creatinine clearance
  - Estimated GFR from the combination of serum creatinine and cystatin C (eGFRcr-cys) following recommendations from the KDIGO 2012 CKD guideline
  - Repeat estimated GFR from eGFRcr
- 5.5: If there are parenchymal, vascular, or urological abnormalities or asymmetry of kidney size on renal imaging, single-kidney GFR should be assessed using radionuclides or contrast agents that are excreted by glomerular filtration (e.g., 99mTc-DTPA).

Selection

- 5.6: GFR $\geq$ 90 mL/min per 1.73 m^2 should be considered as an acceptable level of kidney function for kidney donation.
- 5.7: The decision to approve donor candidates with GFR 60–89 mL/min per 1.73 m^2 should be individualized based on demographic and health profile in relation to the transplant center's acceptable risk threshold.
- 5.8: Donor candidates with GFR <60 mL/min per 1.73 m^2 should not donate.
- 5.9: When asymmetry in GFR, parenchymal abnormalities, vascular abnormalities, or urological abnormalities are present but do not preclude donation, the more severely affected kidney should be used for donation.

Counseling

- 5.10: We suggest that donor candidates be informed that the future risk of developing kidney failure necessitating treatment with dialysis or transplantation is slightly higher because of the donation; however, average absolute risk in the 15 years following donation remains low.

The 2017 KDIGO living donor guideline recommends a two-stage evaluation process, starting with eGFR$_{cr}$ using the CKD-EPI equation as the first step in the evaluation, followed by confirmation of GFR using the most accurate method available at the transplant center, recognizing that in many centers, more than one method may be available. In the United States, OPTN policy requires a clearance measurement for confirmation of GFR. The 2017 KDIGO guideline recommends GFR measurement by urinary or plasma clearance of specific exogenous filtration markers, which are known to be more accurate than mCl$_{cr}$, but allows other methods.

The 2017 KDIGO guideline recommends mGFR $\geq$90 mL/min per 1.73 m^2 as a threshold to routinely accept a donor candidate, mGFR <60 mL/min per 1.73 m^2 as a threshold to routinely decline a donor candidate, and a wide intermediate range of mGFR (60–89 mL/min per 1.73 m^2) in which transplant centers can individualize decisions based on other risk factors. The guideline recommends that all information from GFR estimates and measurements be included in reaching a conclusion on the level of GFR and risk (Fig. 3.6) [19, 37]. Additionally, the guideline recommends that the likelihood of a small increase in ESRD risk should be discussed with donor candidates, and such counseling is now required in OPTN/UNOS policy [18].

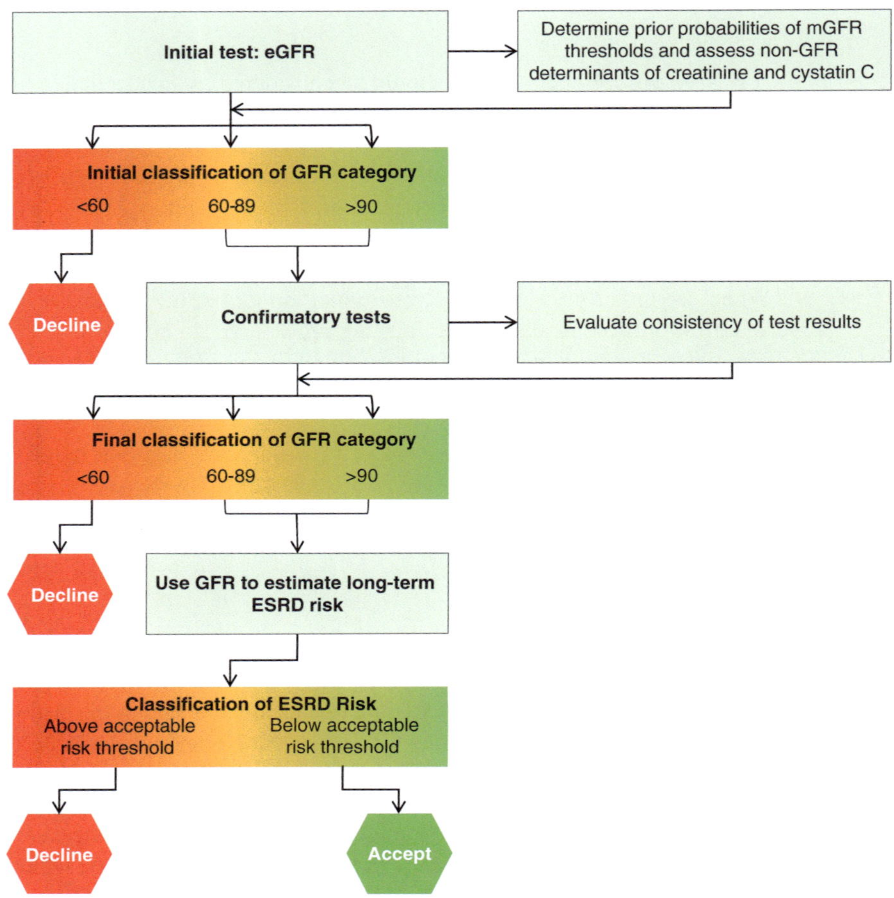

Fig. 3.6 Recommended steps in donor GFR evaluation. Initial test. eGFR$_{cr}$ is the initial test in most candidates. eGFR$_{cys}$ may be the preferred initial test for candidates with variations in non-GFR determinants of serum creatinine, for example, variation in muscle mass or diet (Table 3.1). Interpretation of eGFR should include consideration of the probability that mGFR is above or below threshold for decision-making (http://ckdepi.org/equations/donor-candidate-gfr-calculator/). Very high likelihood that mGFR <60 mL/min per 1.73 m^2 is justification for a decision to decline without further consideration. Confirmatory tests. mGFR and mClcr are required in the United States. Elsewhere, eGFR$_{cr-cys}$ can be acceptable if mGFR and mClcr are not available and eGFR$_{cys}$ was not used as the initial test. Repeat eGFR$_{cr}$ can be acceptable if none of the other confirmatory tests are available, but is not preferred. Inconsistent test results suggest inaccuracy of one or more tests, which should be discarded or repeated. Very high likelihood that mGFR <60 mL/min per 1.73 m^2 is justification for a decision to decline without further consideration. Using GFR to estimate long-term ESRD risk. Long-term estimated risk of ESRD is compared to the transplant center threshold for acceptable risk. Long-term risk in the absence of donation can be computed from demographic and clinical characteristics, including GFR (http://www.transplantmodels.com/esrdrisk/). Additional risk attributable to donation is likely to be 3.5–5.2 times higher than risk in the absence of donation, but there is substantial uncertainty, especially in younger donor candidates, and we suggest caution in decision-making. Postdonation risk above the threshold is justification for a decision to decline. Candidates with risk below the threshold are acceptable to make their own decision whether to donate. *Abbreviations*: *eGFR*$_{cys}$ estimated GFR based on cystatin C, *mGFR* measured GFR, *mCL*$_{cr}$ measured creatinine clearance, *eGFR*$_{cr-cys}$ estimated GFR based on creatinine and cystatin C. (From Garg et al. [45])

Some prior guidelines recommend GFR ≥80 mL/min as a threshold for acceptance, based on the level of GFR in the donor (not adjusted for BSA) that was associated with the best outcomes in the recipient [38]. Alternatively, some guidelines recommend a GFR level within two standard deviations of normal for age and sex. In general, other guidelines do not specify the GFR measurement method to be used, whether the threshold value should be adjusted for BSA or provide standardized reference values based on sex, race, and age [39].

The 2017 KDIGO guideline states that there is insufficient evidence to justify a single threshold value of 80 mL/min not adjusted for BSA nor age-specific thresholds. In contrast, the KDIGO guideline is more consistent with accepted measurement methods and thresholds in general clinical practice and acknowledges that there is variation in GFR measurement methods and uncertainty in the appropriate threshold for decision-making to accept or decline donor candidates. Of note, the intermediate range 60–89 mL/min per 1.73 m^2 would generally include a mCl_{cr} of 80 mL/min as well as previously recommended age and sex thresholds for mGFR.

Assessment of single-kidney ("divided" or "split") GFR is not required in all kidney donor candidates. Many factors determine the preferred kidney to remove for transplantation. If GFR is acceptable, but there are parenchymal, vascular, or urological abnormalities or asymmetry in kidney function, it is preferable to procure and transplant the more severely affected kidney or the kidney with lesser function. The 2017 KDIGO guideline did not make a recommendation regarding criteria for individual kidney GFR as no studies were found meeting criteria for review by the evidence review team. Based on low quality evidence, one prior guideline suggested considering a radionuclide imaging study if the difference between kidney lengths is ≥2 cm and that a difference in function ≥10% between the kidneys may be considered significant [40].Research recommendations include ongoing work to define the accuracy of $eGFR_{cr}$, $eGFR_{cys}$, and $eGFR_{cr-cys}$ for the prediction of mGFR in the evaluation and selection of living donor candidates and to quantify long-term risks, including lifetime risk of ESRD, in living donor candidates and living donors according to predonation GFR.

Albuminuria

Pathophysiology and Measurement

An elevated level of albuminuria is widely accepted as a marker of kidney damage. Elevated albuminuria is associated with a wide range of clinical conditions and is one of the criteria in the definition and staging of CKDs [3]. In diabetic kidney disease and other glomerular diseases, albuminuria is generally elevated before the decline in GFR.

Normal range and variability. Albumin is one of many proteins that can be detected in the urine. Urine protein is composed of small amounts of high molecular weight proteins (principally albumin) whose filtration is normally restricted by the glomeruli, low molecular weight serum proteins that are normally filtered by the glomeruli and reabsorbed by the tubules, and proteins secreted by the urinary tract. Increased urinary protein is generally considered a marker of kidney damage: albuminuria reflects increased permeability of the glomeruli (glomerular proteinuria), and low molecular weight serum proteinuria reflects decreased tubular reabsorption (tubular proteinuria). In addition, protein in the tubules may directly cause kidney damage. Chronic kidney disease due to either glomerular or tubulointerstitial diseases is generally associated with both glomerular and tubular proteinuria (albuminuria and low molecular weight serum proteinuria). Some tubulointerstitial diseases may cause predominantly tubular proteinuria, including Dent disease, toxicity due to heavy metals (cadmium and lead) or aristolochic acid (Balkan and Chinese herb) nephropathy, Sjogren syndrome, multiple myeloma or hereditary diseases associated with Fanconi syndrome, and acute tubular necrosis. Conditions other than kidney disease can also cause proteinuria: low molecular serum proteins may also reflect overproduction (e.g., light chain proteinuria in lymphoproliferative disorders), and high and low molecular weight proteins may arise from increased secretion of urinary tract proteins (due to lower urinary tract diseases).

Urine albumin is the preferred measure of urine protein for assessment of kidney damage. Ongoing efforts are directed to establishing traceability of tests for urine albumin to standardized reference material for serum albumin [41, 42]. Tests for total urine protein cannot be standardized because they are not traceable to a standard reference material due to the varying compositions of urine protein. Tests for some other specific urine proteins are available, such as α1-microglobulin, β2 microglobulin, and monoclonal heavy or light chains (also known as "Bence Jones" proteins).

The normal level of albumin loss rate (hereafter referred to as albumin excretion rate (AER)) in healthy young men and women is less than 10 mg/d. The coefficient of variation for repeated measurements is approximately 30% [43]. Because of the high coefficient of variation, repeated measurements are preferred for assessment of albuminuria. AER rises with age, although the cause of rise is not known and the rate of rise appears widely variable (Fig. 3.7) [44]. Most data are based on cross-sectional studies. As discussed earlier, abnormalities in kidney function and structure are common in the elderly, and there is debate about whether higher AER in older people represents normal aging or disease.

The 2012 KDIGO CKD guideline defines AER >30 mg/d for 3 months or more as satisfying the criteria for CKD [3]. AER <30 mg/d in young men and women is considered normal to mildly increased; AER 30–300 mg/d is defined as moderately increased compared to the young adult level; and AER >300 mg/d is defined as severely increased compared to the young adult level. Approximate ranges for other measures of urine protein are as shown in Table 3.2 [3].

2012 KDIGO CKD guideline recommendations for evaluation. The 2012 KDIGO CKD guideline for the evaluation of albuminuria in the general population recommends two-stage testing (initial testing followed by confirmatory testing as necessary).[3] Initial tests, in order of preference, and the rationale are described below. In

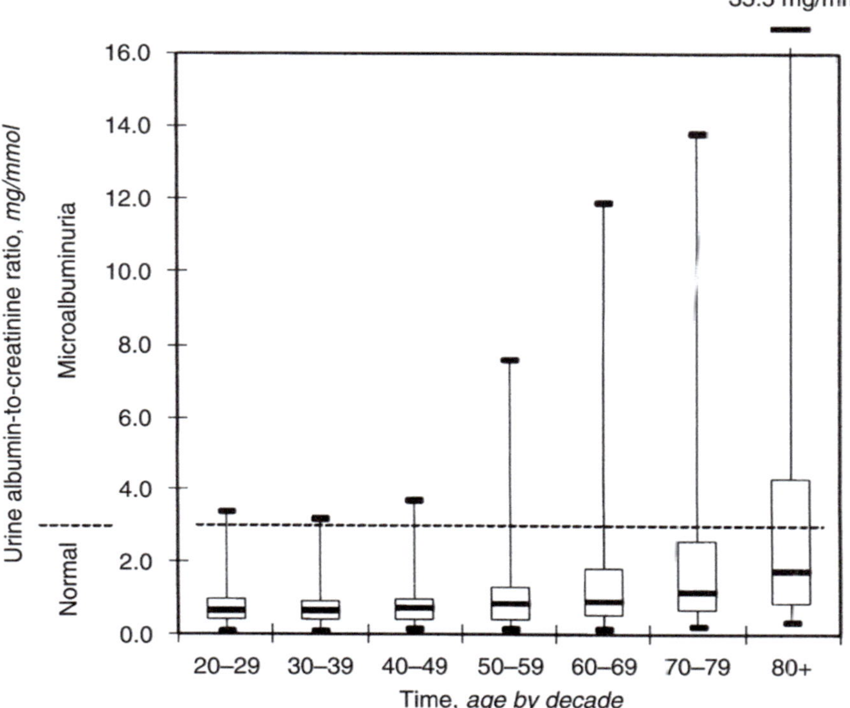

Fig. 3.7 Albuminuria in the US Population. Box plots of random urine albumin-to-creatinine ratio for 14,622 adult participants in National Health and Examination Survey III (1988–1994). The boxes represent the interquartile range (50% of the values). The line across the box indicates the median. The whiskers extend to the 95th and 5th percentiles. (From Garg et al. [44])

all cases, an early morning urine sample is preferred as it minimizes variation due to diurnal variation in albumin excretion and urine concentration.

Urine ACR. The rationale for preferring ACR to albumin concentration is that urine concentration and dilution can vary by more than tenfold among individuals and during the day. The 2012 KDIGO CKD guideline therefore recommends that clinical laboratories measure creatinine when albumin is requested and express the results as ACR in addition to albumin concentration. Indexing urine albumin by urine creatinine concentration overcomes variation due to urine concentration and dilution, but introduces variation by creatinine generation. To overcome variation by creatinine generation, some have proposed estimating the creatinine excretion rate (CER) and multiplying this quantity by ACR to estimate AER [46]. Other factors affecting urine ACR in addition to kidney disease are shown in Table 3.3 [3]. One study reported on the performance of levels of ACR to detect AER of 30 mg/day. The area under the receiver operator curve (AUROC) was 0.93 [47]. An ACR

Table 3.2 Relationship among albuminuria and proteinuria categories

Measure	Categories		
	Normal to mildly increased (A1)	**Moderately increased (A2)**	**Severely increased (A3)**
AER (mg/24 h)	<30	30–300	>300
PER (mg/24 h)	<150	150–500	>500
ACR			
(mg/mmol)	<3	3–30	>30
(mg/g)	<30	30–300	>300
PCR			
(mg/mmol)	<15	15–50	>50
(mg/g)	<150	150–500	>500
Protein reagent strip	Negative to trace	Trace to +	+ or greater

Albuminuria and proteinuria can be measured using excretion rates in timed urine collections, ratio of concentrations to creatinine concentration in spot urine samples, and reagent strips in spot urine samples. Relationships among measurement methods within a category are not exact. For example, the relationships between AER and ACR and between PER and PCR are based on the assumption that average creatinine excretion rate is approximately 1.0 g/d or 10 mmol/d. The conversions are rounded for pragmatic reasons. (For an exact conversion from mg/g of creatinine to mg/mmol of creatinine, multiply by 0.113.) Creatinine excretion varies with age, sex, race, and diet; therefore the relationship among these categories is approximate only. ACR less than 10 mg/g (<1 mg/mmol) is considered normal; ACR 10–30 mg/g (1–3 mg/mmol) is considered "high normal." ACR greater than 2200 mg/g (>220 mg/mmol) is considered "nephrotic range." The relationship between urine reagent strip results and other measures depends on urine concentration.
Abbreviations: *ACR* albumin-to-creatinine ratio, *AER* albumin excretion rate, *PCR* protein-to-creatinine ratio, *PER* protein excretion rate
(From KDIGO 2012 [3])

threshold of 10 mg/g was associated with sensitivity and specificity of 88% for an AER threshold of 30 mg/day. There was minor variation in AUROC based on age, sex, race, and body weight.

Urine PCR. Tests for total urine protein cannot substitute for tests for urine albumin. PCR is less sensitive than ACR, so even negative tests must be confirmed by tests for albumin. Increased PCR suggests increased ACR, but non-albumin protein can cause a positive test, so positive tests should be confirmed by tests for albumin. Patients with elevated PCR and negative tests for albumin may have tubular proteinuria, light chain proteinuria, or urinary tract disease.

Reagent strip urinalysis for total protein with automated reading. Reagent strips allow point-of-care, semiquantitative assessment of total urine protein concentration. Reagent strips ("dipsticks") are more sensitive to albumin than other proteins, but lack specificity. Automated readers are more accurate than manual reading of reagent strips. Reagent strip urinalysis for total protein with manual reading may be used, if the above measures are not available.

Table 3.3 Factors affecting urinary albumin-creatinine ratio

Factor	Examples of Effect
Preanalytical factors	
Transient elevation in albuminuria	• Menstrual blood contamination • Urinary tract infection • Exercise • Upright posture (orthostatic proteinuria) • Other conditions increasing vascular permeability (e.g., septicemia)
Intraindividual variability	• Intrinsic biological variability • Genetic variability
Preanalytical storage conditions	• Degradation of albumin before analysis
Nonrenal causes of variability in creatinine excretion	• Age (lower in children and older people) • Race (lower in white than black people) • Muscle mass (e.g., lower in people with amputations, paraplegia, muscular dystrophy) • Sex (lower in women)
Changes in creatinine excretion	• Nonsteady state for creatinine (AKI)
Analytical factors	
Antigen excess ("prozone") effect	• Samples with very high albumin concentrations may be falsely reported as low or normal using some assays

Samples for urinary albumin (or total protein) measurement may be analyzed fresh, stored at 4 °C for up to 1 week, or stored at -70 °C for longer periods. Freezing at -20 °C appears to result in loss of measurable albumin and is not recommended. When analyzing stored samples, they should be allowed to reach temperature and thoroughly mixed prior to analysis

Abbreviations: *AKI* acute kidney injury

(From KDIGO 2012 [3])

Risk of Kidney Failure Related to Elevated Albuminuria

Risk in the general population. Elevated albuminuria in the general population is associated with a higher risk of complications of CKD, including ESRD, cardiovascular disease, and death. In general populations, compared to a reference ACR of 5 mg/g (0.5 mg/mmol), the RR for complications related to elevated ACR has no apparent threshold when expressed on the log scale [48]. For this reason, 10–29 mg/g is considered "high normal." The risk related to elevated ACR is independent of the eGFR (Fig. 3.3). The association of elevated albuminuria with higher risk of adverse outcomes may be related to other conditions that co-occur with elevated albuminuria, such as hypertension, diabetes, and cardiovascular disease. Elevated albuminuria in older people is associated with increased risk for CKD outcomes, including ESRD, cardiovascular disease, and death. The RR for these outcomes in older people with elevated urine ACR compared to the reference urine ACR is less than the RR in younger people; however, the increment in absolute risk in older people is higher than in younger people [23].

A recent meta-analysis that included 5 million healthy persons from seven US general population cohorts found that each tenfold increase in ACR was associated

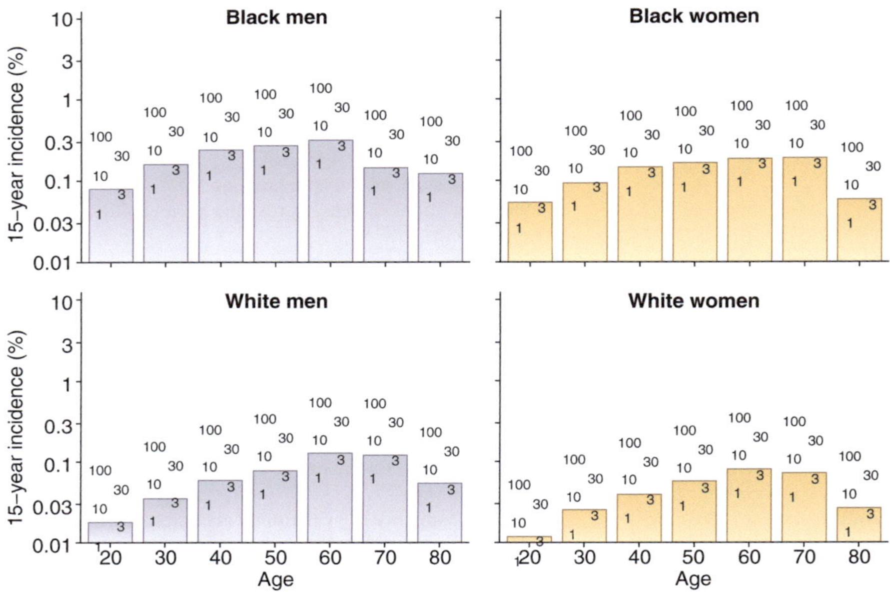

Fig. 3.8 Estimated 15-year Incidence (%) of ESKD in the United States according to baseline albumin-to-creatinine ratio (ACR, mg/g) and demographic profile. The base-case scenario is the following: age-specific eGFR (114, 106, 98, 90, 82, 74, and 66 mL/min per 1.73 m² for ages 20, 30, 40, 50, 60, 70, and 80 years, respectively), systolic blood pressure 120 mmHg, urine ACR 4 mg/g [0.4 mg/mmol], BMI 26 kg/m², and no diabetes mellitus or antihypertensive medication use. These were selected as being representative of recent US living kidney donors where, with the exception of eGFR, there was little variation in health characteristics by age. *Abbreviations*: *eGFR* estimated GFR, *ACR* albumin-creatinine ratio, *BMI* body mass index. (From Grams et al. [24])

with three times the risk of ESRD over a median cohort follow-up of 4–16 years, although the finding was not statistically significant (adjusted hazard ratio (HR): 2.94, 95% CI 0.99–8.75) [24]. The projected 15-year and lifetime risks of ESRD according to differences in ACR, age, sex, and race for healthy persons are displayed graphically in Figs. 3.8 and 3.9 [24]. Key findings are that elevated ACR is associated with higher lifetime risk for ESRD in all subgroups, with higher risk in men than women and blacks than whites. For urine ACR <10 mg/g, lifetime risk for white men and white women was less than 1% at all ages, but exceeded 2% for black men and women younger than 30 and 20 years, respectively. In whites, lifetime risk at ACR 100 mg/g was less than 1% at age older than 50 in men and 40 in women. In blacks, lifetime risk at ACR 30 mg/g was less than 1% at age older than 60 in men and women.

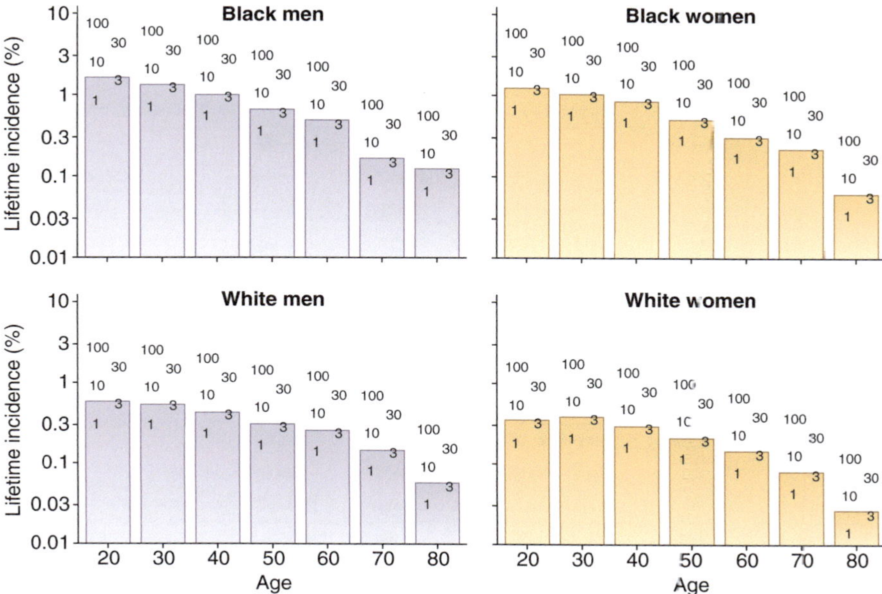

Fig. 3.9 Estimated lifetime incidence (%) of ESKD in the United States according to baseline albumin-to-creatinine ratio (ACR, mg/g) and demographic profile. The base-case scenario is the following: age-specific eGFR (114, 106, 98, 90, 82, 74, and 66 mL/min per 1.73 m² for ages 20, 30, 40, 50, 60, 70, and 80 years, respectively), systolic blood pressure 120 mmHg, urine ACR 4 mg/g [0.4 mg/mmol], BMI 26 kg/m², and no diabetes mellitus or antihypertensive medication use. These were selected as being representative of recent US living kidney donors where, with the exception of eGFR, there was little variation in health characteristics by age. Lifetime risk projections are based on 15 years of follow-up data and calibrated to the incidence of ESKD in the low-risk population and thus are likely imprecise. *Abbreviations*: *eGFR* estimated GFR, *ACR* albumin-creatinine ratio, *BMI* body mass index, *ESKD* end-stage kidney disease. (From Grams et al. [24])

Risk after kidney donation. A systematic review quantified the incidence of proteinuria after kidney donation in 42 studies of 4793 living donors followed for an average of 7 years (range 2–25 years) (Fig. 3.10) [27]. There was substantial variation across the studies. Some reported an incidence of proteinuria over 20%, whereas in others the incidence was less than 5%. The pooled incidence of proteinuria was 12% (95% CI 8–16%). These results were consistent even after restricting to the nine studies which defined proteinuria as >300 mg/day based on 24-hour urine (incidence of proteinuria 10% (95% CI 7–12%).

The risk associated with albuminuria in kidney donors is uncertain, but there is theoretical justification for concern about development of kidney disease after nephrectomy. First, in experimental animals, reduction in renal mass is associated

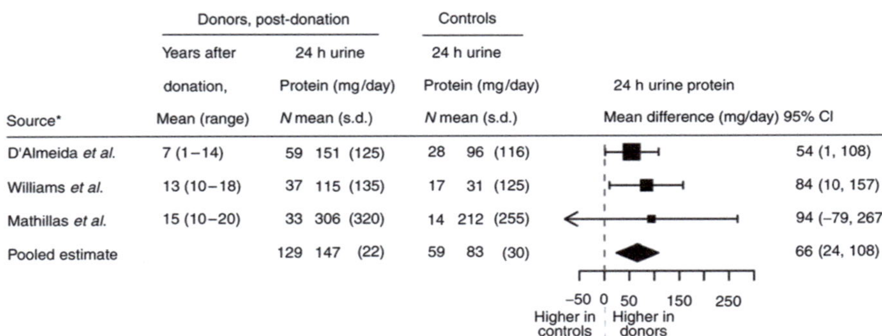

Fig. 3.10 Proteinuria after kidney donation. Controlled studies of proteinuria after kidney donation. The size of each square is inversely proportional to the variability of the study estimate. Studies are arranged by the average number of years after donation. Microalbuminuria was assessed by 24-h urine. Mathematically pooled results are not presented graphically because of statistical heterogeneity between studies. *Abbreviations*: *N* number of participants, *n* number of events. (From Garg et al. [27])

with increased glomerular permeability to albumin followed by other structural and functional abnormalities associated with kidney disease. Second, given that GFR declines after kidney donation, the filtered load of albumin would be expected to decline. Unchanged or higher albuminuria after donation suggests increased albumin filtration per nephron.

Box 3.2: 2017 KDIGO Living Donor Guideline Recommendations Related to Predonation Albuminuria

Measurement
- 6.1: Donor proteinuria should be measured as albuminuria, not total urine protein.
- 6.2. Initial evaluation of albuminuria (screening) should be performed using urine albumin-to-creatinine ratio (ACR) in a random (untimed) urine specimen.
- 6.3 Donor albuminuria should be confirmed using:
  - Albumin excretion rate (AER, mg/day [mg/d]) in a timed urine specimen
  - Repeat ACR if AER cannot be obtained

Criteria for Acceptable Predonation Albuminuria
- 6.4 Urine AER <30 mg/day should be considered as an acceptable level for kidney donation.
- 6.5 The decision to approve donor candidates with AER 30–100 mg/day should be individualized based on demographic and health profile in relation to the transplant center's acceptance risk threshold.
- 6.6 Donor candidates with urine AER >100 mg/d should not donate.

The 2017 KDIGO donor guideline recommends measuring albuminuria and recommends spot urine ACR as the first step in the evaluation. Because of variability in urine ACR and its relationship to urine AER, the guideline recommends confirmation in all cases. The preferred confirmatory test is urine AER, expressed as mg/day. Tests of total urine protein in addition to albumin are not recommended by KDIGO because there are no accepted normal ranges for urine non-albumin protein excretion, disorders associated with predominant tubular proteinuria (tubulointerstitial kidney disease) and overproduction proteinuria (plasma cell or B-lymphocyte disorders) are uncommon, and patients with these disorders usually have other clinical abnormalities that would be discovered during the donor evaluation. Testing for specific urine proteins can be undertaken if significant non-albumin proteinuria is suspected. These assays can be performed at the same time as tests for albuminuria. In the United States, current OPTN policy requires measurement of both total urinary protein and albumin excretion [18].

The 2017 KDIGO living donor guideline recommends an AER threshold of <30 mg/d to routinely accept a donor candidate, which corresponds to normal and mildly increased albuminuria, and recommends an AER threshold of >100 mg/g to routinely decline a donor candidate, which corresponds to the lower range for moderately elevated albuminuria. The guideline recommends individualized decision-making based on other risk factors for AER 30–100 mg/day, which corresponds to the lower range of moderately elevated albuminuria.

The 2017 KDIGO guideline acknowledges that AER 30–100 mg/day meets the criteria for CKD, and past guidelines have strived to exclude donor candidates with CKD. The rationale for not excluding candidates solely on the basis of AER 30–100 mg/day is that the estimated predonation lifetime ESRD risk in older persons with ACR in this range is very low in the absence of decreased GFR and other clinical risk factors [24], and it would not be consistent with the proposed rationale that allows donation from other candidates with similar risk due to other clinical risk factors.

Some past guidelines recommend that living donor candidates have a protein excretion rate (PER) less than 150–300 mg per day, based on the usually accepted normal range, generally without reference to measurement methods. A survey of practices by US transplant centers reported in 2007 found that approximately 76% of programs used a PER in a 24-hour urine collection and that 50% of programs used a threshold of 300–1000 mg, corresponding to moderately increased proteinuria (approximately one-third of these required qualification by other evaluations) [49]. Of note, 36% used a threshold of <150 mg/day, which corresponds roughly to AER <30 mg/d, and includes normal and mildly increased proteinuria.

By comparison, the 2017 KDIGO living donor guideline is more consistent with the recently accepted criterion standard, measurement methods, and thresholds in general clinical practice, but acknowledges that there is variation in ascertainment of albuminuria for screening and uncertainty in the appropriate threshold for decision-making to accept or decline donor candidates. Research recommendations include more work to assess the accuracy of urine ACR compared to AER for evaluation and selection of living donor candidates and quantifying the association of urine albumin with other kidney measures (GFR and kidney size) at the time of donor evaluation and with kidney measures and outcomes (GFR, kidney failure, and others) after donation.

Hematuria

Pathophysiology and Measurement

Normal range and variability. Hematuria can arise at any location in the genitourinary tract and can be classified as symptomatic or asymptomatic, macroscopic (macrohematuria) or microscopic (microhematuria, requiring microscopic evaluation for its detection), persistent or transient, and isolated or accompanied by other abnormalities in the urine (proteinuria or pyuria). Of special concern in the evaluation of otherwise healthy kidney donor candidates is asymptomatic, persistent

Table 3.4 Causes of persistent microhematuria according to location in the urinary tract

Upper urinary tract	Lower urinary tract
Glomerular diseases	• Cystitis, prostatitis, urethritis
• IgA nephropathy	• Urethral stricture
• Alport syndrome (hereditary nephritis)	• Benign bladder and ureteral
• Thin basement membrane disease	tumors/polyps
Non-glomerular diseases	• Bladder cancer/prostate cancer
• Nephrolithiasis	• Schistosomiasis (North Africans)
• Hypercalciuria, hyperuricosuria, or both without nephrolithiasis	
• Pyelonephritis	
• Renal cell cancer/transitional cell cancer	
• Ureteral stricture	
• Arteriovenous malformation	
• Renal tuberculosis	
• Sickle cell trait or disease	

Abbreviations: *IgA* immunoglobulin A

isolated microscopic hematuria. For the purpose of the 2017 KDIGO guideline, microscopic hematuria is defined as isolated when it occurs in an asymptomatic patient who has normal AER, normal GFR, and normal blood pressure [1]. The estimated prevalence of microscopic hematuria varies widely from 0.18% to 16% depending on age and sex distribution of populations studied, methodology of diagnosis (dipstick vs microscopic), and number of screenings performed [50]. The most common causes are urologic conditions (stones, tumors) or glomerular diseases (IgA nephropathy, thin basement membrane nephropathy (TBMN), and Alport syndrome) (Table 3.4) [50–54]. Koushik et al. reported a series of 512 consecutive donors at a US center in which 14 (2.7%) were found to have asymptomatic, persistent microscopic hematuria. Hematuria resolved after treatment for urinary tract infection in two and another two declined donation [55]. Kidney biopsy was performed in ten and showed TBMN (4/10), normal (2/10), nonhomogeneous basement membrane abnormalities (1/10), IgA nephropathy (1/10), and global glomerulosclerosis 7/30 glomeruli in a patient with a family history of Schimke's syndrome (immune-osseous dysplasia), and one patient had hypertensive changes and thin basement membranes.

American Urological Association (AUA) recommendations for evaluation. Persistent microscopic hematuria is most often defined as more than two to five red blood cells (RBC) per high-power field of urinary sediment on two to three separate occasions, unrelated to exercise, trauma, sexual activity, or menstruation [4, 50, 56, 57]. Consensus-based guidelines of the AUA state that a positive dipstick alone does not define microhematuria and evaluation should be based on findings from microscopic examination of urine sediment. A positive dipstick reading warrants microscopic examination to confirm or refute a diagnosis of microhematuria [4]. Causes of a positive dipstick reading in the absence of red blood cells in the urine include hemoglobinuria, myoglobinuria, or a false-positive test.

Recommendations for evaluation of asymptomatic microhematuria in the general population include careful history, physical examination, and laboratory examination for benign causes. Further radiologic and urologic evaluation is recommended once benign etiologies are excluded. These evaluations may include multiphasic computed tomography (CT) urography, without and with intravenous contrast, magnetic resonance urography, noncontrast CT, or magnetic resonance imaging in those who are unable to receive contrast and cystoscopy in patients 35 years or older regardless of history of use of anticoagulation therapy. Urine cytology and urine biomarkers are not recommended as a part of the routine evaluation of asymptomatic microhematuria.

The presence of red blood cell casts is generally thought to indicate a glomerular cause of microhematuria, but the sensitivity and specificity of this finding is not well established. The presence of dysmorphic urinary red blood cells detected by conventional microscopy, phase-contrast microscopy, or automated analyzer is associated with a wide range of sensitivity (from 33% to 100%) and specificity (from 33% to 100%) for glomerular causes of microhematuria. The presence of dysmorphic red blood cells or casts and other clinical information should be assessed in directing the evaluation toward glomerular causes of hematuria (e.g., patient and family history, physical exam, urinary albumin excretion, and level of GFR). However, the presence of dysmorphic red blood cells does not exclude underlying urologic disease [4].

Risk of Kidney Failure Related to Hematuria

Risk in the general population. Isolated microscopic hematuria in young adults is often considered benign, but a population-based study of 1.2 million persons aged 16–25 in Israel showed a small but significant increase in long-term renal risk associated with persistent asymptomatic isolated microscopic hematuria, quantifying ESRD rates of 34.0 vs 2.05 per 100,000 person-years after a mean follow-up of 22 years among those with vs without persistent microscopic hematuria (adjusted HR: 18.5, 95% CI 12.4–27.6) [57]. The prevalence of asymptomatic persistent microscopic hematuria in this study was 0.3%. While participants were required to have S_{cr} values "within the normal range" and 24-hr urine PER <200 mg, this study does not provide information on ESRD risk after comprehensive evaluation and selection including estimated or measured GFR.

Risk in patients with Alport syndrome, TBMN, and IgA nephropathy. Alport syndrome (often termed hereditary nephritis) is a basement membrane disorder arising from mutations in genes encoding type IV collagen. Both X-linked and autosomal recessive Alport syndrome have similar presentation and course with progressive kidney failure. The carrier state may also be associated with adverse kidney disease outcomes. A European study examined 349 female carriers in 195 X-linked families with COL4A5 mutation. Information on proteinuria and kidney function was available for 234 and 288 patients respectively; of these, 75% developed proteinuria (176/234), 18% (51/288) reached ESRD, and another 12% (34/288) developed decreased eGFR [58]. A more recent study identified adverse kidney disease outcomes in 234 Alport carriers (including 29 autosomal recessive and 205 X-linked mutation carriers). ESRD developed in 17.5% at a median age of 49 years; outcomes including ESRD, proteinuria, and decreased eGFR were similar in X-linked and autosomal recessive carriers [59], although the number of autosomal recessive carriers was small. Thus, while data are limited, female carriers of X-linked Alport syndrome (i.e., *COL4A5* mutation) appear to have an increased risk of adverse kidney disease outcomes.

TBMN disease is defined based on pathological description with the only abnormal finding being diffuse thinning of glomerular basement membranes on electron microscopy. Historically, this condition was considered benign with the only finding being isolated microhematuria. Epidemiological studies of TBMN suggest increased risks of hypertension and proteinuria compared to the general population over time, but progression to ESRD is rare and thought to require an additional insult [60, 61]. More recently, many heterozygous mutations of type IV collagen genes COL4A3 and COL4A4 have been identified in patients with TBMN, but these mutations are not present in all families with TBMN. Some consider hematuria and thin basement membrane associated with heterozygous mutation in COL4A3 or COLA4A4 as autosomal dominant Alport syndrome [62]. Heterozygous mutation in COL4A3/COL4A4 is known to be associated with development of focal segmental glomerulosclerosis (FSGS), proteinuria, and progressive kidney disease. In one study of 13 Cypriot families with TBMN, heterozygous mutations in COL4A3 or COL4A4 were identified in ten families (82 individuals); 38% had decline in GFR and 19% developed ESRD during follow-up of up to three decades. The diagnosis of both FSGS and TBMN was made in 15 biopsied cases of these ten families [63]. In another study of 11 large pedigrees, 127/236 at-risk family members carried a heterozygous mutation in COL4A3 or COL4A4. Proteinuria with decline in GFR developed in 33% (42/127) and 14% (18/127) progressed to ESRD at a mean age of 60 years. Renal biopsies in 21 patients showed FSGS; electron microscopy was done in 13/21 cases and showed TBMN in all [64]. In both these studies, there was significant late progression to proteinuria and decline in GFR with highest prevalence in patients older than 70 years [63, 64]. Glomerular basement membrane thinning can also be the only finding in early stages of Alport syndrome, especially in female carriers of X-linked and young male and females with autosomal recessive forms, making it challenging to distinguish TBMN from Alport syndrome [58, 62]. Genetic testing can be helpful in these situations. In patients with isolated hematuria and TBMN, the presence of either proteinuria, family history of CKD, or heterozygous mutation of COL4A3/COLA4 genes may suggest a greater risk for kidney disease progression.

IgA nephropathy that presents with hematuria and minimal proteinuria is often a progressive disease. In a study of 177 Chinese patients with IgA nephropathy, preserved GFR, and proteinuria less than 0.4 g/day, 46% developed increased proteinuria of >1 g/d, 38% developed hypertension, and 24% developed worsening GFR after a median follow-up of 9 years [65]. In another series in Hong Kong, 72 consecutive normotensive patients with IgA nephropathy presenting as hematuria, proteinuria <0.4 g/day and normal GFR were followed for a median of 84 months; 33% developed worsening proteinuria, 26% became hypertensive, and 7% developed decreased GFR [66]. A recent study showed that persistent hematuria in patients with IgA nephropathy is associated with increased risk of kidney failure and remission of hematuria has a favorable effect [67]. Thus, the presence of hematuria in IgA nephropathy appears to be associated with increased risk of progressive kidney disease even in the absence of other clinical findings.

Risk after kidney donation. Data on outcomes of living donor evaluation and donation in persons with Alport syndrome and TBMN are limited to small series with short-term follow-up [55, 61, 68]. Among six female Alport carriers (five X-linked, one autosomal recessive) who donated to their children at several European centers and were followed for an average of 6.7 years, three developed new-onset hypertension and two developed new onset of proteinuria. mCr$_{Cl}$ remained >40 mL/min in all donors at up to 14 years [69]. A center in Korea recently published outcomes in 11 donors with biopsy-proven TBMN who donated from 2007 to 2016. Two donors were lost to follow-up and 9/11 donors had stable eGFR over a mean follow-up period of 41.0 ± 39.1 months. In recipients, one allograft failed due to arterial occlusion, and the remaining allografts maintained preserved kidney function over 57.4 ± 28.6 months of follow-up [61]. This study is limited by the absence of information on hematuria or proteinuria in donors during follow-up. Another Korean series including five living donors with TBMN defined by predonation biopsy reported favorable short-term outcomes, including mean S$_{cr}$ 0.94 ± 0.32 mg/dL and no cases of new-onset hypertension or proteinuria over a mean follow-up of 34.7 ± 42.5 months [68]. In the report by Koushik et al., two of the four candidates with TBMN (age 44 and 53 years) proceeded with donation; after 15 months of follow-up, both donors were free of hypertension and proteinuria, and recipients had "excellent" graft function [55].

Persistent predonation hematuria without defined kidney histopathology has been associated with postdonation proteinuria. In a series of 242 living kidney donors at one center in Japan, persistent predonation hematuria was identified in 8.3%. Persistent hematuria was more common in donors with a family history of IgA nephropathy or Alport syndrome [70]. Ninety-five percent of those with persistent predonation hematuria continued to have persistent hematuria after donation over a median 27 months of follow-up, and persistent hematuria was associated with increased likelihood of persistent proteinuria (dipstick $\geq 1+$) after donation. The risk of persistent postdonation proteinuria was significantly higher in donors with persistent predonation hematuria characterized by dysmorphic red blood cells compared to those without dysmorphic RBC (adjusted odds ratio 12.3 vs 3.8).

Postdonation persistent hematuria with dysmorphic RBC was associated with significant GFR decline over the study period. Kidney biopsy or genetic testing was not performed prior to donation, and it is possible that some donors had early IgA nephropathy with the only finding of persistent hematuria or mutations in the COLA3, COLA4, or COLA5 gene.

Box 3.3: 2017 KDIGO Living Donor Guideline Recommendations Related to Predonation Hematuria

Evaluation
- 7.1:   Donor candidates should be assessed for microscopic hematuria.
- 7.2:   Donor candidates with persistent microscopic hematuria should undergo testing to identify possible causes, which may include:
  - Urinalysis and urine culture to assess for infection
  - Cystoscopy and imaging to assess for urinary tract malignancy
  - 24-hr urine stone panel to assess for nephrolithiasis and/or microlithiasis
  - Kidney biopsy to assess for glomerular disease (e.g., thin basement membrane nephropathy, IgA nephropathy, Alport syndrome)

Donor Selection
- 7.3:   Donor candidates with hematuria from a reversible cause that resolves (e.g., a treated infection) may be acceptable for donation.
- 7.4: Donor candidates with IgA nephropathy should be referred for treatment and should not donate.

The 2017 KDIGO living donor guideline recommends that donor candidates should be screened for microscopic hematuria. The sequence of the evaluation is designed to perform less invasive and less expensive tests prior to more invasive/expensive tests and only if the less invasive and less expensive tests do not preclude donation (Fig. 3.11) [1]. Reversible causes of microscopic hematuria, e.g., treatable urinary tract infection, should generally not preclude donation. Donor candidates with a urological malignancy should be referred for treatment and should not donate. A family history is critical to recognition of possible Alport syndrome or TBMN. Kidney donation may be considered in individuals with microhematuria from TBMN or carriers for autosomal recessive Alport syndrome who do not have COL4A5 mutation, if blood pressure, urinary albumin excretion, and GFR are normal. Donor candidates with IgA nephropathy should be referred for treatment and should not donate.

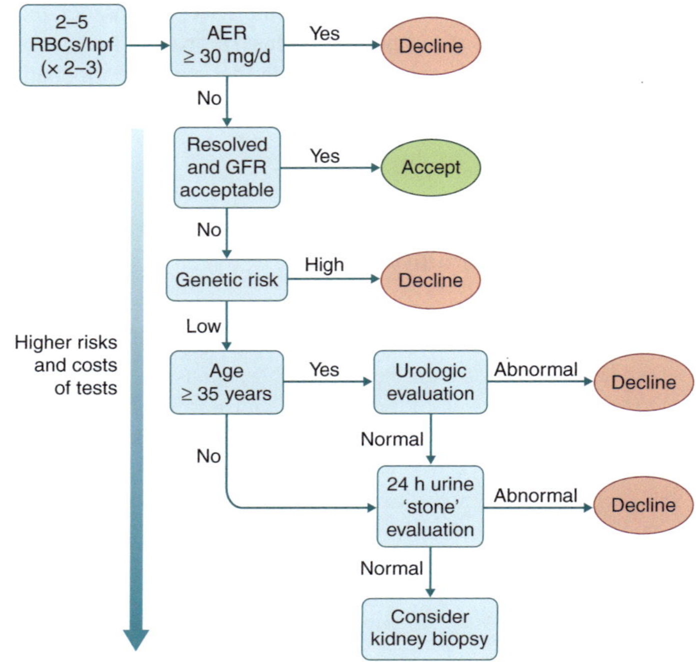

Fig. 3.11 Sequential evaluation of microscopic hematuria in living kidney donor candidates. In general, lower risk and less expensive tests should be performed first, and at each step additional testing should only be performed if necessary. Boxes indicate stopping points in the donor candidate hematuria evaluation. Abbreviations: ABNL abnormal, ACR urine albumin-to-creatinine ratio, hpf high-power field, NL normal, RBC red blood cell. (From with Lentine et al. [1])

The 2017 KDIGO guideline is generally consistent with other guidelines regarding donor evaluation and selection related to hematuria. Other guidelines have recommended that evaluation of donor candidates for causes of hematuria includes urine culture and imaging [40], cystoscopy if age older than 40 years [40], urine cytology, and "complete" urological evaluation [71]. A recent Canadian protocol recommends tests of urine culture, urine cytology, 24-hour urine calcium, metabolic stone workup, and, then if the cause of hematuria is undetermined, cystoscopy and a native kidney biopsy [72]. In the absence of an identified cause, evaluation by kidney biopsy has been advised if hematuria is >1+ [40] or thought to be possibly caused by glomerular diseases [71, 72].

The 2011 British Transplantation Society guidelines offer a "moderate quality" recommendation that "glomerular pathology precludes donation, with the possible exception of thin basement membrane disease" [40]. A Canadian protocol defines IgA nephropathy and Alport syndrome (including carrier status) as exclusions to donation [72].

The 2013 "Expert Guidelines for the Management of Alport Syndrome and Thin Basement Membrane Nephropathy" include several consensus-based recommendations related to live donation selection [73]: (A) "Individuals with TBMN may be kidney donors if they have normal blood pressure (BP), proteinuria, and renal function" and if a biopsy is done and Alport syndrome is excluded." Close monitoring and use of nephroprotective strategies are advised. (B) "Individuals from families with autosomal recessive Alport syndrome who have only one of the causative mutations (parents, offspring, some siblings) may be renal donors if they have normal blood pressure, proteinuria levels, and renal function; if coincidental renal disease has been excluded by renal biopsy; and if X-linked Alport syndrome has been excluded by genetic testing." The document recommends, "discouraging affected mothers of males with X-linked Alport syndrome from renal donation because of their own risk of kidney failure."

The above guidelines do not take age into consideration in donor evaluation for individuals with TBMN or Alport carriers. It may be reasonable to accept an older donor candidate with TBMN or an Alport syndrome carrier if GFR and albuminuria are normal, while a more careful assessment, including genetic testing, may be required in younger patients, since long-term outcomes and implications of different collagen gene mutations in donors are not well known.

Research recommendations related to hematuria include developing prospective studies of living donors with suitable controls and adequate statistical power to assess risk and predictors of risk for ESRD, premature death, health-related quality of life, and other events of importance to donors. It would be important to conduct detailed, prospective, long-term, postdonation follow-up of living donors with infrequent clinical conditions, such as Alport syndrome "carriers," TBMN, incidental IgA deposition in glomeruli and isolated hematuria, or stone formers.

Acknowledgment The authors are grateful to Juhi Chaudhari, MPH, for assistance with manuscript preparation.

References

1. Lentine KL, Kasiske BL, Levey AS, Adams PL, Alberu J, Bakr MA, et al. KDIGO Clinical Practice Guideline on the Evaluation and Care of Living Kidney Donors. Transplantation. 2017;101(8S Suppl 1):S1–s109. https://doi.org/10.1097/tp.0000000000001769

2. Cheng XS, Glassock RJ, Lentine KL, Chertow GM, Tan JC. Donation, Not Disease! A Multiple-Hit Hypothesis on Development of Post-Donation Kidney Disease. Curr Transplant Rep. 2017;4(4):320–6. https://doi.org/10.1007/s40472-017-0171-8

3. Kidney Disease. Improving Global Outcomes (KDIGO), KDIGO 2012 Clinical Practice Guideline for the Evaluation and Management of Chronic Kidney Disease. Kidney Int Suppl. 2013;3(1):1–150. https://doi.org/https://kdigo.org/wp-content/uploads/2017/02/KDIGO_2012_CKD_GL.pdf

4. Davis R, Jones JS, Barocas DA, Castle EP, Lang EK, Leveillee RJ, et al. Diagnosis, evaluation and follow-up of asymptomatic microhematuria (AMH) in adults: AUA guideline. J Urol. 2012;188(6 Suppl):2473–81. https://doi.org/10.1016/j.juro.2012.09.078

5. Wesson L. Physiology of the human kidney. New York: Grune & Stratton; 1969. p. 96–108.

6. Jafar TH, Islam M, Jessani S, Bux R, Inker LA, Mariat C, et al. Level and determinants of kidney function in a South Asian population in Pakistan. Am J Kidney Dis. 2011;58(5):764–72. https://doi.org/10.1053/j.ajkd.2011.06.012

7. Inker LA, Shafi T, Okparavero A, Tighiouart H, Eckfeldt JH, Katz R, et al. Effects of Race and Sex on Measured GFR: The Multi-Ethnic Study of Atherosclerosis. Am J Kidney Dis. 2016;68(5):743–51. https://doi.org/10.1053/j.ajkd.2016.06.021

8. Wang X, Vrtiska TJ, Avula RT, Walters LR, Chakkera HA, Kremers WK, et al. Age, kidney function, and risk factors associate differently with cortical and medullary volumes of the kidney. Kidney Int. 2014;85(3):677–85. https://doi.org/10.1038/ki.2013.359

9. Glodny B, Unterholzner V, Taferner B, Hofmann KJ, Rehder P, Strasak A, et al. Normal kidney size and its influencing factors - a 64-slice MDCT study of 1.040 asymptomatic patients. BMC Urol. 2009;9:19. https://doi.org/10.1186/1471-2490-9-19

10. Emamian SA, Nielsen MB, Pedersen JF, Ytte L. Kidney dimensions at sonography: correlation with age, sex, and habitus in 665 adult volunteers. AJR Am J Roentgenol. 1993;160(1):83–6. https://doi.org/10.2214/ajr.160.1.8416654

11. Levey AS, Stevens LA, Schmid CH, Zhang YL, Castro AF, 3rd, Feldman HI, et al. A new equation to estimate glomerular filtration rate. Ann Intern Med. 2009;150(9):604–12. https://doi.org/10.7326/0003-4819-150-9-200905050-00006

12. Inker LA, Schmid CH, Tighiouart H, Eckfeldt JH, Feldman HI, Greene T, et al. Estimating glomerular filtration rate from serum creatinine and cystatin C. N Engl J Med. 2012;367(1):20–9. https://doi.org/10.1056/NEJMoa1114248

13. Fan L, Inker LA, Rossert J, Froissart M, Rossing P, Mauer M, et al. Glomerular filtration rate estimation using cystatin C alone or combined with creatinine as a confirmatory test. Nephrol Dial Transplant. 2014;29(6):1195–203. https://doi.org/10.1093/ndt/gft509

14. Soveri I, Berg UB, Bjork J, Elinder CG, Grubb A, Mejare I, et al. Measuring GFR: a systematic review. Am J Kidney Dis. 2014;64(3):411–24. https://doi.org/10.1053/j.ajkd.2014.04.010

15. Ognibene A, Grandi G, Lorubbio M, Rapi S, Salvadori B, Terreni A, et al. KDIGO 2012 Clinical Practice Guideline CKD classification rules out creatinine clearance 24 hour urine collection? Clin Biochem. 2016;49(1-2):85–9. https://doi.org/10.1016/j.clinbiochem.2015.07.030

16. Huang N, Foster MC, Lentine KL, Garg AX, Poggio ED, Kasiske BL, et al. Estimated GFR for Living Kidney Donor Evaluation. Am J Transplant. 2016;16(1):171–80. https://doi.org/10.1111/ajt.13540

17. Gaillard F, Flamant M, Lemoine S, Baron S, Timsit MO, Eladari D, et al. Estimated or Measured GFR in Living Kidney Donors Work-up? Am J Transplant. 2016; https://doi.org/10.1111/ajt.13908

18. OPTN (Organ Procurement and Transplantation Network)/UNOS (United Network for Organ Sharing). OPTN Policy 14: Living Donation. Available at: https://optn.transplant.hrsa.gov/governance/policies/. Accessed: 7 Sept 2020.

19. Inker LA, Koraishy FM, Goyal N, Lentine KL. Assessment of Glomerular Filtration Rate and End-Stage Kidney Disease Risk in Living Kidney Donor Candidates: A Paradigm for Evaluation, Selection, and Counseling. Adv Chronic Kidney Dis. 2018;25(1):21–30. https://doi.org/10.1053/j.ackd.2017.09.002

20. Levey AS, de Jong PE, Coresh J, El Nahas M, Astor BC, Matsushita K, et al. The definition, classification, and prognosis of chronic kidney disease: a KDIGO Controversies Conference report. Kidney Int. 2011;80(1):17–28. https://doi.org/10.1038/ki.2010.483

21. Matsushita K, Mahmoodi BK, Woodward M, Emberson JR, Jafar TH, Jee SH, et al. Comparison of risk prediction using the CKD-EPI equation and the MDRD study equation for estimated glomerular filtration rate. JAMA. 2012;307(18):1941–51. https://doi.org/10.1001/jama.2012.3954

22. Shlipak MG, Matsushita K, Arnlov J, Inker LA, Katz R, Polkinghorne KR, et al. Cystatin C versus creatinine in determining risk based on kidney function. N Engl J Med. 2013;369(10):932–43. https://doi.org/10.1056/NEJMoa1214234

23. Hallan SI, Matsushita K, Sang Y, Mahmoodi BK, Black C, Ishani A, et al. Age and association of kidney measures with mortality and end-stage renal disease. JAMA. 2012;308(22):2349–60. https://doi.org/10.1001/jama.2012.16817

24. Grams ME, Sang Y, Levey AS, Matsushita K, Ballew S, Chang AR, et al. Kidney-Failure Risk Projection for the Living Kidney-Donor Candidate. N Engl J Med. 2016;374(5):411–21. https://doi.org/10.1056/NEJMoa1510491

25. Kasiske BL, Anderson-Haag T, Israni AK, Kalil RS, Kimmel PL, Kraus ES, et al. A prospective controlled study of living kidney donors: three-year follow-up. Am J Kidney Dis. 2015;66(1):114–24. https://doi.org/10.1053/j.ajkd.2015.01.019

26. Ibrahim HN, Foley R, Tan L, Rogers T, Bailey RF, Guo H, et al. Long-term consequences of kidney donation. N Engl J Med. 2009;360(5):459–69. https://doi.org/10.1056/NEJMoa0804883

27. Garg AX, Muirhead N, Knoll G, Yang RC, Prasad GV, Thiessen-Philbrook H, et al. Proteinuria and reduced kidney function in living kidney donors: A systematic review, meta-analysis, and meta-regression. Kidney Int. 2006;70(10):1801–10. https://doi.org/10.1038/sj.ki.5001819

28. Blantz RC, Steiner RW. Benign hyperfiltration after living kidney donation. J Clin Invest. 2015;125(3):972–4. https://doi.org/10.1172/jci80818

29. Lenihan CR, Busque S, Derby G, Blouch K, Myers BD, Tan JC. Longitudinal study of living kidney donor glomerular dynamics after nephrectomy. J Clin Invest. 2015;125(3):1311–8. https://doi.org/10.1172/jci78885

30. Fehrman-Ekholm I, Duner F, Brink B, Tyden G, Elinder CG. No evidence of accelerated loss of kidney function in living kidney donors: results from a cross-sectional follow-up. Transplantation. 2001;72(3):444–9. https://doi.org/10.1097/00007890-200108150-00015

31. Fournier C, Pallet N, Cherqaoui Z, Pucheu S, Kreis H, Mejean A, et al. Very long-term follow-up of living kidney donors. Transpl Int. 2012;25(4):385–90. https://doi.org/10.1111/j.1432-2277.2012.01439.x

32. Cherikh WS, Young CJ, Kramer BF, Taranto SE, Randall HB, Fan PY. Ethnic and gender related differences in the risk of end-stage renal disease after living kidney donation. Am J Transplant. 2011;11(8):1650–5. https://doi.org/10.1111/j.1600-6143.2011.03609.x

33. Lentine KL, Segev DL. Understanding and Communicating Medical Risks for Living Kidney Donors: A Matter of Perspective. J Am Soc Nephrol. 2017;28(1):12–24. https://doi.org/10.1681/asn.2016050571

34. Mjoen G, Hallan S, Hartmann A, Foss A, Midtvedt K, Oyen O, et al. Long-term risks for kidney donors. Kidney Int. 2014;86(1):162–7. https://doi.org/10.1038/ki.2013.460

35. Muzaale AD, Massie AB, Wang MC, Montgomery RA, McBride MA, Wainright JL, et al. Risk of end-stage renal disease following live kidney donation. JAMA. 2014;311(6):579–86. https://doi.org/10.1001/jama.2013.285141

36. Massie AB, Muzaale AD, Luo X, Chow EKH, Locke JE, Nguyen AQ, et al. Quantifying Postdonation Risk of ESRD in Living Kidney Donors. J Am Soc Nephrol. 2017;28(9):2749–55. https://doi.org/10.1681/asn.2016101084

37. Levey AS, Inker LA. GFR Evaluation in Living Kidney Donor Candidates. J Am Soc Nephrol. 2017;28(4):1062–71. https://doi.org/10.1681/ASN.2016070790

38. Norden G, Lennerling A, Nyberg G. Low absolute glomerular filtration rate in the living kidney donor: a risk factor for graft loss. Transplantation. 2000;70(9):1360–2. https://doi.org/10.1097/00007890-200011150-00016

39. Zaky ZS, Gebreselassie S, Poggio ED. Evaluation of Kidney Function and Structure in Potential Living Kidney Donors: Implications for the Donor and Recipient. Curr Transpl Rep. 2015;2:12–21. https://dx.doi.org/10.1681%2FASN.2016070790

40. Association, T.B.T.S.a.T.R. The United Kingdom Guidelines for Living Donor Kidney Transplantation. 2011 [cited Third Edition September 7, 2016]. https://doi.org/10.1097/tp.0b013e318247a7b7

41. Miller WG. Urine albumin: Recommendations for standardization. Scand J Clin Lab Invest Suppl. 2008;241:71–2. https://doi.org/10.1080/00365510802150125

42. Miller WG, Bruns DE, Hortin GL, Sandberg S, Aakre KM, McQueen MJ, et al., Current issues in measurement and reporting of urinary albumin excretion. Clin Chem, 2009. 55(1): p. 24-38 https://doi.org/clinchem.2008.106567 [pii] 10.1373/clinchem.2008.106567.

43. Mogensen C. Microalbuminuria and kidney function. Notes on methods, interpretation, and classification. Methods in. diabetes research. 1986;2:611–31.

44. Garg AX, Kiberd BA, Clark WF, Haynes RB, Clase CM. Albuminuria and renal insufficiency prevalence guides population screening: results from the NHANES III. Kidney Int. 2002;61(6):2165–75. https://doi.org/10.1046/j.1523-1755.2002.00356.x

45. Garg AX, Levey AS, Kasiske BL, et al. Application of the 2017 KDIGO Guideline for the Evaluation and Care of Living Kidney Donors to Clinical Practice. Clin J Am Soc Nephrol. 2020;15(6):896-905. https://doi.org/10.2215/cjn.12141019"10.2215/CJN.12141019

46. Inker LA. Albuminuria: time to focus on accuracy. Am J Kidney Dis. 2014;63(3):378–81. https://doi.org/10.1053/j.ajkd.2014.01.002

47. Gansevoort RT, Verhave JC, Hillege HL, Burgerhof JG, Bakker SJ, de Zeeuw D, et al. The validity of screening based on spot morning urine samples to detect subjects with microalbuminuria in the general population. Kidney Int Suppl, 2005(94): p. S28-35 https://doi.org/10.1111/j.1523-1755.2005.09408.x.

48. Matsushita K, van der Velde M, Astor BC, Woodward M, Levey AS, de Jong PE, et al. Association of estimated glomerular filtration rate and albuminuria with all-cause and cardiovascular mortality in general population cohorts: a collaborative meta-analysis. Lancet, 2010. 375(9731): p. 2073-2081. https://doi.org/10.1016/S0140-6736(10)60674-5.

49. Mandelbrot DA, Pavlakis M, Danovitch GM, Johnson SR, Karp SJ, Khwaja K, et al. The medical evaluation of living kidney donors: a survey of US transplant centers. Am J Transplant. 2007;7(10):2333–43. https://doi.org/10.1111/j.1600-6143.2007.01932.x

50. Cohen RA, Brown RS. Microscopic hematuria. New England Journal of Medicine. 2003;348(23):2330–8. https://doi.org/10.1056/nejmcp012694

51. Chow K, Kwan B, Li P, Szeto C. Asymptomatic isolated microscopic haematuria: long-term follow-up. Qjm. 2004;97(11):739–45. https://doi.org/10.1093/qjmed/hch125

52. Kovačević Z, Jovanović D, Rabrenović V, Dimitrijević J, Djukanović J. Asymptomatic microscopic haematuria in young males. International journal of clinical practice. 2008;62(3):406–12. https://doi.org/10.1111/j.1742-1241.2007.01659.x

53. Lee YM, Baek SY, Hong Kim J, Soo Kim D, Seung Lee J, Kim PK. Analysis of renal biopsies performed in children with abnormal findings in urinary mass screening. Acta Paediatrica. 2006;95(7):849–53. https://doi.org/10.1080/08035250600652005

54. Park Y-H, Choi J-Y, Chung H-S, Koo J-W, Kim S-Y, Namgoong M-K, et al. Hematuria and proteinuria in a mass school urine screening test. Pediatric Nephrology. 2005;20(8):1126–30. https://doi.org/10.1007/s00467-005-1915-8

55. Koushik R, Garvey C, Manivel JC, Matas AJ, Kasiske BL. Persistent, asymptomatic, microscopic hematuria in prospective kidney donors. Transplantation. 2005;80(10):1425–9. https://doi.org/10.1097/01.tp.0000181098.56617.b2

56. Sutton JM. Evaluation of hematuria in adults. Jama. 1990;263(18):2475–80. https://doi.org/10.1001/jama.1990.03440180081037

57. Vivante A, Afek A, Frenkel-Nir Y, Tzur D, Farfel A, Golan E, et al. Persistent asymptomatic isolated microscopic hematuria in Israeli adolescents and young adults and risk for end-stage renal disease. Jama. 2011;306(7):729–36. https://doi.org/10.1001/jama.2011.1141

58. Jais JP, Knebelmann B, Giatras I, De Marchi M, Rizzoni G, Renieri A, et al. X-linked Alport syndrome: natural history and genotype-phenotype correlations in girls and women belonging to 195 families: a "European Community Alport Syndrome Concerted Action" study. J Am Soc Nephrol. 2003;14(10):2603–10. https://doi.org/10.1097/01.asn.0000090034.71205.74

59. Temme J, Peters F, Lange K, Pirson Y, Heidet L, Torra R, et al. Incidence of renal failure and nephroprotection by RAAS inhibition in heterozygous carriers of X-chromosomal and autosomal recessive Alport mutations. Kidney international. 2012;81(8):779–83. https://doi.org/10.1038/ki.2011.452

60. Savige J, Rana K, Tonna S, Buzza M, Dagher H, Wang YY. Thin basement membrane nephropathy. Kidney international. 2003;64(4):1169–78. https://doi.org/10.1046/j.1523-1755.2003.00234.x

61. Choi C, Ahn S, Min SK, Ha J, Ahn C, Kim Y, et al. Midterm Outcome of Kidney Transplantation From Donors With Thin Basement Membrane Nephropathy. Transplantation. 2018;102(4):e180–4. https://doi.org/10.1097/tp.0000000000002089

62. Kashtan CE, Ding J, Garosi G, Heidet L, Massella L, Nakanishi K, et al. Alport syndrome: a unified classification of genetic disorders of collagen IV alpha345: a position paper of the Alport Syndrome Classification Working Group. Kidney Int. 2018;93(5):1045–51. https://doi.org/10.1016/j.kint.2017.12.018

63. Voskarides K, Damianou L, Neocleous V, Zouvani I, Christodoulidou S, Hadjiconstantinou V, et al. COL4A3/COL4A4 mutations producing focal segmental glomerulosclerosis and renal failure in thin basement membrane nephropathy. J Am Soc Nephrol. 2007;18(11):3004–16. https://doi.org/10.1681/asn.2007040444

64. Pierides A, Voskarides K, Athanasiou Y, Ioannou K, Damianou L, Arsali M, et al. Clinico-pathological correlations in 127 patients in 11 large pedigrees, segregating one of three heterozygous mutations in the COL4A3/ COL4A4 genes associated with familial haematuria and significant late progression to proteinuria and chronic kidney disease from focal segmental glomerulosclerosis. Nephrol Dial Transplant, 2009. 24(9): p. 2721-9 https://doi.org/10.1027293/ndt/gfp158.

65. Shen P, He L, Huang D. Clinical course and prognostic factors of clinical early IgA nephropathy. Neth J Med. 2008;66(6):242–7. https://pubmed.ncbi.nlm.nih.gov/18689907/

66. Szeto C-C, Lai FM-M, K.-F. To, Wong TY-H, Chow K-M, Choi PC-L, et al. The natural history of immunoglobulin a nephropathy among patients with hematuria and minimal proteinuria. The American journal of medicine. 2001;110(6):434–7. https://doi.org/10.1016/s0002-9343(01)00659-3

67. Sevillano AM, Gutiérrez E, Yuste C, Cavero T, Mérida E, Rodríguez E, et al. Remission of hematuria improves renal survival in IgA nephropathy. J Am Soc Nephrol. 2017;28:3089–99. https://doi.org/10.1681/asn.2017010108

68. Choi S, Sun I, Hong Y, Kim H, Park H, Chung B, et al. The role of kidney biopsy to determine donation from prospective kidney donors with asymptomatic urinary abnormalities. in Transplantation proceedings. 2012. Elsevier. https://doi.org/10.1016/j.transproceed.2011.12.008

69. Gross O, Weber M, Fries JW, Müller G-A. Living donor kidney transplantation from relatives with mild urinary abnormalities in Alport syndrome: long-term risk, benefit and outcome. Nephrology Dialysis Transplantation. 2008;24(5):1626–30. https://doi.org/10.1093/ndt/gfn635

70. Kido R, Shibagaki Y, Iwadoh K, Nakajima I, Fuchinoue S, Fujita T, et al. Persistent glomerular hematuria in living kidney donors confers a risk of progressive kidney disease in donors after heminephrectomy. American Journal of Transplantation. 2010;10(7):1597–604. https://doi.org/10.1111/j.1600-6143.2010.03077.x

71. Organisation SSoNaST. SEN-ONT recommendations for living-donor kidney transplantation. Nefrologia. 2011;30(52):0–105.

72. Richardson R, Connelly M, Dipchand C, Garg AX, Ghanekar A, Houde I, et al. Kidney paired donation protocol for participating donors 2014. Transplantation. 2015;99:S1–S88. https://doi.org/10.1097/tp.0000000000000918

73. Savige J, Gregory M, Gross O, Kashtan C, Ding J, Flinter F. Expert guidelines for the management of Alport syndrome and thin basement membrane nephropathy. Journal of the American Society of Nephrology. 2013;24(3):364–75. https://doi.org/10.1681/asn.2012020148

Evaluation of Renal Anatomy, Structure and Nephrolithiasis in Living Donor Candidates

Emilio D. Poggio, Nasir Khan, Christian Bolanos, Thomas Pham, and Jane C. Tan

Introduction

The assessment of kidney function and anatomy is a critical component in the evaluation of living kidney donor candidates. Evaluation is aimed at assessing whether an individual has sufficient reserve for adequate function in the remaining kidney following donation and whether the kidney planned for procurement is suitable for donation. This assessment complements the traditional clinical practice of living donor evaluation, which focuses on clinical examination, history, and laboratory testing to screen for risk factors associated with development of chronic kidney disease (CKD). In clinical practice, evaluation of donor candidates focuses on bio-markers of kidney function in blood and urine (i.e., glomerular filtration rate (GFR)), presence of albuminuria as discussed in Chap. 3, and delineation of renal anatomy through imaging. More recently, histology of the donated kidney has also been studied in the context of kidney donation. Although assessment of histology, another correlate of renal function, is not routine clinical practice in the evaluation of kidney donor candidates, implantation biopsies may reveal findings with important

E. D. Poggio · N. Khan
Department of Nephrology and Hypertension, Glickman Urological and Kidney Institute, Cleveland Clinic, Cleveland, OH, USA

C. Bolanos · J. C. Tan (✉)
Division of Nephrology, Department of Medicine, Stanford University, Stanford, CA, USA
e-mail: janetan@stanford.edu

T. Pham
Division of Abdominal Transplantation, Department of Surgery, Stanford University, Stanford, CA, USA

© Springer Nature Switzerland AG 2021
K. L. Lentine et al. (eds.), *Living Kidney Donation*,
https://doi.org/10.1007/978-3-030-53618-3_4

implications for donor health and transplant outcomes following donation. These three aspects of the evaluation of kidney health – kidney anatomy, function, and histology – are interrelated.

Since the inception of living donor kidney transplantation as treatment for kidney failure, the assessment of kidney function and anatomy has been a critical component in the evaluation of kidney donor candidates. Advances in medical technology have led to increased resolution in preoperative imaging and incorporation of these techniques into the practice of living donor evaluation. Over the past few decades, radiologic evaluation has shifted from ultrasonography and pyelograms to the near universal adoption of computed tomography (CT) or magnetic resonance imaging (MRI). Such advancements in imaging techniques allow for better accuracy in assessing kidney size, anatomy, vasculature, and volumes. Higher-resolution imaging has also increased the detection of incidental findings previously undetected (e.g., small kidney stones). This information can now be integrated into the broader knowledge of kidney function following donation and transplantation to frame long-term implications for both kidney donors and their recipients.

Histology of the kidney can be assessed using biopsies taken intraoperatively. To date, this practice has been mainly limited to research studies. Recently, multicenter studies using implant biopsies have increased the knowledge of living donor histology. Indeed, some transplant centers now routinely perform kidney donor implant biopsies, and ongoing research derived from this collective effort has shed light on issues pertaining to living donor health and transplant outcomes. Notably, this research has revealed the presence of subclinical but significant features on the histological level to be evident in a subset of donor kidneys despite normal laboratory and imaging studies. Histologic data may have important clinical implications, including with regard to postdonation management and follow-up. Living donors and candidates in the current era are increasingly medically complex, with comorbidities such as mild metabolic abnormalities, obesity, and older age at donation. Sole reliance on laboratory and imaging results may not suffice in accurately predicting donors who may benefit from closer medical surveillance following donation; subtle histological abnormalities may be early markers of CKD and could potentially help identify such donors. In this chapter, we review the current literature on how renal anatomy and histology associate with kidney function in donor candidates.

Kidney Structure and Anatomy

The 2017 Kidney Disease: Improving Global Outcomes (KDIGO) "Guideline on the Evaluation and Care of Living Donors" recommends performance of renal imaging (e.g., CT angiography) in all donor candidates to assess renal anatomy before nephrectomy [1]. Determination of the surgical approach for nephrectomy is discussed in Chap. 13.

Development of the Kidney

During fetal development, two kidneys form on either side of the vertebral column. The kidneys begin development in the pelvis just anterior to the sacrum and assume a more cranial position usually at the level of the first four lumbar vertebrae as the caudal portion of the body elongates. The pelvic kidney derives its blood supply from branches of the distal aorta and common iliac artery. As the kidneys migrate cranially, new branches from the abdominal aorta appear and supply blood to the kidney while the distal branches involute and disappear, with the kidneys ultimately receiving their main blood supply from the abdominal aorta.

Arterial Anatomy

Approximately 70% of adults have kidneys with a single artery and vein originating from the aorta and inferior vena cava, respectively. The remaining 20–30% have two or more arteries and/or veins. Renal artery duplication is twice as common as venous duplications. These supernumerary arteries can enter the hilum or supply the superior or inferior pole directly. Accessory inferior pole arteries are twice as common as ones that supply the superior pole [2]. The left kidney lies closer to the aorta. Thus, the left renal artery is typically shorter in length when compared to the right renal artery.

Segmental arteries can originate from the main renal artery or the aorta itself. When being considered for kidney donation, the surgeon is most concerned with those segmental renal arteries originating from the aorta or within 2–3 cm of the renal artery takeoff from the aorta. Segmental arteries that branch early from the main renal artery may have to be divided separately creating multiple arteries for the transplant. The left renal artery may have branches that supply the left adrenal gland and rarely the left gonad. The right renal artery courses posterior to the inferior vena cava and typically supplies an arterial branch to the right adrenal gland. These branches are typically encountered during a donor nephrectomy and should be taken into consideration. Right kidney accessory arteries that originate from the aorta are found anterior to the vena cava in 5% of patients [3]. This is especially important to note during dissection of the kidney for donation (Fig. 4.1).

Renal Artery Stenosis

Renal artery stenosis (RAS) is most commonly caused by atherosclerosis and fibromuscular dysplasia. Findings of atherosclerotic RAS in a kidney donor will typically deter most centers from proceeding with that particular donor because of concern for disease progression in the remaining kidney. Atherosclerotic RAS is also a common cause of renovascular hypertension. The 2017 KDIGO guideline

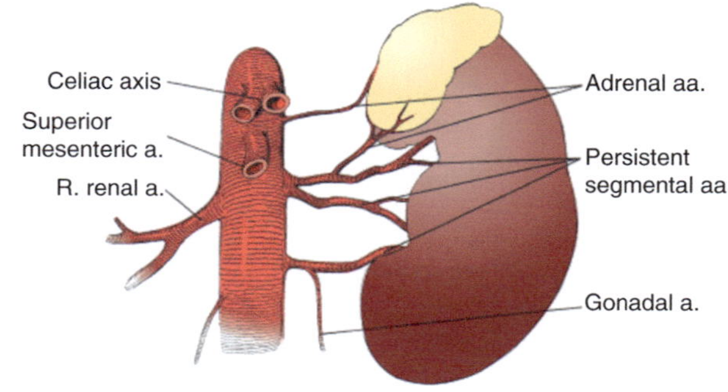

Fig. 4.1 Arterial supply of the left kidney. This illustrates the possible segmental arteries that can arise from the aorta or from the main renal artery. Note the close proximity of the renal artery to the superior mesenteric artery. (From MacLennan et al. [4])

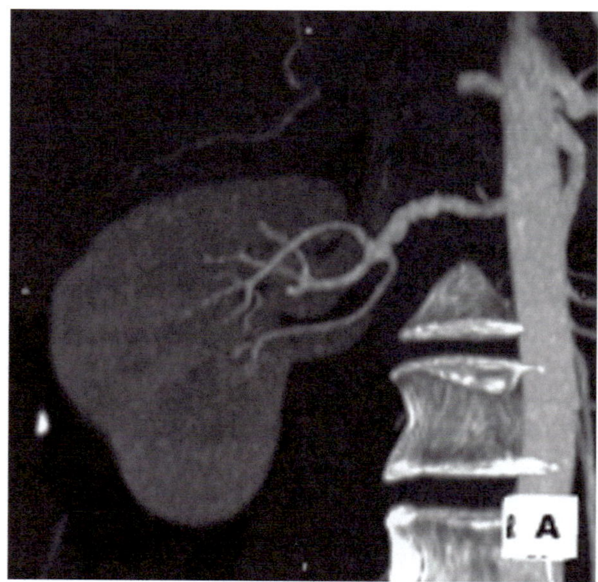

Fig. 4.2 Fibromuscular dysplasia. CT angiogram showing the distinctive beading appearance of the renal artery. (From Quaia et al. [9])

recommends that a donor candidate with atherosclerotic renal artery disease or fibromuscular dysplasia involving the orifices of both renal arteries should not donate [1]. When donation has been approved in the context of unilateral RAS, the stenosis commonly occurs at the renal artery ostium, and so division of the artery distal to this will avoid the stenosis in the transplanted kidney. Case reports have shown acceptable short-term outcomes with some reporting improvement of the donor's baseline hypertension [5].

The second most common cause of RAS after atherosclerosis is fibromuscular dysplasia (FMD). FMD often causes renovascular hypertension and can be present in up to 4.4% of asymptomatic patients [6, 7]. Most cases of FMD involve the medial layer of the artery wherein collagen deposits give the artery a beaded appearance (Fig. 4.2). There have been several reports of approving living donation with FMD with utilization of affected kidneys for transplantation [5, 8]. When donation is considered, it is recommended to use the affected kidney or the kidney with more severe FMD for transplant, leaving the donor kidney with the lesser arterial defect. Donation and transplant should only proceed with careful informed consent of donor and recipient and attention to progression of FMD in the donor's remaining kidney and the transplanted kidney [6].

Renal Vein Anatomy

The left renal vein lies anterior to the aorta and renal artery in the majority of patients. Its average length is 6–10 cm and is greater than twice the length of the right renal vein which averages 2–4 cm. Anomalies of venous drainage occur because of residual veins that persist after embryological development. Most common are the persistence of a left-sided cava and the formation of retro-aortic renal veins. The left gonadal vein and adrenal vein always drain into the left renal vein. Left testicular pain following laparoscopic nephrectomy has been reported in as high as 9.6% of men [10, 11]. Although the etiology may be multifactorial, a proposed cause is the division of the left gonadal vein at or near the pelvic brim. It has been reported that preservation of the gonadal vein with division at the renal vein confluence resolves this problem, but the number of patients studied was small [11]. The posterior lumbar vein almost always drains into the left renal vein and will vary in size and number of veins. The gonadal vein drains directly into the right renal vein in approximately 20% of cases. The right renal vein rarely has any other tributaries as most surrounding branches will drain directly into the vena cava.

Left Kidney Retro-aortic Veins

Left renal vein abnormalities are commonly categorized into four different types (Fig. 4.3) [12]. Type 3 is also known as the circumaortic renal vein and is the most common venous anomaly seen in the left kidney venous system, present in 2–16% of the patients. The posterior retro-aortic portion of the venous ring is usually

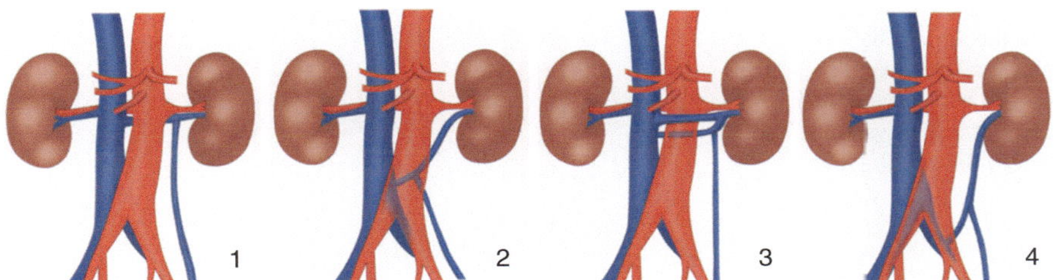

Fig. 4.3 Illustration of the different types of retro-aortic left renal veins. (1) Type 1. Isolated retro-aortic vein in the orthotopic position. (2) Type 2. Retro-aortic vein that inserts into the inferior vena cava at the lumbar level. (3) Type 3. Circumaortic renal vein. (4) Type 4. Insertion of the vein into the left common iliac vein. (From Nam et al. [14])

smaller in size and can be divided during the nephrectomy without consequence to the venous drainage of the kidney. This is because the circumaortic venous ring is the result of a redundancy of the renal vein.

Isolated retro-aortic left renal veins (Types 1, 2, and 4) occur in up to 4% of patients while multiple left renal veins occur in 15% of patients. Most accessory veins of the left kidney are retro-aortic [13]. Isolated retro-aortic veins are not a contraindication to kidney donation. It is important that the donor candidate undergo adequate vascular imaging so that these venous abnormalities are delineated and a surgical plan is in place prior to proceeding with nephrectomy. Retro-aortic veins typically do not alter the recipient operation.

Renal Nutcracker Vein

Nutcracker vein is the result of compression of the distal left renal vein by the superior mesenteric artery and aorta which causes proximal dilation and may result in venous hypertension, hematuria, and variceal formation (Fig. 4.4). The characteristic findings on CT/MRI are beak sign which represents narrowing of the vein as it passes the aortomesenteric junction, well-developed collateral veins in the retroperitoneum and renal hilum, left renal vein diameter ratio cut of 4.9 between the hilum and aortomesenteric junction, and angle between superior mesenteric artery (SMA) and aorta less than 41 degrees [14].

Nutcracker phenomenon is the finding of a nutcracker vein without clinical symptoms. Nutcracker phenomenon in kidney donor candidates is typically found incidentally on kidney imaging. The presence of a nutcracker vein is not a contraindication for donor nephrectomy unless the nutcracker kidney is to remain with the donor. If a nutcracker kidney remains with the donor after the donation, it will compensate for the donated kidney as expected. This compensation will increase blood

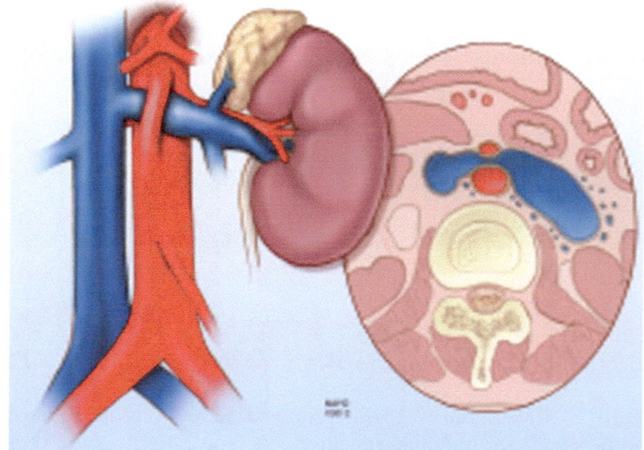

Fig. 4.4 Illustration of a nutcracker renal vein. The renal vein is compressed by the junction of the superior mesenteric artery and the aorta. The proximal renal vein is dilated with development of surrounding varices. (From Said et al. [15])

flow to the kidney which has the potential to worsen the nutcracker vein. It is recommended that if a nutcracker vein is found in the donor candidate, that kidney could be used for transplant.

Ureteral Anatomy

Development of an extra supernumerary kidney is extremely rare and is the result of complete division of a ureteric bud. More common is the duplication of the ureter and renal pelvis because of an incompletely divided ureteric bud which results in a fused kidney. Each kidney then develops a separate ureter which may be duplicated upon entering the bladder or fuse into a single ureter after exiting the renal pelvis. The presence of multiple ureters is not a contraindication to nephrectomy but should be assessed with an operative management plan prior to proceeding with nephrectomy.

Horseshoe Kidney

Horseshoe kidney is the most common renal parenchymal abnormality and is found in approximately 1:500 to 1:1000 individuals [2]. The fusion of kidney most commonly occurs at the inferior poles but may involve both superior and inferior pole. Horseshoe kidneys have used en bloc for deceased donor kidney transplant with good results. Over the past decades, there have been several reports of living kidney donation from individuals with horseshoe kidneys [16, 17]. The case is accomplished by division of the kidneys at the isthmus and then transplantation of the divided kidney in the usual fashion. Although rare overall, utilization of horseshoe kidneys from living donors is considered an option in countries that do not have a well-established deceased donor transplant network [17].

Renal Structure

Kidney Size and Volume

Past studies utilizing ultrasound to assess kidney size and volume in healthy adults showed that the median kidney length of the left and right kidneys are 11.2 cm and 10.9 cm, respectively. Median kidney volumes are 146 cm³ on the left and 134 cm³ on the right. Although differences may not be significant, several studies show that the left kidney is longer in length and typically has greater volume [18, 19]. Men typically have larger kidney volumes than women and are likely related to the larger body surface area (BSA) seen in men. BSA has been shown to directly correlate with renal volume. Renal cortical volume directly relates to the number of nephrons and is a reliable predictor of kidney function [20, 21]. The 2017 KDIGO guideline recommends that when asymmetry in GFR, parenchymal abnormalities, vascular abnormalities, or urological abnormalities are present but do not preclude donation, the more severely affected kidney should be used for donation. What is determined to be a significant difference in function between each kidney is usually determined by the donor evaluation team and varies between transplant centers.

Factors Associated with Kidney Function Pre- and Postdonation

GFR has long been considered as the best clinical marker of kidney function. Assessment of predonation kidney function is discussed in Chap. 3. In otherwise healthy donors with two kidneys of comparable size and function, donor nephrectomy results in the immediate loss of approximately 50% of nephron mass and consequently a similar loss in GFR. However, in healthy individuals, this loss in nephron mass and function is compensated by an increase in GFR of the remaining kidney, which begins in the immediate postnephrectomy period [22] and continues over time [23]. Assuming each kidney represents 50% of the total GFR prior to donation, the remaining kidney compensates with an approximately 10–40% increase above the baseline GFR of the remaining kidney, eventually leaving the donor with approximately 60–70% of the total predonation GFR [24]. As mentioned earlier, there are data to suggest that GFR improvement continues over a rather extended period of time. In one such study with 3 years of follow-up, Kasiske et al. showed that GFR as measured by iohexol renal clearances continues to increase by approximately 1.47 ml/min/1.73 m^2 per year after nephrectomy [25]. Further, as shown in another study with longer follow-up, this trend in GFR increase continues for several subsequent years after nephrectomy [26].

Several baseline clinical factors influence postdonation residual kidney function. Among these, factors such as age, body size, risk factors for kidney disease (e.g., hypertension), family history of kidney disease, and predonation GFR were found to be important correlates of postdonation GFR. As reviewed below, several of these factors also closely relate to kidney mass and histology.

Predonation GFR and age at donation appear to be two key determinants of postdonation kidney function, as demonstrated by Ibrahim et al. [27]. Studies utilizing this large single-center cohort of kidney donors have helped characterize the natural history of kidney health in donors of predominantly Caucasian ethnicity; kidney donors described in the early decades of living donation have overwhelmingly been Caucasian, first-degree relatives of recipients. More recently, other factors such as family history of kidney disease have been established as risk factors for faster decline in kidney function following donation [28]. The onset of progressive decline appears to be delayed by several years after donor nephrectomy [29].

Age-related accelerated decline in GFR probably represents a decrease in "renal reserve capacity," and not a blunting of the compensatory hyperfiltration in response to the loss of nephron mass. Thus, although donors who are older at the time of nephrectomy would have lower absolute GFR levels compared to their younger counterparts, they retain the early nephron-level compensatory function. It appears that the extent of postdonation GFR compensation is dependent in part on predonation GFR. GFR is known to decline with age, and lower levels of GFR after nephrectomy often manifest as "impaired kidney function" in older donors. The GFR loss with age is not uniform but occurs at different rates in aggregate age-stratified populations and is highly variable on an individual level [30]. For instance, the rate of decrease in GFR is 4 ml/min per 1.73 m^2 per decade of life in donors younger than 45 at the time of donation while this decline is more pronounced in older donors [31].

Studies of donor physiology, histology, and morphometry have shown that the magnitude of compensatory rise in GFR after nephrectomy depends to a great degree on the predonation GFR. Using morphometric analyses of implant biopsies and physiologic studies of younger deceased donor ($\leq$ 45 years old) vs. older donor ($\geq$55 years old) kidneys, Tan et al. found that postnephrectomy compensatory GFR response was more closely related to the number of functional glomeruli rather than to hyperfiltration capacity [32]. Older donor kidneys had a lower number of functional glomeruli that translated into lower postnephrectomy GFR. An alternate hypothesis by Rook et al. emphasized that the lower GFR observed in older living donors is a result of the lower "reserve capacity" of the remaining nephrons in the older patients, as quantified by impaired low-dose dopamine-induced hyperfiltration in older donors [33, 34]. In a study by Ohashi et al., the degree of nephrosclerosis/renal micro-vascular disease in implant biopsies, but not the age of the donor per se, correlated with postdonation GFR [35]. Since there is generally a higher degree of nephrosclerosis in older compared to younger subjects, this may explain the lower postnephrectomy GFR in the older donors. This becomes clinically relevant in light of the gradual decline in GFR with age. The standard diagnosis scheme for CKD is based on an estimated GFR (eGFR) of less than 60 ml/min per 1.73 m^2 for $\geq$3 months, with graded increase in CKD stage at lower GFR levels. Older kidney donors frequently have postdonation eGFR lower than 60 ml/min per 1.73 m^2, resulting in labeling as CKD by this widely accepted practice [36]. Historically, this framework of CKD diagnosis staging was derived from large epidemiologic studies of binephric nondonors [37]. Whether and/or to what extent this current definition of CKD is applicable to living donors is a topic of debate.

Other donor characteristics such as obesity may also be important factors associated with postdonation GFR. Rook et al. showed that while predonation reserve capacity was preserved independent of body mass index (BMI), postnephrectomy reserve capacity was significantly blunted in overweight and obese donors compared to donors with BMI < 25 kg/m^2. This observation raises the question of whether obesity translates to increased long-term risk for progressive CKD in donors who remain overweight after donation [33].

Effects of Donor Kidney Size: "Nephron Dose"

Kidneys from healthy individuals contain between 480,000 and 970,000 (860,000 $\pm$ 370,000 nephrons) functioning nephrons per kidney [38]. These estimates were derived from studies in living kidney donors, mostly of Caucasian race. In the setting of living kidney donation, nephron mass can have clinical implications for both donor and recipient. The number of functional nephrons per kidney varies with age, gender, and body size. The sum of the single-nephron GFR across nephron units totals to the GFR for a whole kidney. From a histological standpoint, the kidney is formed by viable nephrons (glomeruli and tubules surrounded by interstitium) and non-functioning glomeruli or nephrosclerosis (interstitial fibrosis, glomerulosclerosis, and arteriosclerosis). These components and their distribution in any given kidney can only be evaluated by histologic examination of biopsy tissue. However, the risk of a kidney biopsy in a healthy individual prior to donation is not justifiable in the usual clinical practice setting of routine donor candidate evaluation. A notable exception is in a strongly motivated donor with incidental microscopic hematuria or mild albuminuria. Thus, alternative surrogate measures are used for assessing nephron dose. Kidney volume is a reasonable surrogate for overall nephron mass (or nephron endowment) in healthy individuals and therefore kidney function assuming that there is no underlying histopathologic disease. Kidney volume as a marker for functioning nephron mass can be estimated using newer reconstructive algorithms of CT or MRI [20]. Notably, like GFR and histology, kidney volume is also determined by many factors including age, body size, and gender.

A strong correlation between kidney volume and GFR was found in a cohort of 119 living kidney donors with calculated kidney volumes by CT and measured iothalamate clearances [20]. This study identified a strong linear correlation between total kidney volume and total GFR. This finding is also supported by other studies showing a significant correlation between single kidney volumes and single kidney GFR as measured by ^{99m}Tc-DTPA kidney scintigraphy [39]. Furthermore, male sex and higher BMI (but not age) correlated with larger kidney volume, while male sex, higher BMI, and younger age correlated with higher GFR [21, 40–42].

As discussed above, after donor nephrectomy, the remaining kidney increases its function to compensate for the loss of renal mass. It has also been hypothesized that this increase in renal function is in part related to an increase in filtration of functional glomeruli in the remaining kidney. The remaining kidney volume increases owing to hypertrophy thought to be from the compensatory functional hyperfiltration seen following donation. This increase in kidney volume following nephrectomy of the contralateral kidney is seen as early as within a week after nephrectomy [43]. Using MRI to assess kidney volume, Song et al. reported an increase in renal volume of 21.3% as early as 3 days after nephrectomy and 24.17% by a week postdonation. In this study, the increase in kidney size directly correlated with higher 1-year GFR but showed a negative correlation with predonation kidney size.

Jeon et al. studied 222 living kidney donors who underwent CT scans predonation and 6 months after donor nephrectomy [21]. Donors also underwent simultaneous GFR measurements using ^{99m}Tc-DTPA kidney scintigraphy. The volume of the remaining kidney increased from an average of 154 ± 26 cc prior to donation to

193 ± 34 cc postdonation, an approximately 28% increase from baseline. An important observation was that younger age was a significant predictor of greater increase in kidney volume on multiple linear regression. This finding suggests that the compensatory increase in kidney function in the remaining kidney after donation is higher in younger donors.

Other smaller studies have shown similar findings with an approximately 25% increase in remaining kidney size within 1 year following donation [44]. In a study of medically complex donors that included donors older than 55 years of age, 11 donors with BMI greater than 35 kg/m^2, and 9 hypertensive donors, CT scan-estimated kidney volumes increased by 29.3 ± 18% after 5 years of donor nephrectomy in all studied donors independent of risk factors [41]. This data suggests that analogous to GFR postdonation, the remnant kidney hypertrophies immediately following donation and continues over time. Based on these studies, one could conclude that there is an approximately 25% increase in remaining kidney size following donation, similar to the gain seen in remaining kidney GFR after donor nephrectomy.

One hypothesis to explain this is that predonation kidney volume and/or the ability to increase kidney volume postdonation is a determinant of postdonation GFR. Several studies have shown a positive correlation between predonation kidney volume and postdonation GFR. Hall et al. published a study of 151 living kidney donors who underwent predonation CT scans and 1 year of follow-up of GFR as estimated using a creatinine-based equation [45]. The investigators found that predonation GFR as well as postdonation GFR were positively correlated with kidney volumes of the retained kidney. In a multivariable analysis, predonation GFR and predonation kidney volume were positively correlated with better 1-year postdonation GFR, while donor age was negatively correlated. Other studies have shown similar findings [42, 46–48].

On the other hand, some studies were unable to show a direct positive correlation between predonation kidney volume and long-term postdonation GFR [21, 49]. Courbedaisse et al. studied 63 living kidney donors who had kidney volumes measured by CT scan and GFR by ^{51}Cr-EDTA renal clearances. The investigators calculated the GFR per volume of the retained kidney and its association with donor GFR 5 years postdonation. Interestingly, along with older age and increased BMI, the donors with higher GFR per kidney showed a negative correlation with postdonation GFR. These results suggest that such donors have limited increase in GFR postdonation, perhaps having reached their near maximal hyperfiltration capacity prior to donation. For the increase in postnephrectomy kidney volume to explain the increase in GFR by the remnant kidney that is observed following donation, the hypertrophy of the kidney needs to reflect an increased filtration in viable nephrons, an effect often referred to as "adaptive or compensatory hyperfiltration."

In summary, just as renal function of the remaining kidney adapts to the loss of the donated kidney, a similar effect occurs with kidney size. Importantly, kidney volume correlates with function, and, therefore, consideration to kidney size should be given when multiple kidney donors are available for a given recipient.

Histology of Implant Biopsies and Relevance to Donor Health

Clinical interest in subclinical histologic abnormalities in living donor candidates has a renewed relevance in our current era of heightened recognition of the potential long-term risks of living donation. Recent epidemiologic studies reported increased risk of ESKD in donors compared to nondonors that can manifest as early as 5–10 years after donation [50, 51]. How to translate these estimates into clinical practice of donor selection, risk stratification, counseling, and follow-up is an area of debate. For example, it is now evident that a small but distinct population of living donors may have increased risk of progressive CKD despite the detailed and careful evaluation that has been practiced. Clinical research in the field of living donor outcomes is challenging due to the low event rate of ESKD along with the long time to event. For instance, a 2014 report identified 102 living donors progressing to ESKD who were subsequently listed for kidney transplantation with a mean time from donation to listing for a renal transplant of 17.6 years [52]. Risk calculators have been developed to better identify populations at increased risk of developing advanced CKD after donation with the goal of improved predonation counseling for decision-making and postdonation counseling for health maintenance [53, 54], but the estimates are based on averages, and limitations to precision for the individual are acknowledged [53].

Predicting living kidney donors who will have adverse renal outcomes is exceedingly challenging. Nonetheless, the confluence of several demographic patterns and clinical practice trends has accentuated the urgency of this area of research. These include (1) ongoing unmet need for organ donors in the context of the organ shortage, (2) trends toward acceptance of donors with isolated medical abnormalities (e.g., those with mild hypertension, higher BMI, and increasing age) based on presumption of safety and in the context of general population trends such as aging and more common obesity.

Studies from renal histopathology of implant biopsies from living donor kidneys taken intraoperatively prior to implantation may refine the identification of the minority of donors at risk for adverse renal outcomes after donation. For instance, donors with subtle histologic abnormalities despite acceptable clinical profile may develop accelerated decline in kidney function compared with those with no histologic abnormality. If so, development of biomarkers of histologic abnormalities may be warranted.

Renal histology often associates with kidney function. However, normal kidney function assessed by the tools currently available does not necessarily predict entirely normal renal histology in otherwise healthy individuals. Subclinical histological abnormalities may be found even in relatively healthy persons, and living kidney donors are no exception. Renal biopsies at time of graft implantation provide a unique opportunity to study renal histology in donors. Recent studies have helped define the association between renal histopathologic features and donor clinical characteristics. It is now clear that underlying pathology and/or histological structural variations in this "healthy" population are not uncommon. The most common histopathologic features observed are glomerulosclerosis, interstitial fibrosis and tubular atrophy (nephrosclerosis), and large glomerular and tubular size (nephron hypertrophy) [55]. As with kidney function and mass, demographic and metabolic attributes associate with histological findings. Risk factors for kidney disease such as hypertension or family history of kidney disease also correlate with histologic abnormalities.

The best studied donor characteristic that associates with structural histological changes in renal parenchyma is age. A robust body of evidence demonstrates a strong linear correlation between age and glomerulosclerosis. In a study by Rule et al., the degree of glomerulosclerosis using both nephron and overall parenchymal scoring systems showed a linear increase with age from 2.7% to 73% in adult kidney donors <30 and 70–77 years of age, respectively [56]. Other donor characteristics such as male sex, higher GFR, degree of albuminuria, family history of kidney disease, and higher BMI were independently associated with nephron hypertrophy as indicated by higher glomerular volume and larger tubular area [57].

In an analysis of the same cohort, Chauhan et al. showed that moderate-to-severe chronic changes in the histology of donors were found in 4.1% of the cases and that this prevalence was higher in donors older than age 60 compared with younger donors (11% vs. 3.5%, p < 0.001). Moderate-to-severe chronic histological abnormalities were also observed in donors with systolic blood pressure of 140 mmHg or greater when compared to normotensive donors (12% vs. 5.7%, p = 0.01) [58]. Short-term follow-up in this study (4 months) showed no difference in postdonation GFR in any group.

Recent studies have used classic histologic, morphometric, and physiologic techniques to (1) describe the range of glomerular and tubulointerstitial histology, (2) measure whole kidney GFR and glomerular volume, and (3) estimate single-nephron GFR and glomerular pressure to understand the early pathophysiologic factors that might ultimately lead to rapid progression to advanced CKD in subgroups of living donors. In a large study of implant biopsies from living donors, Denic et al. identified significant structural and pathological variation in implant biopsies from apparently healthy living kidney donors. These variations fell into one of the two broad categories: nephron hypertrophy (larger nephron size as assessed by the size of the glomeruli or tubule) and nephrosclerosis (ischemic chronic changes due to arteriosclerosis, leading to interstitial fibrosis, glomerulosclerosis and tubular atrophy). Nephron hypertrophy reflects the increased metabolic demand to the reduced number of functional nephrons following kidney donation and is not necessarily pathologic. In contrast, nephrosclerosis reflects a chronic pathologic process. Progressive and severe nephrosclerosis invariably leads to loss of functional nephrons ('nephropenia'), and this can eventually be reflected in renal imaging as renal cysts or decreased cortex-to-medulla ratio.

Age-dependent nephrosclerosis and decrease in the number of functioning nephrons has been well-established in studies of cadaveric kidneys [59, 60]. This phenomenon was also demonstrated in deceased donor kidneys [32] as well as living donor kidneys [61, 62]. Over the past decade, increasingly larger cohorts of implant biopsies of living donors have sharpened the collective resolution of early pathologic findings. Several studies have focused on determining clinical factors associated with poorer renal histology and clinical outcomes following kidney donation. For instance, Choi et al. characterized the histological findings in 121 implant biopsies donors who were followed over 2 years [63]. These findings were compared to the donor characteristics, predonation kidney function, intraoperative factors and perioperative renal function parameters including serum creatinine and GFR calculations in an attempt to identify histological abnormalities that correlate with kidney function in donors at 1-year postdonation. While donor age and preoperative GFR were confirmed as significant factors associated with postdonation donor kidney function, no additional predonation factors associated with 1-year postdonation kidney function. Similarly, Chauhan et al. [58] studied a larger cohort including 1600 donor biopsies over 10 years (2001–2011). They found that moderate-to-severe histologic changes were relatively uncommon (4%, n = 65) and that age and systolic blood pressure were the only significant clinical factors associated with histologic abnormalities. Notably, other routine clinical characteristics of kidney donors such as gender, BMI, diastolic blood pressure, GFR, and urine microalbuminuria did not appear to be associated with abnormal histological findings assessed in this fashion.

In contrast, Fahmy et al. followed a cohort of 310 donors (1997–2012) with a median follow-up time of 6.2 years to study the association between histological attributes of the donor kidneys on implantation biopsies and postdonation eGFR [64]. Of the 310 donor kidneys, 65.8% had some degree of moderate-to-severe histological abnormalities – a much higher incidence than was found in the studies by Choi et al. and Chauhan et al. (roughly one-third with arteriolar hyalinosis and intimal thickening each, 20% with glomerulosclerosis, and 25% with interstitial fibrosis and tubular atrophy (IFTA)). After adjusting for multiple donor demographic and clinical parameters, only IFTA was found to be associated with a postdonation decrease in eGFR by 5 ml/min per $1.73m^2$. These findings corroborated a study by Ohashi et al. which showed that moderate-to-severe chronic histological changes in the donor implant biopsies were associated with a 0.23% decrease in eGFR recovery from immediate postdonation to 2-years postdonation [35]. The eGFR also decreased with older donor age at donation by 3 ml/min per 1.73 m^2 for every decade of age increase, while eGFR increased by 4 ml/min per 1.73 m^2 for every 10 ml/min per 1.73 m^2 increment in preoperative eGFR, suggesting the importance of these two easily quantifiable donor characteristics to predict postdonation recovery of eGFR.

More recently, Issa et al. showed that these structural findings/variations in the kidneys of living donors when assessed using age-related thresholds, better predict postdonation renal function [28]. The substantially larger cohort (n = 1334) of patients in this study allowed for better analysis of multiple patient variables not previously tenable in smaller studies. Thresholds were defined for nephron numbers (by CT imaging and biopsy measures), and for nephrosclerosis (by glomerulosclerosis, degree of arteriosclerosis, IFTA). The investigators used structural parameters to predict postdonation measured GFR, 24-hour urine albumin and hypertension. Larger glomerular size and greater IFTA in the donated kidney associated with low GFR (< 60 ml/min per $1.73m^2$). Further, larger cortex volumes per glomerulus and low estimated number of nephrons were associated with mild microalbuminuria, and arteriosclerosis with was associated with postdonation hypertension. This study suggests that while some donors may harbor early subclinical renal pathology that is undetectable through standard clinical testing prior to donation, the loss of renal mass from nephrectomy may manifest as subtle findings following donation. Longer follow up studies are needed to determine whether progressive CKD, hypertension or other clinical sequalae ensue in such donors.

In the context of the general population obesity epidemic, overweight and obese BMI have also become more common among living donors, although transplant programs vary in acceptance of obese living donors [65], in part due to uncertainty about associated risks [66]. Obesity and metabolic syndrome are associated with kidney disease and renal pathology in the form of glomerulopathy [67, 68]. Patients with higher BMI (> 30 kg/m^2) were shown by Rea et al. to have subtle histologic features (e.g., glomerular hypertrophy, tubular dilatation and less tubular vacuoliza-tion). Whether or not these features translate into more pronounced chronic changes over time in the setting of further compensatory changes with kidney donation is unknown. Meta-analysis based on data from nearly 5 million healthy persons found a modest association of BMI greater than 30 kg/m^2 with increased risk of ESKD over median cohort follow-up of 4–16 years (adjusted HR, 1.16; 95% CI 1.04–1.29) [53]. However, in living donors, the hyperfiltration stress of obesity may be exacer-bated by reduction in kidney mass from donor nephrectomy. In a national registry-based study of U.S. living kidney donors, obese donors had 1.9-fold higher risk of ESKD postdonation compared with non-obese donors, although the absolute risk of ESKD was low (94 per 10,000) [69]. This raises concerns for worse long-term kid-ney outcomes compared with those without metabolic syndrome; however, clear risk thresholds have not yet to be identified.

Contemporary studies of implant biopsies use either wedge biopsies or core biopsies taken intraoperatively. Wedge biopsies are used preferentially because of the larger glomerular sample number and lower risk of bleeding after implantation. However, a recent study examining the glomerular volume and glomerulosclerosis at different depths of the cortex of tissue taken from 812 radical nephrectomy sam-ples [70] showed significant differences in glomerular volume and glomeruloscolero-sis among superficial, middle and deep regions of the cortex. The authors correlated these variations with demographics and diseases to describe a "disease-related" pat-tern of glomerular pathology that was diffuse and less related to cortical depth vs. "age-related" pattern of glomerular pathology that is differentially observed in the superficial cortex.

A recent study of glomerular hyperfiltration provide insight into potential mani-festations of supraphysiologic elevation in GFR. Brenner proposed hyperfiltration's relation to kidney injury – chronic vasodilation in the kidney due to diabetes, pro-tein intake or reduction in kidney mass causes increased single-nephron hyperfiltra-tion. Single-nephron hyperfiltration occurs either through increased glomerular surface area (adaptive), increased glomerular pressure (maladaptive), or a combina-tion of both. Sustained increase in glomerular pressure results in initiation and pro-gression of cellular injury and glomerulosclerosis. Hyperfiltration has been demonstrated in early Type 1 diabetes, obesity, and nephrectomy. The best studied natural history of glomerular hyperfiltration is in diabetic nephropathy. To what extent the increase in GFR observed in early stages of diabetic nephropathy represents pathologic hyperfiltration vs. supranormal GFR has remained unresolved. A recent study investigated whether high measures of GFR in a range presumed to reflect hyperfiltration indicate elevated risk for adverse kidney outcomes in setting of T1DM. Using data form Diabetes Control and Complications Trial (DCCT)/Epidemiology of Diabetes Interventions and Complications (EDIC) Study [71], Molitch et al. studied patients with hyperfiltration (measured GFR > 140 ml/min per 1.73 m^2 to measured the incidence of CKD (eGFR <60) and macroalbuminuria; 110/446 met criteria with a median 28 years follow-up. Surprisingly, patients with hyperfiltration had lower incident CKD. This finding argues against hyperfiltration *per se* as a marker for eventual progression to CKD. This is reassuring for living donors, as the remaining kidney undergoes adaptive hyperfiltration. Because we lack clinical methods to directly measure single-nephron GFR and glomerular pressure in humans, clinical teaching has equated GFR measures with hyperfiltration and the level of the individual nephron. The importance of intraglomerular pressure as a contributor to progression of diabetic kidney disease has been validated by success of therapies that modulate intraglomerular pressure (e.g., RAS inhibitors, Na-glucose cotransporter-2 inhibitors). Thus, we have proposed a multiple-hit hypothesis for the minority of kidney donors with progressive CKD [72]. In other words, kidney donation per se would not initiate a self-perpetuating injury resulting in progressive CKD. However, additional injuries (e.g., diabetes, hypertension) in a kidney donor could initiate a cascade of chronic injury.

In conclusion, renal histology and mass are interrelated and translate into renal function in the setting of health. It is not uncommon to find subtle abnormalities in these renal parameters in the living kidney donor population, and, while this information when available rarely precludes living kidney donation, it might be helpful in improving care postdonation.

Nephrolithiasis and Kidney Donation

Epidemiology and History of Stone Disease in Donor Candidates

It is estimated that 12% of men and 5% of women will develop a symptomatic kidney stone during their lifetime [73]. In the United States, the prevalence of stone disease has almost doubled since the 1960s [73]. The rising incidence and prevalence have been attributed to changes in dietary habits, obesity, and global warming. Historically, kidney stones were more prevalent in men, but the gender gap has been closing [73]. Improvement in imaging techniques has further contributed to the incidental detection of small asymptomatic kidney stones. With increasing prevalence of symptomatic and asymptomatic kidney stones, nephrolithiasis is not an uncommon diagnosis in potential kidney donor candidates.

Nephrolithiasis is a relative contraindication to kidney donation because of the concern for injury in the remaining kidney [74–76]. Although caution is still warranted, kidney donor candidates with small asymptomatic stones or a remote history of stones are increasingly accepted as new reassuring evidence emerges regarding outcomes in donors with normal metabolic workup for risk factors for recurrent stone disease.

Donor Candidates with Clinical Stone Disease

Many transplant programs assess donor candidates with history of kidney stones with imaging studies such as CT angiograms (performed as part of the routine pre-donation anatomical assessment) or urograms. Approximately 3% of donor candidates evaluated for stone disease have passed symptomatic kidney stones in the past, and 5–11% have evidence of stones on renal imaging performed in the routine donor evaluation [77]. The gold standard for radiologic detection of stone disease is CT imaging. Some findings of small calcifications on radiologic imaging tests may be incorrectly identified as a kidney stone. For example, Randall's plaques are small 1–2 mm calcifications found in the renal papillae. These plaques have uncertain prognostic significance.

The 2017 KDIGO guideline recommends that [1]:

- Donor candidates with prior or current kidney stones should be assessed for an underlying cause.
- The acceptance of a donor candidate with prior or current kidney stones should be based on an assessment of stone recurrence risk and knowledge of the possible consequences of kidney stones after donation.

Traditionally, the pathophysiology and natural history of asymptomatic kidney stone formers and symptomatic stone formers are thought to be different. Asymptomatic stones are common and relatively benign; patients often do not have the same comorbidities found in those with symptomatic kidney stones [78].

Clinical trials on the prevention of kidney stone recurrence often use composite outcomes of symptomatic and radiographic recurrence [78]. Symptomatic recurrences are captured by clinical care or as self-report on a survey. Reliance on clinical care records may underestimate recurrence by missing self-managed episodes, whereas self-report surveys may overestimate recurrence by incorrectly attributing pain from other causes to stone passage. Radiographic recurrence estimations based on clinical care records are prone to selection bias and detection bias. The relation between symptomatic and radiographic manifestation of recurrences is illustrated in Fig. 4.5.

There are no large trials on recurrent stone disease or progression of CKD in kidney donors with stone disease prior to donation to provide evidence-based guidelines. However, a recent multicenter study of recurrent stone disease in first-time

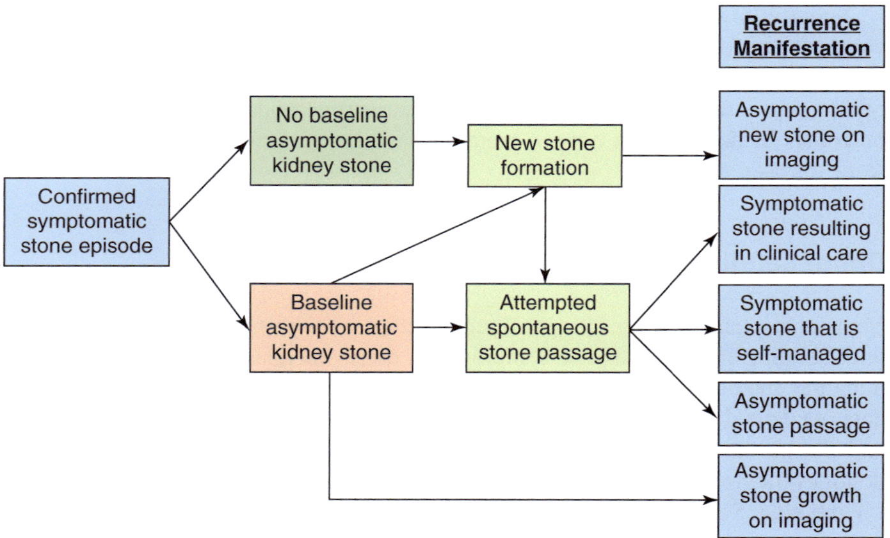

Fig. 4.5 Relationships between various symptomatic and radiographic manifestations of kidney stone recurrence

symptomatic stone formers may be applicable to the living donor population. The mean age and serum creatinine of this cohort were 49 years and 0.9 mg/dl, respectively. Among 175 stone formers, 19% and 25% had symptomatic recurrence detected by clinical care and self-report, respectively [79]. Radiographic recurrence manifested as new stones was 35%, growth of a preexisting stone was 24%, and stone passage was 27%. In this cohort, baseline asymptomatic stones were found in 54%, and 51% had radiographic evidence of stone passage at 5 years. The risk of kidney stones requiring surgical intervention in living kidney donors was assessed in a matched retrospective cohort study [80]. They report no difference in the rate of kidney stones with surgical intervention in donors compared to nondonors (8.3 vs. 9.7 events/10000 person-years; rate ratio 0.85; 95% confidence interval [CI] 0.47–1.53) and no difference in the rate of hospital encounters for kidney stones (12.1 vs. 16.1 events/10000 person-years; rate ratio 0.75; 95% CI 0.45–1.24). These interim results are reassuring for the safety of living kidney donation.

An instructive clinical rule of thumb that was made in this study may be useful in counseling potential living donors with preexisting stone disease, namely the "rule of halves": half of first-time symptomatic stone formers present with a baseline asymptomatic kidney stone, half of these will pass the stone over the next 5 years, and half of these will have symptoms. The baseline asymptomatic kidney stones in the cohort studied above had an average stone size of 3 mm in diameter by CT. This is a size often missed by X-ray or ultrasound [81]. When an asymptomatic stone is detected in a potential living donor, assuming otherwise similar renal size, structure, and vasculature, it is recommended to use the kidney with the stone for kidney donation, to leave the donor with the most normal kidney [1]. This can result

Table 4.1 Guidelines from the American Urological Association (AUA) for Evaluation of Stone Disease. (From [75])

- Screening evaluation with detailed medical and dietary history, serum chemistries (including calcium and uric acid), and urinalysis in patients newly diagnosed with kidney stones
- Obtain an intact parathyroid hormone (PTH) level if primary hyperparathyroidism is suspected
- Stone analysis at least once if stone is available
- Review available imaging studies to quantify stone burden
- Additional metabolic testing in high-risk or interested first-time stone formers and recurrent stone formers
- Metabolic testing consists of one or two 24-hour urine collections obtained on a random diet and analyzed at minimum for total volume, pH, calcium oxalate, uric acid, citrate, sodium, potassium, and creatinine

in symptomatic stone disease in the kidney transplant recipient [82] and is sometimes referred to as "donor-gifted stone." There are reports of nephrolithiasis-related adverse events for recipients of an allograft with a stone left in situ [83]. There are also reports on the safety and success of ex vivo ureteroscopy to remove stones from explanted donor kidneys before transplantation [84].

Potential donors with a history of a single, non-obstructing kidney stone should have a metabolic workup, a 24-hour urine collection (preferably on two occasions) to assess for calcium, oxalate, uric acid, and citrate excretion to exclude any abnormality [1, 85]. Guidelines from the American Urological Association are outlined in Table 4.1 [75].

Stone Disease After Kidney Donation

The main concern for the donor candidate with a history of stones is the recurrence of nephrolithiasis post nephrectomy, with associated risk of obstruction or structural damage to the single kidney, including secondary to associated infections or treatments such as lithotripsy [74, 75]. Considerations for risk of stone recurrence include age, onset and time since symptomatic episode, and family history of kidney stones (Table 4.2) [75]. The cumulative risk of developing recurrent kidney stones is higher in the younger population given their longer projected lifespan.

Potential donors with an absolute contraindication for kidney donation include those with recurrent stones and those at high risk for recurrence, such as those with metabolic abnormalities (e.g., hypercalciuria), chronic diarrhea, malabsorption, gout, cysteine, uric acid, or struvite stones [1]. In counseling donor candidates with a history of kidney stones who are not deemed to be at prohibitive risk, the Recurrence of Kidney Stone (ROKS) score, initially published in 2014 [86] and revised in 2019 [87], may be helpful. This risk calculator is based on demographic and clinical factors and may help in risk stratification of recurrent stone formation, although kidney donors were not included in the initial cohort.

There are few studies with small number of cases involving long-term follow-up of donors with a history of kidney stone, but overall the results suggest that the prevalence of recurrence is between 5% and 9.7%, the stone size is around 2–3 mm,

Table 4.2 Risk factors for recurrent stone disease after kidney donation

Higher lifetime risk of recurrence	• Younger age (<40 years) • Family history of kidney stones • Frequent or recurrent kidney stones
Lower lifetime risk of recurrence	• Older age (>40 years) • No prior symptoms of kidney stones • Kidney stones <15 mm • Solitary and unilateral stones • Remote history of stones >10 years

and there is a very small risk of a stone event on follow-up [88]. One study reported the prevalence of recurrence postdonation is reported at 15 per 100-person years [89]. The longest study, published by Serur et al., which followed 18 donors with asymptomatic kidney stones for 6 years, reported an absence of any symptomatic event in 6 years postdonation.

One retrospective study of 2019 living donor cohort in Canada suggested no difference in the risk of developing a kidney stone after donation in living kidney donors without a predonation history of kidney stones, compared to healthy nondonor controls [80].

Conclusion

We are in an era of increased reliance on living kidney donation. In addition, the culture of donor evaluation has shifted toward increased acceptance of unrelated kidney donors, a rising interest of potential donors with increased demographic and biometric risk factors. Cumulative research on long-term donor outcomes especially among donors with higher risk factors for suboptimal long-term well-being will continue to shape our practices in living donor evaluation and follow-up.

References

1. Lentine KL, Kasiske BL, Levey AS, Adams PL, Alberu J, Bakr MA, et al. KDIGO Clinical Practice Guideline on the Evaluation and Care of Living Kidney Donors. Transplantation. 2017;101(8S Suppl 1):S1–S109. https://doi.org/10.1097/TP.0000000000001769
2. MacLennan GT, Hinman F, Kidney SPH. ureter and adrenal gland. Hinman's atlas of urosurgical anatomy. 2nd ed. Philadelphia: Elsevier Saunders; 2012. p. 151–210.
3. Yeh BM, Coakley FV, Meng MV, Breiman RS, Stoller ML. Precaval right renal arteries: prevalence and morphologic associations at spiral CT. Radiology. 2004;230(2):429–33. https://doi.org/10.1148/radiol.2302021030
4. MacLennan GT. Kidney, ureter and adrenal gland. In: Hinman's atlas of urosurgical anatomy. 2nd ed. Philadelphia: Saunders; 2012. p. 151–210.
5. Reddy VS, Guleria S, Bora GS. Donors with renal artery stenosis: fit to donate. Saudi J Kidney Dis Transpl. 2012;23(3):577–80. https://pubmed.ncbi.nlm.nih.gov/22569449/
6. Andreoni KA, Weeks SM, Gerber DA, Fair JH, Mauro MA, McCoy L, et al. Incidence of donor renal fibromuscular dysplasia: does it justify routine angiography? Transplantation. 2002;73(7):1112–6. https://doi.org/10.1097/00007890-200204150-00018

7. Balzer KM, Grotemeyer D, Pfeiffer T, Voiculescu A, Sandmann W. Fibromuscular dysplasia and renal transplantation. Lancet. 2007;369(9557):187. author reply 188 https://doi.org/10.1016/S0140-6736(07)60101-9

8. Kolettis PN, Bugg CE, Lockhart ME, Bynon SJ, Burns JR. Outcomes for live donor renal transplantation using kidneys with medial fibroplasia. Urology. 2004;63(4):656–9. https://doi.org/10.1016/j.urology.2003.11.026

9. Quaia E, Martingano P, Cavallaro M, Premm M, Angileri R. Normal Radiological Anatomy and Anatomical Variants of the Kidney. In: Radiological Imaging of the Kidney, E. Quaia, Editor. 2014, Springer Berlin Heidelberg. Heidelberg: Berlin. p. 17–74.

10. Kim FJ, Pinto P, Su LM, Jarrett TW, Rattner LE, Montgomery R, et al. Ipsilateral orchialgia after laparoscopic donor nephrectomy. J Endourol. 2003;17(6):405–9. https://doi.org/10.1089/089277903767923209

11. Shirodkar SP, Gorin MA, Sageshima J, Bird VG, Martinez JM, Zarak A, et al. Technical modification for laparoscopic donor nephrectomy to minimize testicular pain: a complication with significant morbidity. Am J Transplant. 2011;11(5):1031–4. https://doi.org/10.1111/j.1600-6143.2011.03495.x

12. Patil AB, Javali TD, Nagaraj HK, Babu S, Nayak A. Laparoscopic donor nephrectomy in unusual venous anatomy - donor and recepient implications. Int Braz J Urol. 2017;43(4):671–8. https://doi.org/10.1590/S1677-5538.IBJU.2016.0309

13. Reed MD, Friedman AC, Nealey P. Anomalies of the left renal vein: analysis of 433 CT scans. J Comput Assist Tomogr. 1982;6(6):1124–6. https://doi.org/10.1097/00004728-198212000-00013

14. Nam JK, Park SW, Lee SD, Chung MK. The clinical significance of a retroaortic left renal vein. Korean J Urol. 2010;51(4):276–80. https://doi.org/10.4111/kju.2010.51.4.276

15. Said SM, Gloviczki P, Kalra M, Oderich GS, Duncan AA, Fleming MD, et al. Renal nutcracker syndrome: surgical options. Semin Vasc Surg. 2013;26(1):35–42. https://doi.org/10.1053/j.semvascsurg.2013.04.006

16. Justo-Janeiro JM, Orozco EP, Reyes FJ, de la Rosa Paredes R, de Lara Cisneros LG, Espinosa AL, et al. Transplantation of a horseshoe kidney from a living donor: Case report, long term outcome and donor safety. Int J Surg Case Rep. 2015;15:21–5. https://doi.org/10.1016/j.ijscr.2015.08.008

17. Kaabak, M.M., N.N. Babenko, A.K. Zokoev, V.V. Khovrin, and T.N. Galyan, Renal Transplantation From a Living Donor With a Horseshoe Kidney. Transplant Direct, 2016. 2(1): p. e53. https://doi.org/10.1097/TXD.0000000000000564.

18. Emamian SA, Nielsen MB, Pedersen JF, Ytte L. Kidney dimensions at sonography: correlation with age, sex, and habitus in 665 adult volunteers. AJR Am J Roentgenol. 1993;160(1):83–6. https://doi.org/10.2214/ajr.160.1.8416654

19. Thakur V, Watkins T, McCarthy K, Beidl T, Underwood N, Barnes K, et al. Is kidney length a good predictor of kidney volume? Am J Med Sci. 1997;313(2):85–9. https://doi.org/10.1097/00000441-199702000-00003

20. Poggio ED, Hila S, Stephany B, Fatica R, Krishnamurthi V, del Bosque C, et al. Donor kidney volume and outcomes following live donor kidney transplantation. Am J Transplant. 2006;6(3):616–24. https://doi.org/10.1111/j.1600-6143.2005.01225.x

21. Jeon HG, Lee SR, Joo DJ, Oh YT, Kim MS, Kim YS, et al. Predictors of kidney volume change and delayed kidney function recovery after donor nephrectomy. J Urol. 2010;184(3):1057–63. https://doi.org/10.1016/j.juro.2010.04.079

22. Velosa JA, Offord KP, Schroeder DR. Effect of age, sex, and glomerular filtration rate on renal function outcome of living kidney donors. Transplantation. 1995;60(12):1618–21. https://pubmed.ncbi.nlm.nih.gov/8545901/

23. Poggio ED, Braun WE, Davis C. The science of Stewardship: due diligence for kidney donors and kidney function in living kidney donation--evaluation, determinants, and implications for outcomes. Clin J Am Soc Nephrol. 2009;4(10):1677–84. https://doi.org/10.2215/CJN.02740409

24. Tan JC, Busque S, Workeneh B, Ho B, Derby G, Blouch KL, et al. Effects of aging on glomerular function and number in living kidney donors. Kidney Int. 2010;78(7):686–92. https://doi.org/10.1038/ki.2010.128

25. Kasiske BL, Anderson-Haag T, Israni AK, Kalil RS, Kimmel PL, Kraus ES, et al. A prospective controlled study of living kidney donors: three-year follow-up. Am J Kidney Dis. 2015;66(1):114–24. https://doi.org/10.1053/j.ajkd.2015.01.019

26. Matas AJ, Vock DM, Ibrahim HN. GFR </=25 years postdonation in living kidney donors with (vs. without) a first-degree relative with ESRD. Am J Transplant. 2018;18(3):625–31. https://doi.org/10.1111/ajt.14525

27. Ibrahim HN, Foley RN, Reule SA, Spong R, Kukla A, Issa N, et al. Renal Function Profile in White Kidney Donors: The First 4 Decades. J Am Soc Nephrol. 2016;27(9):2885–93. https://doi.org/10.1681/ASN.2015091018

28. Issa N, Vaughan LE, Denic A, Kremers WK, Chakkera HA, Park WD, et al. Larger nephron size, low nephron number, and nephrosclerosis on biopsy as predictors of kidney function after donating a kidney. Am J Transplant. 2019; https://doi.org/10.1111/ajt.15259

29. Matas AJ, Berglund DM, Vock DM, Ibrahim HN. Causes and timing of end-stage renal disease after living kidney donation. Am J Transplant. 2018;18(5):1140–50. https://doi.org/10.1111/ajt.14671

30. Denic A, Glassock RJ, Rule AD. Structural and Functional Changes With the Aging Kidney. Adv Chronic Kidney Dis. 2016;23(1):19–28. https://doi.org/10.1053/j.ackd.2015.08.004

31. Poggio, E.D., A.D. Rule, R. Tanchanco, S. Arrigain, R.S. Butler, T. Srinivas, et al., Demographic and clinical characteristics associated with glomerular filtration rates in living kidney donors. Kidney Int, 2009. https://doi.org/ki200911 [pii]10.1038/ki.2009.11.

32. Tan, J.C., B. Workeneh, S. Busque, K. Blouch, G. Derby, and B.D. Myers, Glomerular function, structure, and number in renal allografts from older deceased donors. J Am Soc Nephrol, 2009. 20(1): p. 181-8 https://doi.org/ASN.2008030306 [pii]10.1681/ASN.2008030306.

33. Rook, M., R.J. Bosma, W.J. van Son, H.S. Hofker, J.J. van der Heide, P.M. ter Wee, et al., Nephrectomy elicits impact of age and BMI on renal hemodynamics: lower postdonation reserve capacity in older or overweight kidney donors. Am J Transplant, 2008. 8(10): p. 2077-85 https://doi.org/AJT2355 [pii]10.1111/j.1600-6143.2008.02355.x.

34. Rook M, Hofker HS, van Son WJ, Homan van der Heide JJ, Ploeg RJ, Navis GJ. Predictive capacity of pre-donation GFR and renal reserve capacity for donor renal function after living kidney donation. Am J Transplant. 2006;6(7):1653–9. https://doi.org/10.1111/j.1600-6143.2006.01359.x

35. Ohashi Y, Thomas G, Nurko S, Stephany B, Fatica R, Chiesa A, et al. Association of metabolic syndrome with kidney function and histology in living kidney donors. Am J Transplant. 2013;13(9):2342–51. https://doi.org/10.1111/ajt.12369

36. Tan JC, Ho B, Busque S, Blouch K, Derby G, Efron B, et al. Imprecision of creatinine-based GFR estimates in uninephric kidney donors. Clin J Am Soc Nephrol. 2010;5(3):497–502. https://doi.org/10.2215/CJN.05280709

37. Levey AS, Stevens LA, Schmid CH, Zhang YL, Castro AF 3rd, Feldman HI, et al. A new equation to estimate glomerular filtration rate. Ann Intern Med. 2009;150(9):604–12. https://doi.org/10.7326/0003-4819-150-9-200905050-00006

38. Denic A, Mathew J, Lerman LO, Lieske JC, Larson JJ, Alexander MP, et al. Single-Nephron Glomerular Filtration Rate in Healthy Adults. N Engl J Med. 2017;376(24):2349–57. https://doi.org/10.1056/NEJMoa1614329

39. Diez A, Powelson J, Sundaram CP, Taber TE, Mujtaba MA, Yaqub MS, et al. Correlation between CT-based measured renal volumes and nuclear-renography-based split renal function in living kidney donors. Clinical diagnostic utility and practice patterns. Clin Transplant. 2014;28(6):675–82. https://doi.org/10.1111/ctr.12365

40. Tatar E, Sen S, Harman M, Kircelli F, Gungor O, Sarsik B, et al. The relationship between renal volume and histology in obese and nonobese kidney donors. Eur J Clin Invest. 2015;45(6):565–71. https://doi.org/10.1111/eci.12444

41. Taner T, Iqbal CW, Textor SC, Stegall MD, Ishitani MB. Compensatory hypertrophy of the remaining kidney in medically complex living kidney donors over the long term. Transplantation. 2015;99(3):555–9. https://doi.org/10.1097/TP.0000000000000356

42. Gardan E, Jacquemont L, Perret C, Heudes PM, Gourraud PA, Hourmant M, et al. Renal cortical volume: High correlation with pre- and post-operative renal function in living kidney donors. Eur J Radiol. 2018;99:118–23. https://doi.org/10.1016/j.ejrad.2017.12.013

43. Song T, Fu L, Huang Z, He S, Zhao R, Lin T, et al. Change in renal parenchymal volume in living kidney transplant donors. Int Urol Nephrol. 2014;46(4):743–7. https://doi.org/10.1007/s11255-013-0592-y

44. Chen KW, Wu MW, Chen Z, Tai BC, Goh YS, Lata R, et al. Compensatory Hypertrophy After Living Donor Nephrectomy. Transplant Proc. 2016;48(3):716–9. https://doi.org/10.1016/j.transproceed.2015.12.082

45. Hall IE, Shaaban A, Wei G, Sikora MB, Bourija H, Beddhu S, et al. Baseline Living Donor Kidney Volume and Function Associate with 1-Year Post-Nephrectomy Kidney Function. Clin Transplant. 2019:e13485. https://doi.org/10.1111/ctr.13485

46. Kwon HJ, Kim DH, Jang HR, Jung SH, Han DH, Sung HH, et al. Predictive Factors of Renal Adaptation After Nephrectomy in Kidney Donors. Transplant Proc. 2017;49(9):1999–2006. https://doi.org/10.1016/j.transproceed.2017.09.024

47. Narasimhamurthy M, Smith LM, Machan JT, Reinert SE, Gohh RY, Dworkin LD, et al. Does size matter? Kidney transplant donor size determines kidney function among living donors. Clin Kidney J. 2017;10(1):116–23. https://doi.org/10.1093/ckj/sfw097

48. Lange D, Helck A, Rominger A, Crispin A, Meiser B, Werner J, et al. Renal volume assessed by magnetic resonance imaging volumetry correlates with renal function in living kidney donors pre- and postdonation: a retrospective cohort study. Transpl Int. 2018;31(7):773–80. https://doi.org/10.1111/tri.13150

49. Courbebaisse M, Gaillard F, Tissier AM, Fournier C, Le Nestour A, Correas JM, et al. Association of mGFR of the Remaining Kidney Divided by Its Volume before Donation with Functional Gain in mGFR among Living Kidney Donors. Clin J Am Soc Nephrol. 2016;11(8):1369–76. https://doi.org/10.2215/CJN.12731215

50. Cherikh WS, Young CJ, Kramer BF, Taranto SE, Randall HB, Fan PY. Ethnic and gender related differences in the risk of end-stage renal disease after living kidney donation. Am J Transplant. 2011;11(8):1650–5. https://doi.org/10.1111/j.1600-6143.2011.03609.x

51. Muzaale AD, Massie AB, Wang MC, Montgomery RA, McBride MA, Wainright JL, et al. Risk of end-stage renal disease following live kidney donation. JAMA. 2014;311(6):579–86. https://doi.org/10.1001/jama.2013.285141

52. Gibney EM, King AL, Maluf DG, Garg AX, Parikh CR. Living kidney donors requiring transplantation: focus on African Americans. Transplantation. 2007;84(5):647–9. https://doi.org/10.1097/01.tp.0000277288.78771.c2

53. Grams ME, Sang Y, Levey AS, Matsushita K, Ballew S, Chang AR, et al. Kidney-Failure Risk Projection for the Living Kidney-Donor Candidate. N Engl J Med. 2016;374(5):411–21. https://doi.org/10.1056/NEJMoa1510491

54. Massie AB, Muzaale AD, Luo X, Chow EKH, Locke JE, Nguyen AQ, et al. Quantifying Postdonation Risk of ESRD in Living Kidney Donors. J Am Soc Nephrol. 2017;28(9):2749–55. https://doi.org/10.1681/ASN.2016101084

55. Denic A, Lieske JC, Chakkera HA, Poggio ED, Alexander MP, Singh P, et al. The Substantial Loss of Nephrons in Healthy Human Kidneys with Aging. J Am Soc Nephrol. 2017;28(1):313–20. https://doi.org/10.1681/ASN.2016020154

56. Rule AD, Amer H, Cornell LD, Taler SJ, Cosio FG, Kremers WK, et al. The association between age and nephrosclerosis on renal biopsy among healthy adults. Ann Intern Med. 2010;152(9):561–7. https://doi.org/10.7326/0003-4819-152-9-201005040-00006

57. Elsherbiny HE, Alexander MP, Kremers WK, Park WD, Poggio ED, Prieto M, et al. Nephron hypertrophy and glomerulosclerosis and their association with kidney function and risk factors among living kidney donors. Clin J Am Soc Nephrol. 2014;9(11):1892–902. https://doi.org/10.2215/CJN.02560314

58. Chauhan A, Diwan TS, Franco Palacios CR, Dean PG, Heimbach JK, Chow GK, et al. Using implantation biopsies as a surrogate to evaluate selection criteria for living kidney donors. Transplantation. 2013;96(11):975–80. https://doi.org/10.1097/TP.0b013e3182a2b455
59. Hoy WE, Bertram JF, Denton RD, Zimanyi M, Samuel T, Hughson MD. Nephron number, glomerular volume, renal disease and hypertension. Curr Opin Nephrol Hypertens. 2008;17(3):258–65. https://doi.org/10.1097/MNH.0b013e3282f 9b1a500041552-200805000-00004 [pii]
60. Nyengaard JR, Bendtsen TF. Glomerular number and size in relation to age, kidney weight, and body surface in normal man. Anat Rec. 1992;232(2):194–201. https://doi.org/10.1002/ar.1092320205
61. Lenihan CR, Busque S, Derby G, Blouch K, Myers BD, Tan JC. Longitudinal study of living kidney donor glomerular dynamics after nephrectomy. J Clin Invest. 2015;125(3):1311–8. https://doi.org/10.1172/JCI78885
62. Lenihan CR, Busque S, Derby G, Blouch K, Myers BD, Tan JC. The association of predonation hypertension with glomerular function and number in older living kidney donors. J Am Soc Nephrol. 2015;26(6):1261–7. https://doi.org/10.1681/ASN.2014030304
63. Choi AI, Rodriguez RA, Bacchetti P, Bertenthal D, Hernandez GT, O'Hare AM. White/black racial differences in risk of end-stage renal disease and death. Am J Med. 2009;122(7):672–8. https://doi.org/10.1016/j.amjmed.2008.11.021
64. Fahmy LM, Massie AB, Muzaale AD, Bagnasco SM, Orandi BJ, Alejo JL, et al. Long-term Renal Function in Living Kidney Donors Who Had Histological Abnormalities at Donation. Transplantation. 2016;100(6):1294–8. https://doi.org/10.1097/TP.0000000000001236
65. Naik AS, Cibrik DM, Sakhuja A, Samaniego M, Lu Y, Shahinian V, et al. Temporal trends, center-level variation, and the impact of prevalent state obesity rates on acceptance of obese living kidney donors. Am J Transplant. 2018;18(3):642–9. https://doi.org/10.1111/ajt.14519
66. Davis CL, Cooper M. The state of U.S. living kidney donors. Clin J Am Soc Nephrol. 2010;5(10):1873–80. https://doi.org/10.2215/CJN.01510210
67. Abrass CK. Overview: obesity: what does it have to do with kidney disease? J Am Soc Nephrol. 2004;15(11):2768–72. https://doi.org/10.1097/01.ASN.0000141963.04540.3E
68. Kambham N, Markowitz GS, Valeri AM, Lin J, D'Agati VD. Obesity-related glomerulopathy: an emerging epidemic. Kidney Int. 2001;59(4):1498–509. https://doi.org/10.1046/j.1523-175 5.2001.0590041498.x
69. Locke JE, Reed RD, Massie A, MacLennan PA, Sawinski D, Kumar V, et al. Obesity increases the risk of end-stage renal disease among living kidney donors. Kidney Int. 2017;91(3):699–703. https://doi.org/10.1016/j.kint.2016.10.014
70. Denic A, Ricaurte L, Lopez CL, Narasimhan R, Lerman LO, Lieske JC, et al. Glomerular Volume and Glomerulosclerosis at Different Depths within the Human Kidney. J Am Soc Nephrol. 2019;30(8):1471–80. https://doi.org/10.1681/ASN.2019020183
71. Molitch ME, Gao X, Bebu I, de Boer IH, Lachin J, Paterson A, et al. Early Glomerular Hyperfiltration and Long-Term Kidney Outcomes in Type 1 Diabetes: The DCCT/ EDIC Experience. Clin J Am Soc Nephrol. 2019;14(6):854–61. https://doi.org/10.2215/CJN.14831218
72. Cheng XS, Glassock RJ, Lentine KL, Chertow GM, Tan JC. Donation, Not Disease! A Multiple-Hit Hypothesis on Development of Post-Donation Kidney Disease. Curr Transplant Rep. 2017;4(4):320–6. https://doi.org/10.1007/s40472-017-0171-8
73. Stamatelou KK, Francis ME, Jones CA, Nyberg LM, Curhan GC. Time trends in reported prevalence of kidney stones in the United States: 1976-1994. Kidney Int. 2003;63(5):1817–23. https://doi.org/10.1046/j.1523-1755.2003.00917.x
74. Lorenz EC, Lieske JC, Vrtiska TJ, Krambeck AE, Li X, Bergstralh EJ, et al. Clinical characteristics of potential kidney donors with asymptomatic kidney stones. Nephrol Dial Transplant. 2011;26(8):2695–700. https://doi.org/10.1093/ndt/gfq769
75. Hughes, P. and I. Caring for Australians with Renal, The CARI guidelines. Kidney stones epidemiology. Nephrology (Carlton), 2007. 12 Suppl 1: p. S26-30 https://doi.org/10.1111/j.1440-1797.2006.00724.x.

76. Kasiske BL, Ravenscraft M, Ramos EL, Gaston RS, Bia MJ, Danovitch GM. The evaluation of living renal transplant donors: clinical practice guidelines. Ad Hoc Clinical Practice Guidelines Subcommittee of the Patient Care and Education Committee of the American Society of Transplant Physicians. J Am Soc Nephrol. 1996;7(11):2288–313. https://pubmed.ncbi.nlm.nih.gov/8959619/

77. Ennis J, Kocherginsky M, Schumm LP, Worcester E, Coe FL, Josephson MA. Trends in kidney donation among kidney stone formers: a survey of US transplant centers. Am J Nephrol. 2009;30(1):12–8. https://doi.org/10.1159/000197115

78. Fink HA, Wilt TJ, Eidman KE, Garimella PS, MacDonald R, Rutks IR, et al. Medical management to prevent recurrent nephrolithiasis in adults: a systematic review for an American College of Physicians Clinical Guideline. Ann Intern Med. 2013;158(7):535–43. https://doi.org/10.7326/0003-4819-158-7-201304020-00005

79. D'Costa MR, Haley WE, Mara KC, Enders FT, Vrtiska TJ, Pais VM, et al. Symptomatic and Radiographic Manifestations of Kidney Stone Recurrence and Their Prediction by Risk Factors: A Prospective Cohort Study. J Am Soc Nephrol. 2019;30(7):1251–60. http://doi.org/10.1681/ASN.2018121241.

80. Thomas SM, Lam NN, Welk BK, Nguan C, Huang A, Nash DM, et al. Risk of kidney stones with surgical intervention in living kidney donors. Am J Transplant. 2013;13(11):2935–44. https://doi.org/10.1111/ajt.12446

81. Kanno T, Kubota M, Funada S, Okada T, Higashi Y, Yamada H. The Utility of the Kidneys-ureters-bladder Radiograph as the Sole Imaging Modality and Its Combination With Ultrasonography for the Detection of Renal Stones. Urology. 2017;104:40–4. https://doi.org/10.1016/j.urology.2017.03.019

82. Kim IK, Tan JC, Lapasia J, Elihu A, Busque S, Melcher ML. Incidental kidney stones: a single center experience with kidney donor selection. Clin Transplant. 2012;26(4):558–63. https://doi.org/10.1111/j.1399-0012.2011.01567.x

83. Strang AM, Lockhart ME, Amling CL, Kolettis PN, Burns JR. Living renal donor allograft lithiasis: a review of stone related morbidity in donors and recipients. J Urol. 2008;179(3):832–6. https://doi.org/10.1016/j.juro.2007.10.022

84. Olsburgh J, Thomas K, Wong K, Bultitude M, Glass J, Rottenberg G, et al. Incidental renal stones in potential live kidney donors: prevalence, assessment and donation, including role of ex vivo ureteroscopy. BJU Int. 2013;111(5):784–92. https://doi.org/10.1111/j.1464-410X.2012.11572.x

85. Organ Procurement and Transplantation Network (OPTN) / United Network for Organ Sharing (UNOS). Policy 14: Living Donation. Available at: https://optn.transplant.hrsa.gov/governance/policies/. Accessed: 7 Sept 2020.

86. Rule AD, Lieske JC, Li X, Melton LJ 3rd, Krambeck AE, Bergstralh EJ. The ROKS nomogram for predicting a second symptomatic stone episode. J Am Soc Nephrol. 2014;25(12):2878–86. https://doi.org/10.1681/ASN.2013091011

87. Vaughan LE, Enders FT, Lieske Jc, et al. Predictors of Symptomatic Kidney Stone Recurrence After the First and Subsequent Episodes. Mayo Clin Proc 2019;9(2):202–210. https://doi.org/10.1016/j.mayocp.2018.09.016.

88. Delmonico F, S. Council. of the Transplantation, A Report of the Amsterdam Forum On the Care of the Live Kidney Donor: Data and Medical Guidelines. Transplantation. 2005;79(6 Suppl):S53–66. https://pubmed.ncbi.nlm.nih.gov/15785361/

89. Ferraro PM, Curhan GC, D'Addessi A, Gambaro G. Risk of recurrence of idiopathic calcium kidney stones: analysis of data from the literature. J Nephrol. 2017;30(2):227–33. https://doi.org/10.1007/s40620-016-0283-8

Evaluation of Hypertension in Living Donor Candidates

5

Mona D. Doshi and Sandra J. Taler

Introduction

Early in the practice of living donation, hypertension was considered an exclusion criterion for kidney donation [1]. Previous practice may in part reflect application of older definitions of hypertension which used higher thresholds of blood pressure levels for diagnosis, above which there is clear evidence for target organ damage [2, 3]. A number of epidemiological studies and treatment trials support stability of renal function in non-black participants with mild hypertension (blood pressure below 165 mm Hg systolic and 106 mm Hg diastolic) and when there is no diabetes, urinary tract abnormalities, or albuminuria [4–8]. Recommended BP thresholds for the diagnosis and treatment of hypertension have declined over the past 40 years for the US population culminating in the 2017 American College of Cardiology (ACC)/ American Heart Association (AHA) hypertension guideline threshold of 130/80 mmHg which was based on data from randomized controlled trials of hypertension treatment to lower targets [9]. The recommendation of a lower threshold for hypertension diagnosis is intended to educate the public to adopt lifestyle changes earlier that might prevent cardiovascular disease progression and providers to begin treatment sooner to prevent morbidity and mortality in persons at high cardiovascular risk [10]. However, the evolving diagnostic criteria have also created a dilemma in the kidney transplant community regarding blood pressure acceptance criteria for otherwise healthy living donor candidates where granular data are lacking for lower

M. D. Doshi (✉)
Division of Nephrology, Department of Medicine, University of Michigan, Ann Arbor, MI, USA
e-mail: doshimd@med.umich.edu

S. J. Taler
Division of Nephrology and Hypertension, College of Medicine, Mayo Clinic, Rochester, MN, USA
e-mail: taler.sandra@mayo.edu

© Springer Nature Switzerland AG 2021
K. L. Lentine et al. (eds.), *Living Kidney Donation*,
https://doi.org/10.1007/978-3-030-53618-3_5

blood pressure thresholds, as reflected in differing opinions by international guidelines and US experts and centers [11, 12].

Based on trends to diagnose hypertension at lower thresholds and with the knowledge that aging promotes increases in blood pressure, one can make the argument that an older donor with mild elevations in blood pressure might be at similar or lower risk than a young donor with normal blood pressure levels. With advancing age of potential kidney transplant recipients and with them, their potential kidney donors, along with cohort-based evidence of safety [13], it has become acceptable to consider older individuals with isolated medical abnormalities such as controlled stage 1 (previously defined as blood pressue 140–159/90–99 mm Hg) hypertension, who are otherwise in good health, as acceptable donor candidates. This practice has been adopted by many centers based on the early Mayo Clinic experience wherein donor candidates older than 40 years with hypertension controlled to target levels, using lifestyle modifications combined with one or two antihypertensive medications, and with otherwise normal kidney function and normal urinary albumin excretion, were accepted for donation [13, 14]. For these donors, follow-up within the first year after donation confirmed acceptable kidney function and improved blood pressure levels. However, it is important to note the inclusion criteria for the reported donor cohort and not overly extrapolate to include hypertension in younger persons, black individuals, or in association with multiple cardiovascular risk factors, where risks remain uncertain.

Evaluation

Blood Pressure Assessment Prior to Donation

Accurate blood pressure measurement is one of the most important steps in donor evaluation [11]. High blood pressure can result in subtle scarring (nephrosclerosis) and may limit renal functional compensation postdonation [15, 16]. Blood pressure measured in the clinic may not be reflective of an individual's true blood pressure, which may be higher in the office (termed "white coat" hypertension) or higher out of the office (termed "masked" hypertension). White coat hypertension has been reported in 20–35% of donor candidates and may reflect anxiety around the time of evaluation and incorrectly exclude them from donation [17, 18]. Most studies suggest that individuals with white coat hypertension have lower risk of cardiovascular events than those with sustained hypertension, although recent evidence from a large Spanish registry and a meta-analysis suggest a comparable mortality risk [19, 20]. Alternatively, masked hypertension, where donor candidates with normal office blood pressure have hypertension by ambulatory testing, occurs less frequently, in approximately 3% [21]. Masked hypertension is associated with greater cardiovascular risk and mortality than seen in individuals with sustained hypertension [19, 22] and therefore should be treated. If not recognized, the donor candidate may be incorrectly accepted for donation without full consideration of risk and without ensuring adequate blood pressure control.

Table 5.1 Definition of hypertension by measurement modality as per the KDIGO Living Donor guideline and ACC/AHA Hypertension Guideline

	KDIGO Living Donor Guideline [11]	ACC/AHA Hypertension Guideline [10]
Year	2017 (based on 2003 JNC-7 [27])	2017
Clinic BP		
Normal	<120/80 mmHg	<120/80 mmHg
Prehypertension/elevated BP	120–139/80–89	120–129/<80 mmHg
Stage 1 hypertension	140–149/90–99 mmHg[a]	130–139/80–89 mmHg[b]
Stage 2 hypertension	≥160/100 mmHg	≥140/90 mmHg[c]
24-hr ABPM		
Daytime	≥135/85 mmHg	≥130/80 mmHg
Nighttime	≥120/75 mmHg	≥110/65 mmHg

Abbreviations: ABPM ambulatory blood pressure monitoring; *BP* blood pressure.

[a]Start antihypertensive medication except in patients with chronic kidney disease or diabetes who would be treated at a lower level

[b]Start antihypertensive medication based on presence of prior cardiovascular events or disease, diabetes mellitus, chronic kidney disease, or a 10-year estimated risk for cardiovascular events ≥10%

[c]Start antihypertensive medication except in patients with chronic kidney disease, diabetes, prior cardiovascular events or disease, or with 10-year estimated risk for cardiovascular events ≥10% who would be treated at a lower level

All potential donors should have their blood pressure checked multiple times. In the United States, Organ Procurement and Transplantation Network (OPTN) policy requires that the donor evaluation includes blood pressure measurement on at least two occasions, either via the auscultatory method, by automated machines in the office, or by 24-hour or overnight ambulatory blood pressure monitoring (ABPM) [23]. Regardless of the modality of measurement, it is important to abide by standardized techniques and use validated equipment to obtain accurate measurements. In some cases, different methods of measurement may have different recommended thresholds to define hypertension (Table 5.1). Below we discuss each method in detail, including their merits and limitations, and the associated blood pressure thresholds for defining hypertension.

Office Blood Pressure Assessment

Office blood pressure measurement is the most widely used method to assess blood pressure in clinical practice and is used in some clinical trials. Blood pressure can be measured manually via the auscultatory method or using automated machines by clinic staff. Newer automated machines are designed to take an initial measurement with a clinic staff in the room with the patient and then take two to five additional measurements with the patient left alone in the room to reduce white coat response [10, 24]. As demonstrated in a recent meta-analysis, automated office blood pressure measurements may be 10–15 mm Hg lower systolic than manual office measurements; thus, fewer individuals would be misdiagnosed as having hypertension based on this measurement modality, and more will meet current lower blood pressure goals [25].

Regardless of the method, it is important to ensure that an appropriate sized cuff is used (bladder should encircle at least 80% of the arm circumference) on the bared arm, and the donor candidate should rest for 5 minutes, seated in a chair with arm supported at heart level prior to measurements. The equipment should be regularly inspected and calibrated for accuracy. Clinic staff should be trained and regularly retrained to ensure that the blood pressure measurements are taken correctly. Current guidelines favor use of automated office blood pressure devices (programmed to take multiple measurements at one sitting), which offer strong agreement with day-time ABPM measurements [10] over manual measurements.

While measuring office-based blood pressure is inexpensive and easily available, the readings are more likely to be affected by a donor candidate's anxiety leading to white coat hypertension or may miss masked hypertension. ABPM, performed by using a wearable device to take and record multiple measurements over a longer time period, is preferred as it detects individuals with white coat hypertension who might otherwise be excluded as donors and identifies those with masked hypertension who should not be accepted without improvement in blood pressure control [26].

While blood pressure readings lower than 140/90 mmHg have traditionally been considered acceptable for donation based on prior guidelines such as the Joint National Committee Guideline on Prevention, Detection, Evaluation, and Treatment of High Blood Pressure (JNC) 7 [27], as mentioned above, recommended thresholds to define hypertension in the general population have declined. The 2017 US hypertension guideline, developed by the ACC/AHA in collaboration with nine additional professional organizations, now defines hypertension as blood pressure $\geq$ 130/80 mmHg [10]. As prior absolute thresholds for excluding an individual donor candidate may have depended on age, weight, race, and other risk factors – or more recently a combined risk profile for future kidney and/or heart disease – the appropriate impact of this revised definition on donor candidate acceptance is unclear [11]. The 2017 Kidney Disease: Improving Global Outcomes (KDIGO) "Clinical Practice Guideline on the Evaluation and Care of Living Kidney Donors" recommends that for a given donor candidate, each risk should be assessed both individually and in combination with other risk factors to consider total risk using acceptance thresholds established at the individual transplant center [11]. It is important to recognize and explain to donor candidates that this difference in hypertension definition thresholds may impact the diagnoses they receive by other providers, similar to the controversies related to the definition of chronic kidney disease based on estimated glomerular filtration rate (eGFR) levels in donors.

Ambulatory Blood Pressure Monitoring (ABPM)

The use of 24-hour ABPM reduces the impact of patient anxiety and reader bias on blood pressure measurements. ABPM provides multiple readings, obtained every 10 to 30 minutes during the course of the day while the individual is performing daily activities and every 20 to 60 minutes at night. This modality provides mean blood pressure over the entire 24-hour monitoring period and averages of day and nighttime readings. In addition, ABPM provides information on blood pressure variability, including nocturnal dipping, and response to environmental stress. There should normally be evidence of nocturnal dipping, defined as a 10–20% fall in blood pressure readings at night when compared to daytime readings. Although not considered an absolute contraindication to donation, individuals with "non-dipping" ABPM patterns are reported to be at a 27% higher risk for cardiovascular events than individuals with nocturnal dipping [28].

Blood pressure thresholds to define hypertension via 24-hour ABPM have also declined, and the 2017 ACC/AHA guideline defines hypertension when one or more of these criteria exist; the 24-hour average blood pressure is $\geq$125/75 mmHg, the daytime average is $\geq$130/80 mmHg, and/or the nighttime average is $\geq$110/65 mmHg [10]. Table 5.1 compares the definition of hypertension adopted in the KDIGO Living Donor guideline [11], as based on the 2003 JNC-7 guideline, and the 2017 ACC/AHA hypertension guideline [10] using office and ABPM measurements.

ABPM is considered the gold standard and preferred method of measuring blood pressure with stronger correlation with cardiovascular mortality. While efforts to routinely utilize this technology were previously limited by the higher cost and lack of easy availability at some centers, there are now national service companies able to arrange for ABPM remotely at reasonable cost, avoiding the need for investment in the devices. ABPM should be performed in the following clinical contexts:

1. Office blood pressure readings of $\geq$130/80 mmHg or higher than values considered to be acceptable for a given donor candidate based on age and other risk factors for kidney disease. Some programs may use lower blood pressure thresholds for younger individuals.
2. Older candidates who are more likely to develop hypertension and for whom it carries greater risk for morbidity and mortality in the shorter term.
3. Prior diagnosis of hypertension currently treated with medication to verify adequate control prior to donation.
4. When presence or absence of hypertension is indeterminate (high normal or variable).
5. Prior history of gestational hypertension.

Table 5.2 compares methods for measuring blood pressure.

Review of Medications

All medications used by donor candidates must be carefully reviewed with consideration of the indication for use. In some cases, antihypertensive agents such as beta-blockers may be used for migraine prophylaxis or tachycardia and not for hypertension. While measuring blood pressure in a donor candidate with a history of hypertension and on drug treatment, it is important to inquire about timing of medication intake. Donor candidates should be counseled about the potential impact

Table 5.2 Advantages and limitations of types of blood pressure assessment

	Single office measurement	Automated office measurements (multiple)	ABPM (18–24 hour)
Advantages	• Inexpensive • Widely available	• Multiple readings checked without a provider in the room eliminates white coat effect, comparable to daytime ABPM	• Multiple readings in the patient's own settings • Higher correlation with cardiovascular outcomes • Eliminates white coat effect • Detects masked hypertension
Limitations	• Not accurate if not performed correctly • White coat effect • May miss masked hypertension	• Moderate cost for device and need for additional measurement time • May miss masked hypertension	• Expensive • Not widely available in every transplant center but can use mail-order service to send ABPM machine to the donor directly • User discomfort and inconvenience

of certain medications such as decongestants, weight loss pills, and stimulants on blood pressure. A careful history regarding smoking, alcohol use, use of over-the-counter medications such as nonsteroid anti-inflammatory agents, supplements, and weight changes should be taken [11, 23].

Selection of Donor Candidates Based on Blood Pressure Readings

While the ideal kidney donor has normal blood pressure, selected individuals with hypertension may be considered suitable to donate once it is established that blood pressure is controlled to normal levels with a limited medication requirement and if additional risks to their kidney health are acceptable (Fig. 5.1). Individuals with a prior history of myocardial infarction, stroke, or other cardiovascular events are typically not considered donor candidates, regardless of blood pressure. Furthermore, individuals with evidence for hypertension-associated target organ damage such as left ventricular hypertrophy, diastolic dysfunction, or microalbuminuria should not be accepted [11, 23]. Among those without clearly defined hypertension, the absolute thresholds for blood pressure readings and potential for acceptance if blood pressure is controlled depend on their comprehensive risk profile for kidney disease, considering factors such as age, race, body mass index (BMI), history of smoking, and the presence of metabolic syndrome. The 2017 KDIGO guideline emphasizes the evaluation of a potential donor's candidacy based on overall demographic and health profile [11]. Several risk calculators have been developed to determine future risk of kidney failure including consideration of hypertension [29–31]. These calculators combine data regarding multiple risk factors and predict future risk of kidney failure, but there remains controversy about the accuracy of their predictions due to lack of long-term follow-up [32].

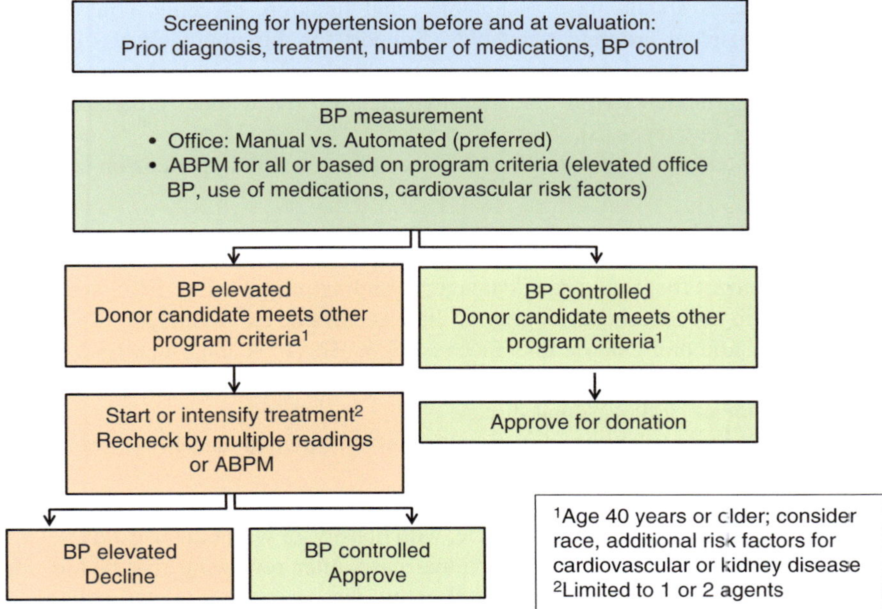

Fig. 5.1 Algorithm for hypertension evaluation in living kidney donor candidates. *Abbreviations: ABPM* ambulatory blood pressure monitoring, *BP* blood pressure

There are some situations such as with a donor candidate with borderline blood pressure who prefers to alter their lifestyle and not take medication, where the donor candidate must understand there is a potential future need to take antihypertensive medication if their blood pressure is elevated after donation or if they are not able to maintain lifestyle modification such as weight control. Decisions on when to initiate antihypertensive medication therapy may be difficult if overall cardiovascular risk is low, particularly since cardiovascular disease risk calculators do not consider kidney function or kidney donation in their calculations.

Special Considerations

Donor Candidates with Hypertension

Donor candidates with a history of well-controlled hypertension on one to two agents, one of which is typically a diuretic, are generally considered suitable for donation under the following circumstances: age 50 years or older, white race and in the absence of target organ damage such as left ventricular hypertrophy on electrocardiogram (ECG) or echocardiogram, diastolic dysfunction, albuminuria (i.e., urinary albumin excretion rate > 30 mg/day), or hypertensive retinopathy. These donor candidates should have acceptable renal function, glycemic control, and BMI, per transplant program thresholds. Support for this approach was derived from a review of control group outcomes in early placebo controlled hypertension trials where participants with moderate hypertension but without proteinuria had generally good outcomes [8].

Additional testing to be ordered in donor candidates with hypertension includes the following:

1. 18–24-hour ABPM to verify good blood pressure control
2. Assessment for target organ damage, including retinal exam, ECG, and consideration of an echocardiogram if there is elevated ECG voltage
3. HbA1c and oral glucose tolerance testing if HbA1c is abnormal, lipid panel, and uric acid to evaluate for other comorbidities that may increase overall risk of kidney or cardiovascular disease
4. Attention to availability of medical follow-up care and medical insurance

Considering donor candidates with hypertension outside of these criteria (e.g., those age 40–49 years, of non-white race, with obesity, or with other cardiovascular risk factors) may be done on an individual basis after reviewing risk factors for kidney and cardiovascular disease and after full discussion of potential risks with the donor candidate and the selection committee.

If a donor candidate is diagnosed with hypertension during their evaluation and they otherwise meet acceptance criteria, treatment should be initiated and adequate blood pressure control confirmed based on several readings taken over several weeks or by repeated ABPM prior to accepting them for donation [11]. Donor candidates with hypertension should be counseled about potential worsening of hypertension after donation [11], which, if left untreated, could result in end-organ damage. It must be emphasized that individuals with hypertension who donate a kidney require regular postdonation follow-up (which may be with their primary care provider) and should adopt and maintain healthy lifestyle practices.

Additional Considerations

Female donor candidates should be asked about prior hypertensive disorders of pregnancy (e.g., gestational hypertension, preeclampsia, or eclampsia) as part of the routine evaluation history [11]. Donor candidates with a remote history of preeclampsia or gestational hypertension may be acceptable for donation if they fulfill all other criteria for donation including the presence of acceptable renal function. Women with childbearing potential should be counseled about the effects donation may have on future pregnancies, including the possibility of a greater likelihood of being diagnosed with gestational hypertension or preeclampsia [33]. Detailed blood pressure evaluation should be performed using ABPM monitoring.

Donor candidates with a history of hypertension thought to be related to or exacerbated by obesity (including those who have undergone bariatric surgery) may be

Table 5.3 Contraindications to living kidney donation based on blood pressure

Absolute
• Uncontrolled hypertension or hypertension requiring three or more agents to achieve control
• Controlled hypertension with target organ damage evidenced by ECG or echocardiogram showing left ventricular hypertrophy, diastolic dysfunction, or hypertensive heart disease or retinal exam showing hypertensive changes or urinalysis showing microalbuminuria
• Prior myocardial infarction, stroke, or transient ischemic attack
Relative
• Hypertension in individuals with other risk factors for renal and/or cardiovascular disease – e.g., family history of kidney or cardiovascular disease in first-degree relatives, obesity, hypercholesterolemia, prediabetes, or active smoking
• A decision regarding acceptance may depend on the specific risk factors, their severity, and the transplant program's acceptable risk threshold
• Hypertension in individuals who lack medical insurance and who have barriers to follow-up with a primary care provider for treatment

acceptable for donation if their blood pressure is normal after a weight loss goal is achieved (e.g., to BMI <30 kg/m²) and sustained for some time or is controlled with medication, if they otherwise meet program acceptance criteria. The evaluation of donor candidates who have had prior bariatric surgery, particularly intestinal bypass or Roux-en-Y gastric bypass, should include assessment for risk of nephrolithiasis (e.g., serum oxalate level and 24-hour urine stone profile) [11].

The application of blood pressure to donor selection is summarized in Table 5.3.

Impact of Donor Nephrectomy on Blood Pressure, Risk for Cardiovascular Events, and Kidney Survival

Blood pressure has been reported to increase after donation in several small studies [34]. It is unclear if this is related to donation-associated loss of nephron mass and function, changes in vascular tone or volume status, and/or due to aging, weight gain, or heightened scrutiny at donor follow-up. The existing evidence has been limited by small sample sizes and low ascertainment rates. While use of antihypertensive medications was lower in a cohort of privately insured donors compared to age- and sex matched non-donors [35], a meta-analysis of mostly white donors who were normotensive at donation showed a rise in systolic blood pressure by 6 mmHg and diastolic blood pressure by 4 mmHg over non-donor healthy controls at 7 years postdonation [34]. An administrative claims linkage study of 1278 Canadian donors also showed higher incidence of claims-based hypertension diagnosis in living donors compared to matched non-donors who were screened for good health at baseline; however there was no increase in risk of death or major cardiovascular events, and the authors suggested that the higher detection rates may have been a result of bias in monitoring [36]. A recent report from the Wellness and Health Outcomes in LivE Donor (WHOLE-Donor) multicenter study of 1295 living kidney donors reported higher rates of self-reported hypertension by donors over a median 6-year follow-up compared to self-reported antihypertensive medication use in control subjects enrolled in the ARIC study or self-reported hypertension in subjects enrolled in the CARDIA study over a median of 23 years [16]. Hypertension incidence was higher in the donors including 23% of white donors and 42% of black donors compared to 8% and 9% of white and black non-donor controls, respectively. Kidney donation was associated with a 19% higher risk of hypertension, regardless of race, with the expected increase in eGFR following donation noted to plateau at development of hypertension. While the data were collected in different eras with potential impact of differing definitions for hypertension and there were fewer controls than donors, these studies suggest higher incidence of hypertension following donation, endorsing the importance of BP follow-up. However, they do not enlighten outcomes for donors with hypertension prior to donation.

There is racial variation in postdonation development of hypertension with greater risk in African Americans and Hispanics than white donors [35, 37, 38]. This is similar to racial disparities seen in prevalence of hypertension in the general population. Several small trials have reported on cohorts in which many donors were unaware of the development of hypertension after donation [37, 38]. An analysis of US registry data for donors age 50 or older reported those with hypertension had a greater risk of developing ESRD at 15 years postdonation (0.8%), compared to older donors without hypertension (0.2%) [39, 40]. This risk estimate is similar to other published estimates for all donors of 30.8 per 10,000 and estimates for donors stratified by age, and the risk for donors 50–59 years was 54.6/10,000 and for 60 years and older was 70.2/10,000. There was no difference in mortality between those with and without hypertension. In this context, the absolute risk increase for ESRD in hypertensive donors is small. It is appropriate to counsel these individuals and emphasize the importance of long-term treatment and follow-up.

Among living donors, kidney function per se may impact the likelihood of postdonation hypertension. A study examining linked US registry data with pharmaceutical claims and laboratory data from electronic health records found a graded increase in odds of antihypertensive medication use after donation with lower postdonation estimated GFR, such that a postdonation eGFR of <30 mL/min/1.73 m^2 was associated with 2.5 times the likelihood of antihypertensive medication use (versus $\geq$75 mL/min/1.73 m^2) [41]. Other significant correlates of postdonation antihypertensive medication use included older age at donation, black race, obesity, first-degree donor–recipient relationship, presence of "prehypertension" at donation, and time elapsed since donation.

Impact of Donor Nephrectomy on Future Pregnancies

Female donors with childbearing potential should be counseled about the effects donation may have on future pregnancies, including a greater likelihood of being diagnosed with gestational hypertension or preeclampsia [33]. Several small studies assessed the impact of donation on outcomes of subsequent pregnancies. Garg et al. reviewed 85 living donors matched to 510 non-donors by age, race, income, urban or rural residence, and previous pregnancy numbers in Canada [33]. This study reported an increased risk of the combined outcome of preeclampsia and gestational hypertension (OR 2.4, 95% CI 1.2–5.0) in kidney donors compared to healthy non-donors, but when outcomes were assessed individually, the difference was not statistically significant [33]. In a case-control series from the United States, where 59 female donors who became pregnant after donation were compared to age- and race- matched non-donors, donors overall did not demonstrate a higher incidence of gestational hypertension or preeclampsia, but there was a higher incidence in primiparous young donors (<30 years) [42]. A study using data from the Norwegian Birth Registry that examined pregnancy outcomes in 326 kidney donors compared to a control group of randomly sampled births reported no increased risk of gestational hypertension or preeclampsia in the main analysis but reported higher incidence in multiparous donors [43]. In all these studies there was no difference in length of stay, preterm delivery, need for Caesarian section or low birthweight between the groups, suggesting that the preeclampsia or gestational hypertension that develops in donors is likely to be a mild form. There is no data on pregnancy outcomes specifically in non-white donors.

Blood Pressure Care for Donors After Donation

As observed in general Western populations, approximately half of the kidney donor population will likely develop hypertension at 10–40 years after donation, with onset typically earlier in African American than white donors [37, 44]. Postdonation risk of hypertension is higher for older individuals, those with a family history of hypertension, higher BMI, higher fasting blood sugars, and smokers [44]. All donors should be advised to receive annual medical follow-up to monitor blood pressure and measures of kidney health (e.g., eGFR and albuminuria measurement) and to follow healthy lifestyle habits including regular exercise, healthy diet, and abstinence from tobacco. Donors should also be advised to avoid routine use of NSAIDs and decongestants.

Special counseling of donors with hypertension: In addition to the above recommendations, donors with hypertension should be advised to limit salt intake. One study showed that use of angiotensin-converting enzyme (ACE) inhibitor or angiotensin receptor blockers in prior donors who had developed hypertension was associated with lower risk of eGFR <45 mL/min and end-stage renal disease [44]. There are limited data related to the need for 24-hour or abbreviated (shortened monitoring periods such as 18 hours) ABPM testing postdonation. Donors should commit to long-term follow-up, including maintenance of adequate medical insurance to cover the costs of medications and follow-up care to monitor blood pressure control and assessment and treatment of possible complications if they arise.

Need for Additional Studies

The lower threshold for defining hypertension established in the 2017 ACC/AHA blood pressure guideline defines blood pressure of 120–129/<80 mmHg as elevated and 130–139/80–89 mmHg as stage 1 hypertension. It is unclear if these thresholds should be applied to decisions for acceptance of living kidney donor candidates. While these newer thresholds increase the prevalence of hypertension in donor candidates and application to donor candidacy may exclude some otherwise acceptable candidates, the lower thresholds improve the sensitivity of clinic blood pressure and lower the prevalence of missed hypertension [26]. As obesity and hypertension rates are rising in the general population, similar trends are seen in donor candidates [45, 46] and may only worsen with time. There is an urgent need for a national US donor registry, especially for those with hypertension and obesity to assess long-term impacts of kidney donation on renal and cardiovascular outcomes. The Living Donor Collective pilot project is an effort to establish a national long-term registry of living donors in the United States [47] .

Case Discussions

The following case scenarios illustrate application of the principles of this chapter to clinical practice.

Case 1

A 45-year-old white woman takes an oral contraceptive pill daily and uses ibuprofen occasionally. She has no prior history of hypertension, cardiovascular disease, or kidney disease. Her BMI is 24.6 kg/m².

Her blood pressure (BP) is measured by several methods:

- Automated office BP (average of five readings): 140/92 mm Hg, heart rate (HR) 93 beats per minute (BPM)
- Trained nurse BP measurement: 136–144/88–90 mm Hg, both arms
- 18-hour ABPM daytime mean: 148/91 mm Hg, HR 85 bpm; night time mean: 142/84 mm Hg, HR 73 bpm

The **ABPM results** are shown (Fig. 5.2).

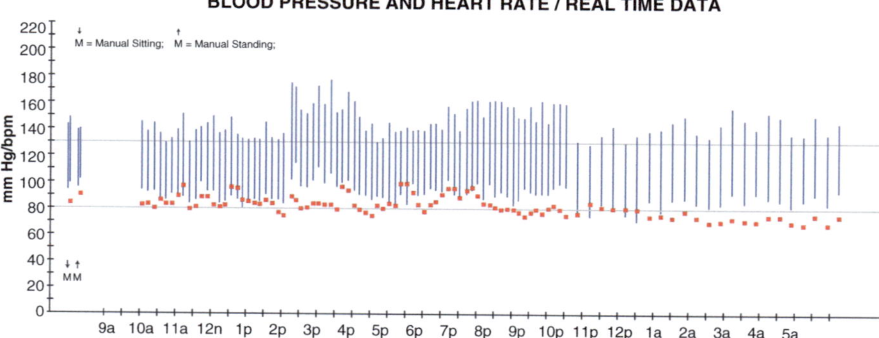

Fig. 5.2 Initial overnight ABPM tracing for Case 1. Time by clock hour is on x-axis. Systolic and diastolic BP is shown on y-axis by the top and bottom of each vertical line. Red squares indicate heart rate. BP is in millimeters mercury (mm Hg); HR is in beats per minute (bpm)

Her **laboratory results** include the following:

- Fasting blood sugar: 95 mg/dL
- Hgb A1c: 5.3%
- Lipid levels: Total cholesterol 210 mg/dL, HDL 52 mg/dL, LDL 122 mg/dL, triglycerides 179 mg/dL
- Creatinine clearance: 133 mL/min per 1.73 m^2
- Iothalamate glomerular filtration rate (GFR): 133 mL/min per 1.73 m^2
- 24-hour urine microalbumin and protein excretion: within normal limits

As she has clear evidence for hypertension, she is treated with lisinopril 5 mg daily.

She is advised to discontinue nonsteroidal anti-inflammatory agent (NSAID) use. It is suggested that she consider alternative contraception related to her age and hypertension.

After 6 weeks of treatment, a repeat ABPM is obtained.

- ABPM daytime mean: 121/76 mm Hg, HR 81 bpm; nighttime mean – 110/72 mm Hg, HR 76 bpm

The ABPM results are shown (Fig. 5.3).

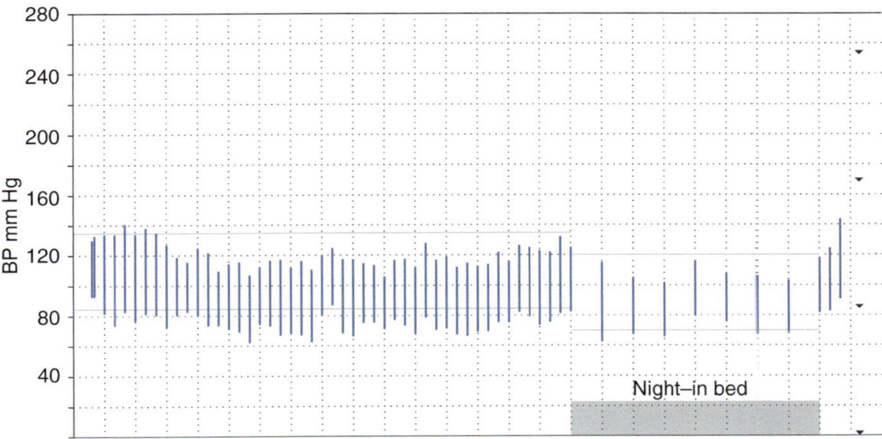

Fig. 5.3 Follow-up overnight ABPM tracing for Case 1 after 6 weeks on medical treatment. Time by clock hour is on x-axis. Systolic and diastolic BP is shown on y-axis by the top and bottom of each vertical line. BP is in millimeters mercury (mm Hg)

Recommendations and decision: With the addition of a single antihypertensive agent at low dose and some lifestyle changes, her BP is controlled. Considering her body weight, lipid measurements, glucose metabolism, and kidney function, there are no other findings of concern. There is no evidence for target organ damage related to her hypertension, which requires treatment whether or not she becomes a kidney donor. The candidate is approved for donation.

Case 2

A 45-year-old white man reports occasional use of a combination tablet of aspirin/ acetaminophen/caffeine for headaches. He has no prior history of hypertension, cardiovascular disease, or kidney disease. His BMI is 30.2 kg/m².

His BP is measured by several methods:

- Automated office BP (average of five readings): 127/92 mm Hg, HR 77 bpm
- Trained nurse BP measurement: 122–140/100–106 mm Hg, both arms
- ABPM daytime mean: 139/85 mm Hg, HR 72 bpm; nighttime mean: 123/75 mm Hg, HR 68 bpm

The **ABPM results** are shown (Fig. 5.4).

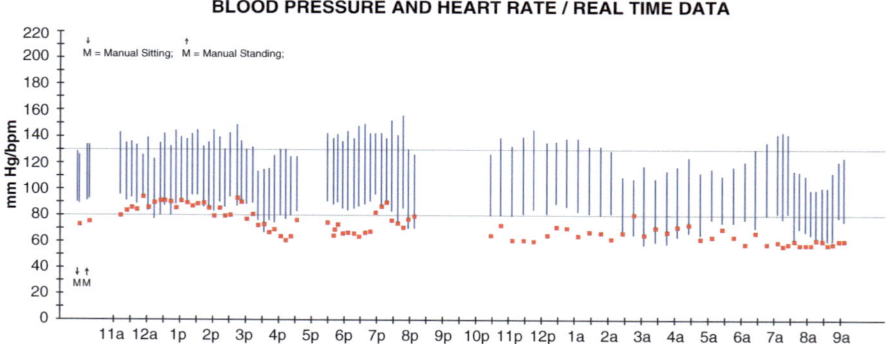

Fig. 5.4 Overnight ABPM tracing for Case 2. Time by clock hour is on x-axis. Systolic and diastolic BP is shown on y-axis by the top and bottom of each vertical line. Red squares indicate heart rate. BP is in millimeters mercury (mm Hg); HR is in beats per minute (bpm)

His **laboratory results** include the following:

- Fasting blood sugar: 101 mg/dL.
- Hgb A1c 5.1%.
- Lipid levels: Total cholesterol 144 mg/dL, HDL 38 mg/dL, LDL 61 mg/dL, triglycerides 223 mg/dL.
- Creatinine clearance: 116 mL/min per 1.73 m^2.
- Iothalamate GFR: 117 mL/min per 1.73 m^2,
- Urinalysis: normal.
- 24-hour urine microalbumin excretion: 42 mg (>30 mg, elevated).
- Other testing: Mild enlargement of cardiac silhouette on chest x-ray. ECG shows borderline concentric left ventricular wall thickness and dilated aortic root.

Recommendations and decision: In addition to hypertension, he has grade 1 obesity and mild hypertriglyceridemia. He is excluded from donation due to the presence of hypertensive target organ damage, including early left ventricular hypertrophy and albuminuria. He is advised to seek treatment from a primary care provider.

Case 3

A 59-year-old white man has been taking irbesartan 75 mg daily for 1 year for hypertension. He has no history of cardiovascular events or kidney disease. His BMI is 25.2 kg/m^2.

His BP is measured by several methods:

- Automated office BP (average of five readings): 146/94 mm Hg, HR 77 bpm
- Trained nurse BP measurement: 126/66 mm Hg, both arms
- ABPM daytime mean: 122/78 mm Hg, HR 78 bpm; nighttime mean: 106/66 mm Hg, HR 61 bpm. Note the drop in BP at 7:30 pm, lying down, which impacts automated mean values

The **ABPM results** are shown (Fig. 5.5).

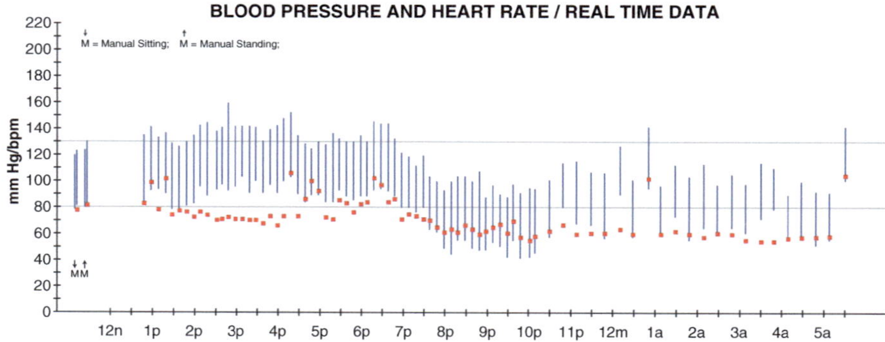

Fig. 5.5 Initial overnight ABPM tracing for Case 3. Time by clock hour is on x-axis. Systolic and diastolic BP is shown on y-axis by the top and bottom of each vertical line. Red squares indicate heart rate. BP is in millimeters mercury (mm Hg); HR is in beats per minute (bpm)

His **laboratory results** include the following:

- Lipid levels: Total cholesterol 205 mg/dL, HDL 64 mg/dL, LDL 130 mg/dL, triglycerides 56 mg/dL
- Creatinine clearance: 100 mL/min per 1.73 m^2
- Iothalamate GFR: 96 mL/min/1.73 m^2
- 24-hour urine microalbumin and protein excretion: within normal limits

He is treated with an increase in irbesartan dose to 150 mg daily.
After 6 weeks at the higher dosage, a repeat ABPM is obtained.

- ABPM daytime mean: 119/79 mmHg, HR 68 bpm; nighttime mean: 110/70 mmHg, HR 60 bpm

The **ABPM results** are shown (Fig. 5.6).

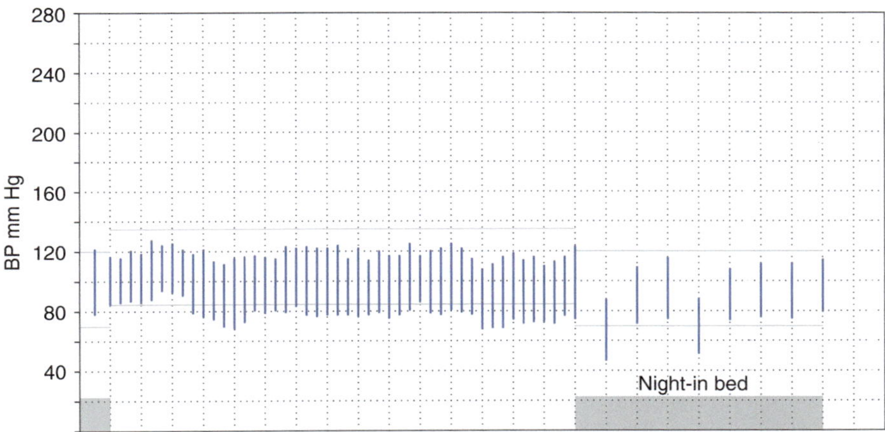

Fig. 5.6 Follow-up overnight ABPM tracing for Case 3 after 6 weeks on medical treatment at higher dosage. Time by clock hour is on x-axis. Systolic and diastolic BP is shown on y-axis by the top and bottom of each vertical line. BP is in millimeters mercury (mm Hg)

Recommendations and decision: With an increase in the dose of his current single antihypertensive agent, his BP is controlled. While he is advised to work with his primary care physician on lowering his cholesterol and triglyceride levels, he is at a good weight and has good kidney function. There is no evidence for target organ damage related to his hypertension, which requires effective treatment whether or not he becomes a kidney donor. The candidate is approved for donation.

Case 4

A 57-year-old white woman has no prior history of hypertension, but her BP runs 130–140 mm Hg systolic checked at store machines. Her BMI is 29.3 kg/m².

Her BP is measured by several methods:

- Automated office BP (average of five readings): 141/88 mm Hg, HR 84 bpm
- Trained nurse BP measurement: 134–136/70–74 mm Hg, both arms
- ABPM daytime mean: 144/79 mm Hg, HR 80 bpm; nighttime mean: 127/64 mm Hg, HR 64 bpm

The **ABPM results** are shown (Fig. 5.7).

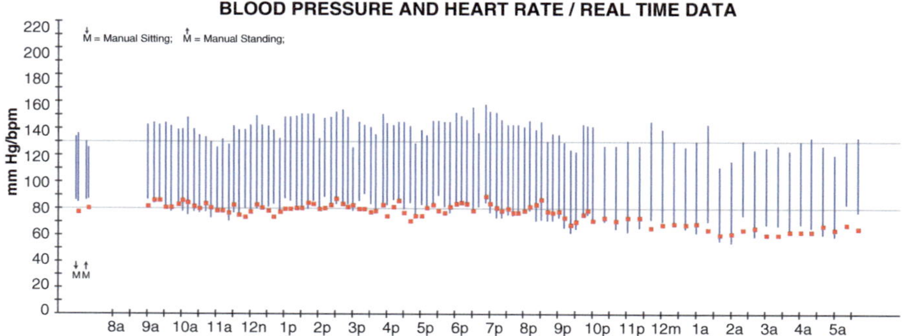

Fig. 5.7 Overnight ABPM tracing for Case 4. Time by clock hour is on x-axis. Systolic and diastolic BP is shown on y-axis by the top and bottom of each vertical line. Red squares indicate heart rate. BP is in millimeters mercury (mm Hg); HR is in beats per minute (bpm)

His **laboratory results** include the following:

- Fasting blood sugar: 108 mg/dL
- Hgb A1c: 5.5%
- Lipid levels: Total cholesterol 199 mg/dL, HDL 46 mg/dL, LDL 127 mg/dL, triglycerides 130 mg/dL
- Creatinine clearance: 92 mL/min per 1.73 m^2
- Iothalamate GFR: 120 mL/min per 1.73 m^2
- 24-hour urine microalbumin excretion: 61 mg (>30 mg, elevated)

Recommendations and decision: As she has clear evidence of hypertension, she is started on losartan 25 mg daily. The presence of microalbuminuria is a sign of target organ damage and, if persistent, would exclude her from donation. She discontinues the medication after 2 weeks and does not wish to try an alternative medication. As she is not able to accept needed hypertension treatment, she is excluded from donation.

References

1. Delmonico F, Council of the Transplantation Society. A report of the Amsterdam forum on the care of the live kidney donor: data and medical guidelines. Transplantation. 2005;79(6 Suppl):S53–66. https://pubmed.ncbi.nlm.nih.gov/15785361/.
2. Veterans Administration Cooperative Study Group. Effects of treatment on morbidity in hypertension. Results in patients with diastolic blood pressures averaging 115 through 129 mm Hg. JAMA. 1967;202(11):1028–34. https://pubmed.ncbi.nlm.nih.gov/4862069/.
3. Veterans Administration Cooperative Study Group. Effects of treatment on morbidity in hypertension. II. Results in patients with diastolic blood pressure averaging 90 through 114 mm Hg. JAMA. 1970;213(7):1143–52. https://pubmed.ncbi.nlm.nih.gov/4862069/.
4. Klag MJ, Whelton PK, Randall BL, Neaton JD, Brancati FL, Ford CE, et al. Blood pressure and end-stage renal disease in men. N Engl J Med. 1996;334(1):13–8. https://doi.org/10.1056/NEJM199601043340103.

5. Hsu CY. Does non-malignant hypertension cause renal insufficiency? Evidence-based perspective. Curr Opin Nephrol Hypertens. 2002;11(3):267–72. https://doi.org/10.1097/00041552-200205000-00001.
6. Perry HM Jr, Miller JP, Fornoff JR, Baty JD, Sambhi MP, Rutan G, et al. Early predictors of 15-year end-stage renal disease in hypertensive patients. Hypertension. 1995;25(4 Pt 1):587–94. https://doi.org/10.1161/01.hyp.25.4.587.
7. Tozawa M, Iseki K, Iseki C, Kinjo K, Ikemiya Y, Takishita S. Blood pressure predicts risk of developing end-stage renal disease in men and women. Hypertension. 2003;41(6):1341–5. https://doi.org/10.1161/01.HYP.0000069699.92349.8C.
8. Beevers DG, Lip GY. Does non-malignant essential hypertension cause renal damage? A clinician's view. J Hum Hypertens. 1996;10(10):695–9. https://pubmed.ncbi.nlm.nih.gov/9004097/.
9. Wright JT Jr, Williamson JD, Whelton PK, Snyder JK, Sink KM, et al. A randomized trial of intensive versus standard blood-pressure control. N Engl J Med. 2015;373(22):2103–15. https://doi.org/10.1056/NEJMoa1511939.
10. Whelton PK, Carey RM, Aronow WS, Casey DE Jr, Collins KJ, Dennison Himmelfarb C, et al. 2017 ACC/AHA/AAPA/ABC/ACPM/AGS/APhA/ASH/ASPC/NMA/PCNA guideline for the prevention, detection, evaluation, and management of high blood pressure in adults: a report of the American College of Cardiology/American Heart Association task force on clinical practice guidelines. Circulation. 2018;138(17):e484–594. https://doi.org/10.1161/CIR.0000000000000596.
11. Lentine KL, Kasiske BL, Levey AS, Adams PL, Alberu J, Bakr MA, et al. KDIGO clinical practice guideline on the evaluation and care of living kidney donors. Transplantation. 2017;101(8S Suppl 1):S1–S109. https://doi.org/10.1097/TP.0000000000001769.
12. Taler SJT, Textor SC. Living kidney donor criteria based on blood pressure, body mass index, and glucose: age-stratified decision-making in the absence of hard data. Curr Transplant Rep. 2016;3:33. https://doi.org/10.1007/s40472-016-0091-z.
13. Textor SC, Taler SJ, Larson TS, Prieto M, Griffin M, Gloor J, et al. Blood pressure evaluation among older living kidney donors. J Am Soc Nephrol. 2003;14(8):2159–67. https://doi.org/10.1097/01.asn.0000077346.92039.9c.
14. Textor SC, Taler SJ, Driscoll N, Larson TS, Gloor J, Griffin M, et al. Blood pressure and renal function after kidney donation from hypertensive living donors. Transplantation. 2004;78(2):276–82. https://doi.org/10.1097/01.tp.0000128168.97735.b3.
15. Denic A, Alexander MP, Kaushik V, Lerman LO, Lieske JC, Stegall MD, et al. Detection and clinical patterns of nephron hypertrophy and nephrosclerosis among apparently healthy adults. Am J Kidney Dis. 2016;68(1):58–67. https://doi.org/10.1053/j.ajkd.2015.12.029.
16. Holscher CM, Haugen CE, Jackson KR, Garonzik Wang JM, Waldram MM, Bae S, et al. Self-reported incident hypertension and long-term kidney function in living kidney donors compared with healthy nondonors. Clin J Am Soc Nephrol. 2019;14(10):1493–9. https://doi.org/10.2215/CJN.04020419.
17. DeLoach SS, Meyers KE, Townsend RR. Living donor kidney donation: another form of white coat effect. Am J Nephrol. 2012;35(1):75–9. https://doi.org/10.1159/000335070.
18. Ommen ES, Schroppel B, Kim JY, Gaspard G, Akalin E, de Boccardo G, et al. Routine use of ambulatory blood pressure monitoring in potential living kidney donors. Clin J Am Soc Nephrol. 2007;2(5):1030–6. https://doi.org/10.2215/CJN.01240307.
19. Banegas JR, Ruilope LM, de la Sierra A, Vinyoles E, Gorostidi M, de la Cruz JJ, et al. Relationship between clinic and ambulatory blood-pressure measurements and mortality. N Engl J Med. 2018;378(16):1509–20. https://doi.org/10.1056/NEJMoa1712231.
20. Cohen JB, Lotito MJ, Trivedi UK, Denker MG, Cohen DL, Townsend RR. Cardiovascular events and mortality in white coat hypertension: a systematic review and meta-analysis. Ann Intern Med. 2019;170(12):853–62. https://doi.org/10.7326/M19-0223.
21. Burkard T, Mayr M, Winterhalder C, Leonardi L, Eckstein J, Vischer AS. Reliability of single office blood pressure measurements. Heart. 2018;104(14):1173–9. https://doi.org/10.1136/heartjnl-2017-312523.

22. Bobrie G, Clerson P, Menard J, Postel-Vinay N, Chatellier G, Plouin PF. Masked hypertension: a systematic review. J Hypertens. 2008;26(9):1715–25. https://doi.org/10.1097/HJH.0b013e3282fbcedf.
23. Organ Procurement and Transplantation Network (OPTN)/United Network for Organ Sharing (UNOS). Policy 14: Living Donation. Available at: https://optn.transplant.hrsa.gov/governance/policies/. Accessed: 7 Sept 2020.
24. Myers MG, Godwin M, Dawes M, Kiss A, Tobe SW, Kaczorowski J. Measurement of blood pressure in the office: recognizing the problem and proposing the solution. Hypertension. 2010;55(2):195–200. https://doi.org/10.1161/HYPERTENSIONAHA.109.141879.
25. Roerecke M, Kaczorowski J, Myers MG. Comparing automated office blood pressure readings with other methods of blood pressure measurement for identifying patients with possible hypertension: a systematic review and meta-analysis. JAMA Intern Med. 2019;179(3):351–62. https://doi.org/10.1001/jamainternmed.2018.6551.
26. Armanyous S, Ohashi Y, Lioudis M, Schold JD, Thomas G, Poggio ED, et al. Diagnostic performance of blood pressure measurement modalities in living kidney donor candidates. Clin J Am Soc Nephrol. 2019;14(5):738–46. https://doi.org/10.2215/CJN.02780218.
27. Chobanian AV, Bakris GL, Black HR, Cushman WC, Green LA, Izzo JL Jr, et al. The seventh report of the joint National Committee on prevention, detection, evaluation, and treatment of high blood pressure: the JNC 7 report. JAMA. 2003;289(19):2560–72. https://doi.org/10.1001/jama.289.19.2560.
28. Salles GF, Reboldi G, Fagard RH, Cardoso CR, Pierdomenico SD, Verdecchia P, et al. Prognostic effect of the nocturnal blood pressure fall in hypertensive patients: the ambulatory blood pressure collaboration in patients with hypertension (ABC-H) meta-analysis. Hypertension. 2016;67(4):693–700. https://doi.org/10.1161/HYPERTENSIONAHA.115.06981.
29. Grams ME, Sang Y, Levey AS, Matsushita K, Ballew S, Chang AR, et al. Kidney-failure risk projection for the living kidney-donor candidate. N Engl J Med. 2016;374(5):411–21. https://doi.org/10.1002/lt.24714.
30. Massie AB, Muzaale AD, Luo X, Chow EKH, Locke JE, Nguyen AQ, et al. Quantifying postdonation risk of ESRD in living kidney donors. J Am Soc Nephrol. 2017;28(9):2749–55. https://doi.org/10.1056/NEJMoa1510491.
31. Ibrahim HN, Foley RN, Reule SA, Spong R, Kukla A, Issa N, et al. Renal function profile in white kidney donors: the first 4 decades. J Am Soc Nephrol. 2016;27(9):2885–93. https://doi.org/10.1681/ASN.2016101084.
32. Ibrahim, H.N., R.N. Foley, S.A. Reule, R. Spong, A. Kukla, N. Issa, et al., Renal Function Profile in White Kidney Donors: The First 4 Decades. J Am Soc Nephrol, 2016;27(9):2885–93. https://doi.org/10.1681/ASN.2015091018.
33. Steiner RW. Amending a historic paradigm for selecting living kidney donors. Am J Transplant. 2019;19(9):2405–6. https://doi.org/10.1111/ajt.15469.
34. Garg AX, Nevis IF, McArthur E, Sontrop JM, Koval JJ, Lam NN, et al. Gestational hypertension and preeclampsia in living kidney donors. N Engl J Med. 2015;372(2):124–33. https://doi.org/10.1056/NEJMoa1408932.
35. Boudville N, Prasad GV, Knoll G, Muirhead N, Thiessen-Philbrook H, Yang RC, et al. Meta-analysis: risk for hypertension in living kidney donors. Ann Intern Med. 2006;145(3):185–96. https://doi.org/10.7326/0003-4819-145-3-200608010-00006.
36. Lentine KL, Schnitzler MA, Xiao H, Saab G, Salvalaggio PR, Axelrod D, et al. Racial variation in medical outcomes among living kidney donors. N Engl J Med. 2010;363(8):724–32. https://doi.org/10.1056/NEJMoa1000950.
37. Garg AX, Prasad GV, Thiessen-Philbrook HR, Ping L, Melo M, Gibney EM, et al. Cardiovascular disease and hypertension risk in living kidney donors: an analysis of health administrative data in Ontario, Canada. Transplantation. 2008;86(3):399–406. https://doi.org/10.1097/TP.0b013e31817ba9e3.
38. Nogueira JM, Weir MR, Jacobs S, Haririan A, Breault D, Klassen D, et al. A study of renal outcomes in African American living kidney donors. Transplantation. 2009;88(12):1371–6. https://doi.org/10.1097/TP.0b013e3181c1e156.

39. Al Ammary F, Luo X, Muzaale AD, Massie AB, Crews DC, Waldram MM, et al. Risk of ESKD in older live kidney donors with hypertension. Clin J Am Soc Nephrol. 2019. https://doi.org/10.2215/CJN.14031118.
40. Muzaale AD, Massie AB, Wang MC, Montgomery RA, McBride MA, Wainright JL, et al. Risk of end-stage renal disease following live kidney donation. JAMA. 2014;311(6):579–86. https://doi.org/10.1001/jama.2013.285141.
41. Lentine KL, Holscher CM, Naik AS, Lam NN, Segev DL, Garg AX, et al. Postdonation eGFR and new-onset antihypertensive medication use after living kidney donation. Transplant Direct. 2019;5(8):e474. https://doi.org/10.1097/TXD.0000000000000913.
42. Davis S, Dylewski J, Shah PB, Holmen J, You Z, Chonchol M, et al. Risk of adverse maternal and fetal outcomes during pregnancy in living kidney donors: a matched cohort study. Clin Transpl. 2019;33(1):e13453. https://doi.org/10.1111/ctr.13453.
43. Reisaeter AV, Roislien J, Henriksen T, Irgens LM, Hartmann A. Pregnancy and birth after kidney donation: the Norwegian experience. Am J Transplant. 2009;9(4):820–4. https://doi.org/10.1111/j.1600-6143.2008.02427.x.
44. Sanchez OA, Ferrara LK, Rein S, Berglund D, Matas AJ, Ibrahim HN. Hypertension after kidney donation: incidence, predictors, and correlates. Am J Transplant. 2018;18(10):2534–43. https://doi.org/10.1111/ajt.14713.
45. Naik AS, Cibrik DM, Sakhuja A, Samaniego M, Lu Y, Shahinian V, et al. Temporal trends, center-level variation, and the impact of prevalent state obesity rates on acceptance of obese living kidney donors. Am J Transplant. 2018;18(3):642–9. https://doi.org/10.1111/ajt.14519.
46. Taler SJ, Messersmith EE, Leichtman AB, Gillespie BW, Kew CE, Stegall MD, et al. Demographic, metabolic, and blood pressure characteristics of living kidney donors spanning five decades. Am J Transplant. 2013;13(2):390–8. https://doi.org/10.1111/j.1600-6143.2012.04321.x.
47. Kasiske BL, Asrani SK, Dew MA, Henderson ML, Henrich C, Humar A, et al. The living donor collective: a scientific registry for living donors. Am J Transplant. 2017;17(12):3040–8. https://doi.org/10.1111/ajt.14365.

Evaluation of Metabolic and Cardiovascular Risks in Living Donor Candidates

6

Margaux N. Mustian, Vineeta Kumar, and Jayme E. Locke

Introduction

Kidney transplantation is the preferred treatment for suitable patients with end-stage kidney disease (ESKD), and living donor transplantation in particular provides superior posttransplant outcomes, compared with deceased donor transplantation [1]. In response to the organ shortage for kidney transplantation worldwide, as well as demographic changes in the general population including aging and the obesity epidemic [2], expansion of living kidney donation has been explored, including acceptance of donor candidates with isolated medical abnormalities, such as hypertension or obesity [3–8]. As of the late 2000s, over 20% of living kidney donors were reported to have a medical abnormality [9, 10], and the majority of living kidney donors were either categorized as overweight or obese [11]. In the United States, the proportion of living kidney donors classified as overweight or obese has continued to increase over the last few decades and accounted for 66% of donors in 2016 [2]. In Australia and New Zealand, nearly one-third of candidates who went on to become living kidney donors from 2004 to 2012 had either a relative or absolute medical contraindication to donation compared to national guidelines [12].

While careful acceptance of medically complex donor candidates may be an appropriate strategy to increase opportunities for living donor transplantation, protecting donor safety is always a critical consideration. When assessing postdonation outcomes, Ibrahim et al. found that living kidney donation was safe among carefully selected donors, with patient survival and risk of ESKD similar to that among

M. N. Mustian · J. E. Locke (✉)
Department of Surgery, University of Alabama at Birmingham, Birmingham, AL, USA
e-mail: mmustian@uabmc.edu; jlocke@uabmc.edu

V. Kumar
Department of Medicine, University of Alabama at Birmingham, Birmingham, AL, USA
e-mail: vkumar@uabmc.edu

© Springer Nature Switzerland AG 2021
K. L. Lentine et al. (eds.), *Living Kidney Donation*,
https://doi.org/10.1007/978-3-030-53618-3_6

nondonor controls [13]. Segev et al. assessed long-term outcomes among a large national cohort of US living kidney donors, compared with healthy controls from the National Health and Nutrition Examination Survey (NHANES), and found that donors and their matched nondonor controls had similar patient survival at a median of 6.3 years [14]. Importantly, the investigators included all living kidney donors from the national registry (in contrast to the single-center, predominantly white race University of Minnesota cohort) and compared donors with "healthy" nondonor controls. However, some donor subgroups had an increased risk for both perioperative and long-term mortality *compared to other donors*, including older (versus younger) donors and those with (versus without) hypertension.

In 2014, Muzaale et al. reported that kidney donors had an increased risk of ESKD at a median of 7.6 years follow-up, compared with matched healthy nondonors from NHANES III [15]. In subgroup analyses, the cumulative incidence of ESKD varied considerably by age, race, and sex, ranging from 17.4 per 10,000 for donors aged 40–49 to 70.2 per 10,000 for donors age 60 years or older [15]. Importantly, over the course of the study, only 99 of the 96,217 living kidney donors developed ESKD [15]. Subsequent work by this group also demonstrated that many of the cases of ESKD secondary to diabetes or hypertension occurred late following donation, with a 7.7-fold increased risk of diabetic ESKD and a 2.6-fold increased risk of ESKD secondary to hypertension in the later years (10–25 years) following donation, compared with earlier years (<10 years) [16]. Furthermore, Locke et al. demonstrated that donors with obesity had an 86% increased risk of developing ESKD, compared with nonobese donors [17].

Living donor characteristics may also impact transplant outcomes among recipients [18–22]. Several donor characteristics, including age, body mass index (BMI), and smoking history, have been incorporated into a living donor profile index, which mirrors the index used for the assessment of deceased donor kidney quality [23]. This tool aids in prediction of recipient graft survival and may aid in selection when multiple donor candidates are available. The benefit derived from increased access to living donor kidney transplantation through the acceptance of medically complex donors must be weighed against potential short-term and/or longer-term risks to the donors. A thorough and comprehensive donor selection process is critical, particularly among medically complex donor candidates.

Evaluation for Metabolic and Cardiovascular Risk Factors

After a potential living kidney donor contacts the transplant center for candidate evaluation, a medical evaluation ensues to assess for the presence of medical, familial, and psychosocial conditions that could place the donor candidate at an increased risk of adverse events, such as perioperative complications or long-term health outcomes such as chronic kidney disease (CKD) or ESKD [24]. All donor candidates must have a general history and physical examination, focused on risk factors associated with the development of kidney disease. As part of the assessment of cardiovascular and metabolic risks, donor candidates should be queried regarding personal and family history of hypertension, dyslipidemia, diabetes mellitus, gestational diabetes, and gestational hypertension. Medication use should be assessed, including prescription and nonprescription agents. Habits, including history of smoking and use of other tobacco or nicotine products, are important elements of the candidate history.

For further assessment of metabolic or cardiovascular risks, the evaluation should include assessment of blood pressure, with at least two different measurements or 24-hour ambulatory blood pressure monitoring [25]. Potential donors should have height and weight measurements to calculate BMI [25]. In addition to assessment of kidney function, laboratory evaluation should include fasting blood glucose and a lipid panel [25]. For donor candidates at increased risk for diabetes (e.g., due to family history of diabetes, history of gestational diabetes, obesity, or elevated fasting glucose), hemoglobin A1c or an oral glucose tolerance test should be measured [24]. US policy requires performance of an electrocardiogram in all donor candidates. Those with cardiovascular risk factors may also warrant further cardiac evaluation, such as echocardiography or stress testing [25].

Special Considerations in Medically Complex Donors

Obesity

Measurement
BMI should be calculated for all donor candidates, and individuals should be classified based on World Health Organization criteria, which define obesity as BMI greater than or equal to 30 kg/m^2, or race-specific categories. Currently, there is no consensus within the transplant community regarding the appropriate BMI cutoff for living kidney donation. This controversy likely in part relates to lack of data to support a given BMI threshold for donor exclusion.

Outcomes Data
One study demonstrated that otherwise healthy Caucasian donors with obesity have good overall short-term outcomes following donor nephrectomy, such as length of stay, although the rate of wound complications, including postoperative infections, seromas and hernias, was higher in obese donors [26]. Linkage of US registry and administrative data from an academic consortium found BMI >30 kg/m^2 associated with 55% increase in risk of severe (Clavien classification 4 or 5) perioperative complications (adjusted HR 1.55, $P = 0.0005$) [27]. Several studies have observed increased operative time for donor nephrectomies among obese compared to non-obese donors [26, 28, 29]. By comparison, a systematic review of eight donor nephrectomy studies found no association of BMI and perioperative complications [30].

With regard to postdonation kidney function, one reason for concern among obese donor candidates relates to the knowledge that obesity is associated with kidney changes and remodeling in the absence of donation. Even in the presence of elevated or normal glomerular filtration rates (GFR), kidneys among obese individuals have been found to have increased transcapillary hydraulic pressure differences in addition to structural changes resulting from hyperfiltration [31, 32]. Among patients who underwent uninephrectomy for indications other than donation, obesity was associated with proteinuria and chronic renal failure following nephrectomy [33].

Meta-analysis based on data from nearly 5 million healthy persons found a modest association of BMI greater than 30 kg/m^2 with increased risk of ESKD over median cohort follow-up of 4–16 years (adjusted HR, 1.16; 95% CI 1.04–1.29) [34]. However, in living donors, the hyperfiltration stress of obesity may be exacerbated by reduction in kidney mass from donor nephrectomy [35, 36]. In a cohort of living kidney donors with long-term outcomes obtained from the Centers for Medicare and Medicaid Services (CMS) claims data linkages, Locke et al. found that obese donors had 1.9 gold higher risk of ESKD postdonation compared with nonobese donors, although the absolute risk of ESKD was low (94 per 10,000) [17] (Fig. 6.1).

Some studies of renal outcomes in living donors examined not only the presence of obesity but also the distribution of adiposity. Using cross-sectional imaging, Pek et al. defined visceral obesity as greater than or equal to 100 cm^2 at the umbilicus and found that donors with visceral obesity had a more severe decline in postdonation estimated GFR [37]. When comparing computed tomography measurements (including waist circumference, subcutaneous adiposity, visceral adiposity, and renal hilar adiposity) and calculated BMI, Chakkera et al. found that BMI was more strongly correlated with glomerulomegaly at a mean follow-up of 7 months afterdonation [38]. However, the authors also noted that at this short-term follow-up, kidney function, as evidenced by GFR and albuminuria, was similar across all BMI categories [38].

Obesity is also a risk factor for the development of medical conditions which may further increase the risk of CKD over time, such as diabetes and hypertension. In a single-center study of predominantly Caucasian living kidney donors at one US center (1975 through 2014), Serrano et al. found that obese donors had greater than

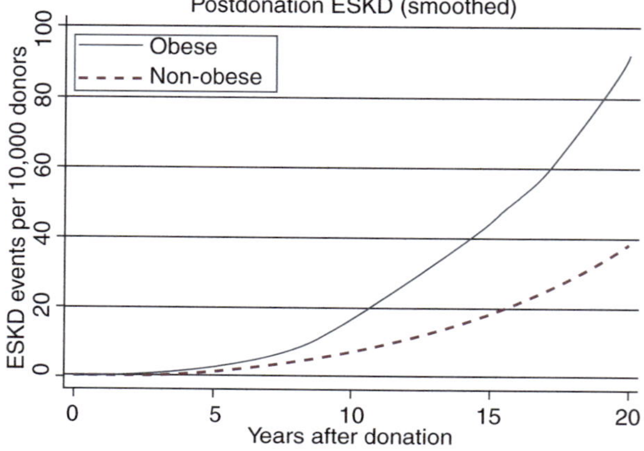

Fig. 6.1 Cumulative incidence of postdonation end-stage kidney disease among living kidney donors by obesity status at time of donation. (From Locke et al. [17])

a threefold increased risk of developing diabetes mellitus (aHR 3.14) and a 75% increased risk of developing hypertension after donation, compared to nonobese donors [39]. Analysis of linked national US donor registry data with records from a pharmacy claims warehouse (2007–2016) found that overweight and obese BMI at donation was associated with two (adjusted HR, 2.23; 95% CI 1.62–3.06) and four times (adjusted HR 4.59 95% CI 3.36–6.27) the likelihood of antidiabetic medication use over 9 years postdonation, respectively [40].

Current Recommendations for Selection

With regard to applications for current clinical practice, in Australia, a BMI of 30 kg/m^2 is often used as a relative contraindication that may preclude living donation [12, 41]. However, in the United States, while some centers use a threshold of 30 kg/m^2, other centers extend this threshold to 35 kg/m^2 [24]. A 2006–2007 survey of living kidney donor programs in the United States reported that up to 50% of the surveyed programs used a BMI of 35 kg/m^2 as their threshold for donor exclusion [5]. A threshold BMI of 35 kg/m^2 has also been adopted in several international guidelines [42–44]. The 2005 Amsterdam Forum on the Care of the Living Kidney Donor suggested that potential donors with BMI of 35 kg/m^2 should be discouraged from donating, particularly in the presence of comorbid disease [42]. The forum also endorsed weight loss recommendations for obese donor candidates in addition to healthy lifestyle education [42]. The 2017 Kidney Disease: Improving Global Outcomes (KDIGO) Clinical Practice Guideline on the Evaluation and Care of Living Kidney Donors recommended that the decision to approve donor candidates with obesity should be individualized based on other demographic and health characteristics, including lifetime projected ESKD risk, and should be viewed within the context of each center's acceptable threshold for postdonation risk [43]. The guideline also advocated for more research to better quantify obesity-related risks in donors to ground acceptance practices.

Weight management postdonation is also critical. As such, weight loss interventions predonation should not simply focus on changes in weight, but rather behavioral changes and sustainable lifestyle modifications. Issa et al. found that weight gain postdonation was also associated with the development of hypertension and type 2 diabetes mellitus [45]. The 2017 KDIGO guideline highlights the need for studies of the effectiveness of predonation interventions including counseling and weight or lifestyle changes on long-term donor outcomes as a research priority. Living kidney donor follow-up afterdonation is essential, particularly among medically complex donors in order to optimize their long-term health and minimize negative sequelae.

Glucose Intolerance

Measurement

In addition to reviewing the medical and family history of the donor candidate, glucose tolerance should be assessed via measurement of fasting blood glucose and/

or hemoglobin A1C. The 2017 KDIGO guideline recommends that those with a family history of diabetes in a first-degree relative, a history of gestational diabetes, or an elevated fasting glucose undergo further laboratory testing with a 2-hour glucose tolerance test or hemoglobin A1C [43]. While the presence of type 1 diabetes mellitus is an absolute contraindication to living kidney donation, living kidney donor candidates with prediabetes or older candidates with well-controlled type 2 diabetes mellitus on single agents may be acceptable for donation based on individualized risk assessment [43].

Outcomes Data

In the general population, it is well established that diabetes is a strong risk factor for CKD and ESKD [46]. Furthermore, Plantinga et al. found a high prevalence of CKD among NHANES cohort participants with prediabetes (fasting glucose 100–125 mg/dL) or those with undiagnosed diabetes (fasting glucose $\geq$126 mg/dL) [47]. Individuals with prediabetes also have an increased likelihood of developing diabetes, CKD, and cardiovascular disease [46]. However, the implications of diabetes risk factors, prediabetes, or well-controlled type 2 diabetes for living donor health outcomes are controversial and may vary with other demographic and health factors, such as age.

One small study demonstrated that living kidney donors with abnormal fasting glucose had no significant short-term increased risk of impaired kidney failure [48]. Recently, a large cohort study found that late postdonation ESKD was commonly reported as being secondary to diabetes or hypertension [16]. While this study was not able to quantify risk in relation to baseline factors such as glucose tolerance, this finding supports the need for careful donor selection and counseling regarding long-term postdonation risks in the setting of medical abnormalities [43]. Another study emphasized the importance of prevention of glucose impairment among potential living kidney donors through lifestyle modifications [49].

Gestational diabetes is associated with an increased risk for development of type 2 diabetes, with a large systematic review and meta-analysis demonstrating a greater than sevenfold increased risk (RR 7.43; 95% CI 4.79–11.51) [24, 50]. A history of gestational diabetes should prompt further workup and counseling prior to living kidney donation. Specifically, a history of gestational diabetes necessitates a 2-hour glucose tolerance test, and if this follow-up testing is abnormal, the candidate should not be approved for donation [24].

The development of diabetes afterdonation has been associated with other complications. In an analysis of 4362 living kidney donors, Ibrahim et al. found that postdonation diabetes mellitus was associated with an increased risk of developing hypertension (aHR 2.19; 95% CI 1.74–2.75) and proteinuria (aHR 2.65; 95% CI 1.89–3.70) [51]. These findings again highlight the importance of postdonation follow-up and access to appropriate healthcare.

Current Recommendations for Selection

With regard to implications for current associated practice, European guidelines have advocated for an individualized assessment of donor candidates with type 2 diabetes or prediabetes, stating that candidates with well-controlled glucose and no evidence of end-organ damage may be considered for donation [44, 52]. Others have advocated that prediabetes should preclude donation [53, 54]. The 2017 KDIGO guideline recommends that the decision to approve donor candidates with prediabetes or type 2 diabetes should be individualized based on demographic and health profile in relation to the transplant program's acceptable risk threshold. The guideline also recommends that donor candidates with prediabetes or type 2 diabetes should be counseled that their condition may progress over time and may lead to end-organ complications.

Dyslipidemia and Metabolic Syndrome

Measurement

Metabolic syndrome is defined as three or more of the following components: elevated triglycerides (greater than 150 mg/dL), decreased high-density lipoprotein (less than 50 mg/dL for men and 40 mg /dL for women), abnormal blood pressure (130/85 mmHg or higher), abdominal obesity (waist circumference of 35 inches or more in women or 40 inches in men), and impaired fasting glucose (fasting blood glucose of 100 mg/dL or higher). Measurement of a lipid panel in the donor candidate evaluation is recommended in several guidelines as part of cardiovascular risk assessment [43, 44, 53].

Outcomes Data

Metabolic syndrome is a risk factor for the development of cardiovascular disease in the general population and has also been shown to predict development of CKD [55]. For example, metabolic syndrome has been found to be associated with an increased incidence of stage 3b CKD among an elderly cohort (age 70 years or greater) [56]. Furthermore, among living donor kidney transplant recipients, Yoon et al. found that several donor factors were associated with delayed graft function, including elevated triglycerides, obesity, and hyperglycemia [57]. When assessing short-term outcomes among living kidney donors, another study found that living kidney donors at 1-year postdonation had increased prevalence of obesity and increased statin use compared to predonation, but longer-term outcomes and cardiovascular disease were not assessed [58]. With regard to outcome implications of lipid levels, a study of ESKD risk among 5 million healthy persons designed to inform living donor candidate selection found no associations of total cholesterol or low-density lipoprotein (LDL) levels with ESKD risk over median cohort follow-up of 4–16 years [34].

Current Recommendations for Selection

Lipid values are not routinely used in isolation to determine candidacy for living kidney donation, but rather should be considered in the context of the potential donor's other comorbid conditions and risk factors [43]. One consensus statement considered components of metabolic syndrome to be relative contraindications to donation [53]. These recommendations reflect some practice patterns, as several single-center studies from Mexico and the United States reported that obesity, impaired fasting glucose, or metabolic syndrome served as primary causes of donor exclusion [59, 60]. The 2017 KDIGO guideline recommends that decision to approve donor candidates with dyslipidemia should be individualized based on demographic and health profile in relation to the transplant program's acceptable risk threshold.

Hypertension

Measurement

Blood pressure assessment is an important component of the living donor candidate evaluation. Standardized blood pressure measurements should be performed in clinic on two separate occasions or by ambulatory blood pressure monitoring [43]. Blood pressure should be classified by guidelines for the general population in the country or region where donation is planned. The acceptance of donor candidates with hypertension varies across transplant centers, secondary to uncertain applicability of general population data to donors and limited data from the living donor population [24].

Outcomes Data

The frequency and outcomes of hypertension may vary with demographic characteristics. Data from the "Reasons for Geographic And Racial Differences in Stroke" study, a large cross-sectional analysis predominantly consisting of participants from the southeastern United States, found prehypertension in 62.9% of African Americans, compared with 54.1% of white participants [61]. Chu et al. demonstrated that age at donation was a significant predictor for hypertension development postdonation [62]. Importantly, while blood pressure may rise with aging, donation may accelerate a rise in blood pressure and need for antihypertensive treatment over expectations with normal aging; the 2017 KDIGO guideline recommends disclosure of this risk to donor candidates.

In the general population, the relationship between hypertension and the development of ESKD [63, 64] and propagation of cardiovascular disease risk [65, 66] is well established. A meta-analysis of data from nearly 5 million healthy persons found that every 20 mm Hg increase in systolic blood pressure was associated with a 42% increase (adjusted HR 1.42; 95% CI 1.27–1.58) in the risk of ESKD over median cohort follow-up of 4–16 years [34]. There is concern that donation nephrectomy may accelerate the progression of kidney function decline in hypertensive patients, due to hyperfiltration [24]. With regard to available data on risks among living kidney donors, Segev et al. found that donors with hypertension had increased risks of perioperative mortality, compared with normotensive donors (36.7 per 10,000 donors vs. 1.3 per 10,000 donors), based on linked donor registry and national death record data [14]. Donors with systolic blood pressure of 140 mm Hg or greater also had a greater than threefold increased risk for mortality at 9 years postdonation (aHR 3.3; 95% CI 1.1–9.7), compared with donors who had systolic blood pressure of 120 mm Hg or less [14]. A recent linkage of donor registry and ESKD records found that among donors age 50 or older, those with predonation hypertension had higher risk of ESKD, but not mortality, at 15 years postdonation [67]. However, the absolute risk of ESKD was small (0.8% vs. 0.2%).

Current Recommendations for Selection

Many centers will assess hypertension in the context of other comorbidities or risk factors to determine candidacy for donation. Uncontrolled hypertension or hypertension coupled with evidence of end-organ dysfunction (characterized by evidence of left ventricular hypertrophy, albuminuria, or changes of hypertensive retinopathy on fundoscopic exam) is considered a contraindication to donation by US Organ Procurement and Transplantation Network (OPTN) policy [68]. The 2017 KDIGO guideline recommends that candidates with hypertension that can be controlled to systolic blood pressure less than 140 mm Hg and diastolic blood pressure less than 90 mm Hg using one or two antihypertensive agents, who do not have evidence of target organ damage, may be acceptable for donation. The guideline recommends that the decision to approve donor candidates with hypertension should be individualized based on demographic and health profile in relation to the transplant program's acceptable risk threshold [43].

Follow-up and continued care of the living kidney donor is critical postdonation, as a large national cohort study of Scientific Registry of Transplant Recipients (SRTR) data identified new-onset hypertension among 3% of living donors without predonation hypertension within 2 years of donation [69]. Please see Chap. 5 for a comprehensive discussion of hypertension in the living donor candidate evaluation.

Tobacco Use

Measurement

All donor candidates should be asked about their history of smoking, and use of other tobacco and nicotine products, including whether use is current or prior. Use should be quantified in terms of frequency and duration (e.g., assessment of pack-years for smoking).

Outcomes Data

Tobacco use in the general population is associated with an increased risk for the development of cardiovascular disease [70, 71], with increased duration and quantity of tobacco use typically corresponding to increased risk. Cigarette smoking also plays a role in the development of microvascular kidney disease through accelerated atherosclerosis, and tobacco use has been associated with the onset and progression of CKD [72, 73]. Meta-analysis of data from nearly 5 million persons identified from seven general population cohorts, performed to support living donor evaluation, found that, compared with nonsmokers over median cohort follow-up of 4–16 years, current smokers had a 76% increase in the risk of ESKD (adjusted HR 1.76; 95% CI 1.29–2.41) and past smokers had a 45% increase in risk (adjusted HR

1.45; 95% CI 1.23–1.71) [34]. Smoking is also associated with perioperative surgical complications, including pulmonary complications and poor wound healing [74].

Risks associated with tobacco use have been documented in the living kidney donor population. Yoon et al. found that both former and current smokers had lower estimated GFR postdonation compared with never smokers, despite similar predonation estimates of kidney function [75]. The authors also demonstrated that increasing pack-years was correlated with declining estimated GFR postdonation [75]. Additionally, donors with a smoking history of 12 pack-years or more had a sevenfold increased risk for development of CKD postdonation (OR 7.5; 95% CI 1.97–28.61) [75].

Tobacco use affects both living kidney donors and their recipients. Heldt et al. found that among kidney transplant recipients, donor smoking status was significantly associated with less improvement in renal function after transplant, quantified as a smaller percent decline in serum creatinine postoperatively [76]. Similarly, smoking donors were found to have a larger rise in postdonation serum creatinine at follow-up, compared with nonsmokers [76]. Underwood et al. found that donor smoking at evaluation was associated with increased transplant recipient mortality (HR 1.93; 95% CI 1.27–2.94) [77].

Current Recommendations for Selection

The 2017 KDIGO guideline recommends individualized assessment donor candidates with respect to smoking history, accounting for the potential donors' other cardiovascular risks [43]. Other guidelines have recommended requirement of smoking cessation prior to donation, ranging from 4 weeks to 6 months predonation [42, 78]. Others advocate for smoking cessation but do not clearly delineate exclusion criteria for donation based on continued tobacco use [44]. We counsel donor candidates on the risks of smoking and use of tobacco and nicotine products, including vaping. We also encourage those who use tobacco products to quit and to commit to lifelong abstinence and suggest determining suitability for donation in light of their other perioperative, renal, and cardiovascular risk factors.

Cardiovascular Risk

Measurement

As previously stated, donor candidate evaluation of cardiovascular risk includes assessing risk factors for cardiovascular disease, such as obesity, hypertension, impaired glucose tolerance, dyslipidemia, and smoking history. Additionally, electrocardiograms and chest X-rays are usually obtained in the donor screening process and mandated in the United States by OPTN policy [25]. Recommendations regarding further cardiac testing, such as echocardiograms or stress testing, are not clearly delineated in most living kidney donor guidelines [25].

Outcomes Data

In assessing cardiovascular risk among living kidney donors, Garg et al. demonstrated living kidney donors had similar major cardiovascular risks compared with nondonor controls, at a median follow-up of nearly 7 years [79]. Reese et al. observed similar incidence of a combined outcome of cardiovascular disease or death among older donors (age ≥ 55 years), compared with matched healthy controls, over a median of 7.8 years follow-up [80]. However, at longer-term follow-up of 15 years, Mjøen et al. found an increased risk of cardiovascular death (aHR 1.40; 95% CI 1.03–1.91) for living kidney donors, compared with healthy nondonor controls in Norway [81]. Therefore, it appears that cardiovascular risks for living kidney donors are similar to that of healthy nondonors in the short term, but may worsen over time [25]. These findings highlight the importance of careful donor selection and health optimization prior to donation, as well as afterdonation, to ensure that living kidney donors maintain cardiovascular health.

Current Recommendations for Selection

The Amsterdam forum recommends following the American Heart Association guidelines, in which low-risk patients require no further cardiac workup preoperatively [25, 82]. Similarly, the 2017 KDIGO guideline recommends that donor candidates should receive guideline-based evaluation and management used for other noncardiac surgeries [43]. The British Transplantation Society recommends that potential living kidney donors with impaired exercise capacity (<4 metabolic equivalents), evidenced by inability to walk up a flight of stairs warrant further cardiac evaluation [25, 52]. Likewise, Canadian protocols require additional cardiac testing for living donor candidates with increased cardiac risk factors, such as advanced age, hypertension, hyperlipidemia, or history of tobacco use [25, 83].

Apolipoprotein L1 Gene

Measurement

Genetic testing represents another screening tool that may aid in the evaluation, selection, and/or counseling of some living donor candidates. Approximately 13% of African Americans possess two renal risk variants in the apolipoprotein L1 (*APOL1*) gene, a genotype that has been associated with increased risk of ESKD, outside of the setting of kidney donation [84]. However, not all individuals with two renal risk variants will develop ESKD, suggesting that there is a "second hit" involved in the development of renal failure [84]. In fact, the risk of kidney disease among these individuals is about 15% over the course of their lifetimes. Nonetheless, there is a concern that donor nephrectomy may serve as the second insult or that starting with lower baseline functional reserve due to GFR loss from donation surgery further increases their likelihood of ESKD in living donors with high-risk *APOL1* genotypes [24].

Outcomes Data

In a study among young adults, Locke et al. projected the 25-year risk of developing CKD, defined as estimated GFR <60 ml/min per 1.73 m^2,and found that young African Americans with two *APOL1* risk variants had the highest risk of CKD [85]. However, the addition of other risk factors, such as impaired fasting glucose or family history of hypertension or diabetes, further increased the long-term risks [85]. Therefore, full assessment of potential donors, particularly for African Americans, may include both modifiable risk factors in addition to genetic information.

Current Recommendations for Selection

At this time, *APOL1* genotyping of living kidney donor candidates is not routinely performed at all transplant centers, but is currently performed at some centers [24]. A 2016 American Society of Transplantation Expert Conference recommended counseling African American potential donors regarding the relationship between *APOL1* and development of renal failure and offering genetic testing offered as part of the evaluation process for those who wish to undergo testing [84]. The 2017 KDIGO guideline recommends that *APOL1* genotyping may be offered to donor candidates with sub-Saharan African ancestors [43]. The guideline recommends informing donor candidates that having two *APOL1* allele risk variants increases the lifetime risk of kidney failure but that the precise kidney failure risk for an affected individual after donation cannot currently be quantified. The KDIGO guideline also emphasizes the need for ongoing research to define the role of *APOL1* genotyping in the living donor candidate evaluation, a topic being addressed in new initiatives such as the National Institutes of Health (NIH)-sponsored APOL1 Long-term Kidney Transplantation Outcomes Network (APOLLO) study and the Living Donor Extended Time Outcomes (LETO) study [86].

In an *American Journal of Kidney Diseases* Core Curriculum article on evaluation of kidney donors, Sawinksi and Locke described a strategy for the evaluation of potential donors (Fig. 6.2) [24]. They proposed that in the absence of obesity, smoking history, family history of hypertension or diabetes, or impaired fasting glucose, donor candidates should be approved for donation (pending other medical/psychosocial clearance). However, in the presence of one non-modifiable risk factor (i.e., family history of diabetes) among African American potential donors, *APOL1* testing should be pursued if available and with zero or one renal risk variant supporting consideration for donation. The presence of two *APOL1* renal risk variants would be considered "high risk." For potential donors with modifiable risk factors, behavioral modifications should be encouraged, but may not necessarily preclude donation. The use of *APOL1* genotyping in the donor candidate evaluation is discussed further in Chap. 8, Genetic Kidney Disease.

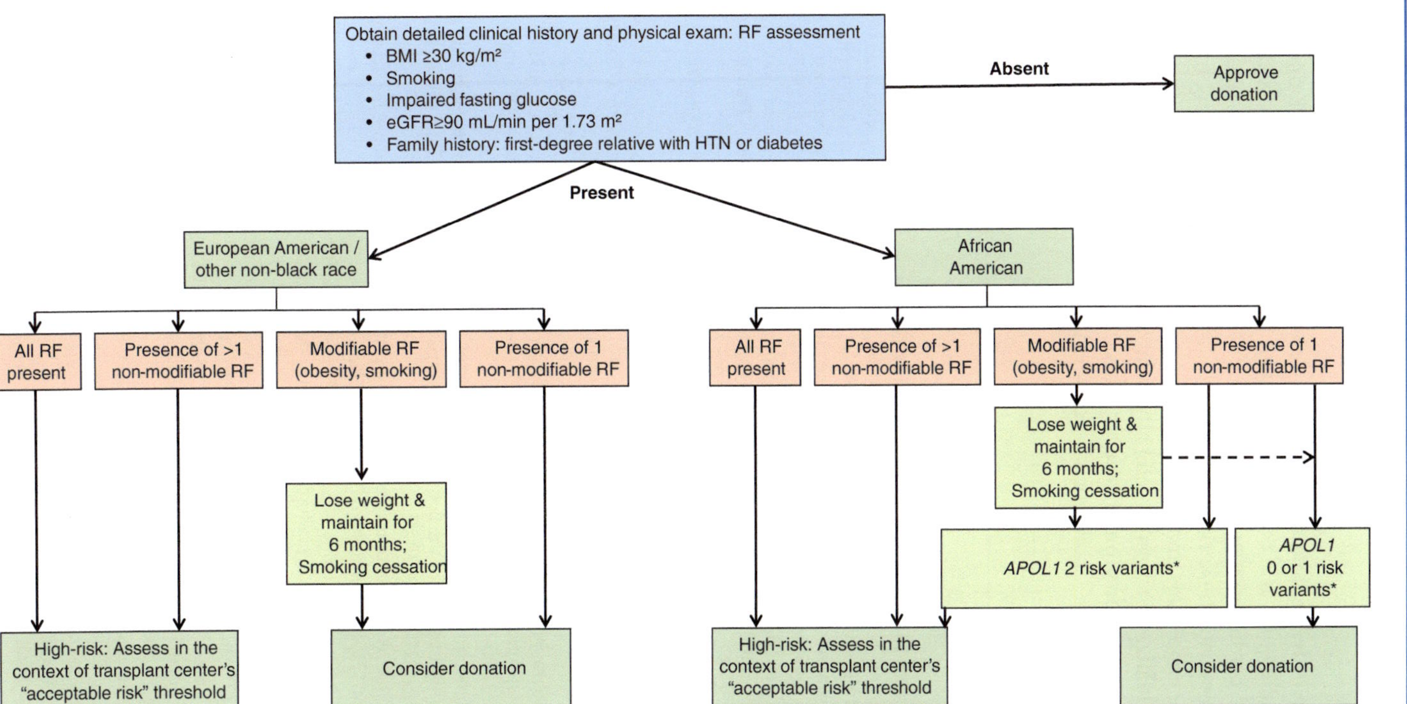

Fig. 6.2 Algorithm for selection of young living kidney donor candidates [24]. *Abbreviations*: *APOL1* apolipoprotein L1, *HTN* hypertension, *RF* risk factor

Conclusion

The evaluation of living donor candidates to determine suitability for kidney donation can be challenging. It is the responsibility of the transplant team to assess donor candidates for cardiovascular and metabolic risks prior to donation and to adequately communicate those risks to potential donors. Especially among medically complex donor candidates, many decisions related to final candidacy determination require individualization. Some medically complex living donor candidates can be safely accepted for donation. However, adequate communication of risks and informed consent is paramount, coupled with individualized, shared decision-making.

References

1. Wang JH, Skeans MA, Israni AK. Current status of kidney transplant outcomes: dying to survive. Adv Chronic Kidney Dis. 2016;23(5):281–6. https://doi.org/10.1053/j.ackd.2016.07.001.
2. Naik AS, Cibrik DM, Sakhuja A, Samaniego M, Lu Y, Shahinian V, et al. Temporal trends, center-level variation, and the impact of prevalent state obesity rates on acceptance of obese living kidney donors. Am J Transplant. 2018;18(3):642–9. https://doi.org/10.1111/ajt.14519.
3. Textor SC, Taler SJ, Driscoll N, Larson TS, Gloor J, Griffin M, et al. Blood pressure and renal function after kidney donation from hypertensive living donors. Transplantation. 2004;78(2):276–82. https://doi.org/10.1097/01.Tp.0000128168.97735.B3.
4. Matas AJ. Transplantation using marginal living donors. Am J Kidney Dis. 2006;47(2):353–5. https://doi.org/10.1053/j.ajkd.2005.11.025.
5. Mandelbrot DA, Pavlakis M, Danovitch GM, Johnson SR, Karp SJ, Khwaja K, et al. The medical evaluation of living kidney donors: a survey of US transplant centers. Am J Transplant. 2007;7(10):2333–43. https://doi.org/10.1111/j.1600-6143.2007.01932.x.
6. Taler SJ, Messersmith EE, Leichtman AB, Gillespie BW, Kew CE, Stegall MD, et al. Demographic, metabolic, and blood pressure characteristics of living kidney donors spanning five decades. Am J Transplant. 2013;13(2):390–8. https://doi.org/10.1111/j.1600-6143.2012.04321.x.
7. Niemi M, Mandelbrot DA. The outcomes of living kidney donation from medically complex donors: implications for the donor and the recipient. Curr Transplant Rep. 2014;1(1):1–9. https://doi.org/10.1007/s40472-013-0001-6.
8. Caliskan Y, Yildiz A. Evaluation of the medically complex living kidney donor. J Transplant. 2012;2012:450471. https://doi.org/10.1155/2012/450471.
9. Reese PP, Feldman HI, McBride MA, Anderson K, Asch DA, Bloom RD. Substantial variation in the acceptance of medically complex live kidney donors across US renal transplant centers. Am J Transplant. 2008;8(10):2062–70. https://doi.org/10.1111/j.1600-6143.2008.02361.x.
10. Davis CL, Cooper M. The state of U.S. living kidney donors. Clin J Am Soc Nephrol. 2010;5(10):1873–80. https://doi.org/10.2215/cjn.01510210.
11. Sachdeva M, Rosen LM, Varghese J, Fishbane S, Molmenti EP. Weight trends in United States living kidney donors: analysis of the UNOS database. World J Transplant. 2015;5(3):137–44. https://doi.org/10.5500/wjt.v5.i3.137.
12. Clayton PA, Saunders JR, McDonald SP, Allen RD, Pilmore H, Saunder A, et al. Risk-factor profile of living kidney donors: the Australia and New Zealand dialysis and transplant living kidney donor registry 2004–2012. Transplantation. 2016;100(6):1278–83. https://doi.org/10.1097/tp.0000000000000877.
13. Ibrahim HN, Foley R, Tan L, Rogers T, Bailey RF, Guo H, et al. Long-term consequences of kidney donation. N Engl J Med. 2009;360(5):459–69. https://doi.org/10.1056/NEJMoa0804883.

14. Segev DL, Muzaale AD, Caffo BS, Mehta SH, Singer AL, Taranto SE, et al. Perioperative mortality and long-term survival following live kidney donation. JAMA. 2010;303(10):959–66. https://doi.org/10.1001/jama.2010.237.

15. Muzaale AD, Massie AB, Wang MC, Montgomery RA, McBride MA, Wainright JL, et al. Risk of end-stage renal disease following live kidney donation. JAMA. 2014;311(6):579–86. https://doi.org/10.1001/jama.2013.285141.

16. Anjum S, Muzaale AD, Massie AB, Bae S, Luo X, Grams ME, et al. Patterns of end-stage renal disease caused by diabetes, hypertension, and glomerulonephritis in live kidney donors. Am J Transplant. 2016;16(12):3540–7. https://doi.org/10.1111/ajt.13917.

17. Locke JE, Reed RD, Massie A, MacLennan PA, Sawinski D, Kumar V, et al. Obesity increases the risk of end-stage renal disease among living kidney donors. Kidney Int. 2017;91(3):699–703. https://doi.org/10.1016/j.kint.2016.10.014.

18. Lin J, McGovern ME, Brunelli SM, Gaccione P, Malek S, Tullius SG, et al. Longitudinal trends and influence of BMI mismatch in living kidney donors and their recipients. Int Urol Nephrol. 2011;43(3):891–7. https://doi.org/10.1007/s11255-011-9921-1.

19. Berger JC, Muzaale AD, James N, Hoque M, Wang JM, Montgomery RA, et al. Living kidney donors ages 70 and older: recipient and donor outcomes. Clin J Am Soc Nephrol. 2011;6(12):2887–93. https://doi.org/10.2215/cjn.04160511.

20. Issa N, Stephany B, Fatica R, Nurko S, Krishnamurthi V, Goldfarb DA, et al. Donor factors influencing graft outcomes in live donor kidney transplantation. Transplantation. 2007;83(5):593–9. https://doi.org/10.1097/01.tp.0000256284.78721.ba.

21. Patel S, Cassuto J, Orloff M, Tsoulfas G, Zand M, Kashyap R, et al. Minimizing morbidity of organ donation: analysis of factors for perioperative complications after living-donor nephrectomy in the United States. Transplantation. 2008;85(4):561–5. https://doi.org/10.1097/TP.0b013e3181643ce8.

22. Chen GD, Gu JL, Zhang XD, Qiu J, Wang CX, Chen LZ. Donor factors predictive for poor outcomes of living donor kidney transplantation. Transplant Proc. 2013;45(4):1445–8. https://doi.org/10.1016/j.transproceed.2012.11.015.

23. Massie AB, Leanza J, Fahmy LM, Chow EK, Desai NM, Luo X, et al. A risk index for living donor kidney transplantation. Am J Transplant. 2016;16(7):2077–84. https://doi.org/10.1111/ajt.13709.

24. Sawinski D, Locke JE. Evaluation of kidney donors: core curriculum 2018. Am J Kidney Dis. 2018;71(5):737–47. https://doi.org/10.1053/j.ajkd.2017.10.018.

25. Lam NN, Lentine KL, Garg AX. Renal and cardiac assessment of living kidney donor candidates. Nat Rev Nephrol. 2017;13:420. https://doi.org/10.1038/nrneph.2017.43.

26. Heimbach JK, Taler SJ, Prieto M, Cosio FG, Textor SC, Kudva YC, et al. Obesity in living kidney donors: clinical characteristics and outcomes in the era of laparoscopic donor nephrectomy. Am J Transplant. 2005;5(5):1057–64. https://doi.org/10.1111/j.1600-6143.2005.00791.x.

27. Lentine KL, Lam NN, Axelrod D, Schnitzler MA, Garg AX, Xiao H, et al. Perioperative complications after living kidney donation: a national study. Am J Transplant. 2016;16(6):1848–57. https://doi.org/10.1111/ajt.13687.

28. Jacobs SC, Cho E, Dunkin BJ, Bartlett ST, Flowers JL, Jarrell B, et al. Laparoscopic nephrectomy in the markedly obese living renal donor. Urology. 2000;56(6):926–9. https://doi.org/10.1016/S0090-4295(00)00813-X.

29. Chow GK, Prieto M, Bohorquez HE, Stegall MD. Hand-assisted laparoscopic donor nephrectomy for morbidly obese patients. Transplant Proc. 2002;34(2):728. https://doi.org/10.1016/S0041-1345(02)02626-X.

30. Lafranca JA, Hagen SM, Dols LF, Arends LR, Weimar W, Ijzermans JN, et al. Systematic review and meta-analysis of the relation between body mass index and short-term donor outcome of laparoscopic donor nephrectomy. Kidney Int. 2013;83(5):931–9. https://doi.org/10.1038/ki.2012.485.

31. Mascali A, Franzese O, Nistico S, Campia U, Lauro D, Cardillo C, et al. Obesity and kidney disease: beyond the hyperfiltration. Int J Immunopathol Pharmacol. 2016;29(3):354–63. https://doi.org/10.1177/0394632016643550.

32. Chagnac A, Weinstein T, Korzets A, Ramadan E, Hirsch J, Gafter U. Glomerular hemodynamics in severe obesity. Am J Physiol Renal Physiol. 2000;278(5):F817–22. https://doi.org/10.1152/ajprenal.2000.278.5.F817.

33. Praga M, Hernandez E, Herrero JC, Morales E, Revilla Y, Diaz-Gonzalez R, et al. Influence of obesity on the appearance of proteinuria and renal insufficiency after unilateral nephrectomy. Kidney Int. 2000;58(5):2111–8. https://doi.org/10.1111/j.1523-1755.2000.00384.x.

34. Grams ME, Sang Y, Levey AS, Matsushita K, Ballew S, Chang AR, et al. Kidney-failure risk projection for the living kidney-donor candidate. N Engl J Med. 2016;374(5):411–21. https://doi.org/10.1056/NEJMoa1510491.

35. Brenner BM, Lawler EV, Mackenzie HS. The hyperfiltration theory: a paradigm shift in nephrology. Kidney Int. 1996;49(6):1774–7. https://doi.org/10.1038/ki.1996.265.

36. Hostetter TH, Olson JL, Rennke HG, Venkatachalam MA, Brenner BM. Hyperfiltration in remnant nephrons: a potentially adverse response to renal ablation. Am J Physiol. 1981;241(1):F85–93. https://doi.org/10.1152/ajprenal.1981.241.1.F85.

37. Pek GXW, Ngoh CLY, Teo BW, Vathsala A, Goh BYS, Yong CHR, et al. Visceral obesity in Asian living kidney donors significantly impacts early renal function after donor nephrectomy. World J Urol. 2019;37:2231–6. https://doi.org/10.1007/s00345-018-2566-2.

38. Chakkera HA, Chang YH, Thomas LF, Avula RT, Amer H, Lerman LO, et al. Obesity correlates with glomerulomegaly but is not associated with kidney dysfunction early after donation. Transplant Direct. 2015;1(1):1–6. https://doi.org/10.1097/txd.0000000000000510.

39. Serrano OK, Sengupta B, Bangdiwala A, Vock DM, Dunn TB, Finger EB, et al. Implications of excess weight on kidney donation: long-term consequences of donor nephrectomy in obese donors. Surgery. 2018;164(5):1071–6. https://doi.org/10.1016/j.surg.2018.07.015.

40. Lentine KL, Koraishy FM, Sarabu N, Naik AS, Lam NN, Garg AX, et al. Associations of obesity with antidiabetic medication use after living kidney donation: an analysis of linked national registry and pharmacy fill records. Clin Transplant. 2019;33:e13696. https://doi.org/10.1111/ctr.13696.

41. Kaisar MO, Nicol DL, Hawley CM, Mudge DW, Johnson DW, Preston JM, et al. Change in live donor characteristics over the last 25 years: a single centre experience. Nephrology (Carlton). 2008;13(7):646–50. https://doi.org/10.1111/j.1440-1797.2008.01039.x.

42. Delmonico FJJoM, Philosophy, Council of the Transplantation Society. A report of the Amsterdam forum on the care of the live kidney donor: data and medical guidelines. Transplantation. 2005;79:S53–66, 26:368. https://pubmed.ncbi.nlm.nih.gov/15785361/.

43. Lentine KL, Kasiske BL, Levey AS, Adams PL, Alberu J, Bakr MA, et al. KDIGO clinical practice guideline on the evaluation and care of living kidney donors. Transplantation. 2017;101(8S Suppl 1):S1–S109. https://doi.org/10.1097/tp.0000000000001769.

44. Abramowicz D, Cochat P, Claas FH, Heemann U, Pascual J, Dudley C, et al. European renal best practice guideline on kidney donor and recipient evaluation and perioperative care. Nephrol Dial Transplant. 2015;30(11):1790–7. https://doi.org/10.1093/ndt/gfu216.

45. Issa N, Sanchez OA, Kukla A, Riad SM, Berglund DM, Ibrahim HN, et al. Weight gain after kidney donation: association with increased risks of type 2 diabetes and hypertension. Clin Transpl. 2018;32(9):e13360. https://doi.org/10.1111/ctr.13360.

46. Narayan KM, Boyle JP, Thompson TJ, Sorensen SW, Williamson DF. Lifetime risk for diabetes mellitus in the United States. JAMA. 2003;290(14):1884–90. https://doi.org/10.1001/jama.290.14.1884.

47. Plantinga LC, Crews DC, Coresh J, Miller ER 3rd, Saran R, Yee J, et al. Prevalence of chronic kidney disease in US adults with undiagnosed diabetes or prediabetes. Clin J Am Soc Nephrol. 2010;5(4):673–82. https://doi.org/10.2215/cjn.07891109.

48. Chandran S, Masharani U, Webber AB, Wojciechowski DM. Prediabetic living kidney donors have preserved kidney function at 10 years after donation. Transplantation. 2014;97(7):748–54. https://doi.org/10.1097/01.TP.0000438625.91095.8b.

49. Guthoff M, Nadalin S, Fritsche A, Konigsrainer A, Haring HU, Heyne N. The medically complex living kidney donor: glucose metabolism as principal cause of donor declination. Ann Transplant. 2016;21:39–45.

50. Bellamy L, Casas J-P, Hingorani AD, Williams D. Type 2 diabetes mellitus after gestational diabetes: a systematic review and meta-analysis. Lancet. 2009;373(9677):1773–9. https://doi.org/10.1016/S0140-6736(09)60731-5.

51. Ibrahim HN, Berglund DM, Jackson S, Vock DM, Foley RN, Matas AJ. Renal consequences of diabetes after kidney donation. Am J Transplant. 2017;17(12):3141–8. https://doi.org/10.1111/ajt.14416.

52. Andrews PA, Burnapp L, Manas D, Bradley JA, Dudley C. Summary of the British Transplantation Society/Renal Association U.K. guidelines for living donor kidney transplantation. Transplantation. 2012;93(7):666–73. https://doi.org/10.1097/TP.0b013e318247a7b7.

53. AST/ASTS/NATCO/UNOS Joint Societies Work Group: Evaluation of the living kidney donor—a consensus document from the AST/ASTS/NATCO/UNOS Joint Societies Work Group. Presented at the Joint Societies Work Group of the Joint Societies Steering Committee; September 27–28, 2010, Rockville, MD.

54. Boudville N, Isbel N. The CARI guidelines. Donors at risk: impaired glucose tolerance. Nephrology (Carlton). 2010;15 Suppl 1:S133–6. https://doi.org/10.1111/j.1440-1797.2009.01222.x.

55. Chen J, Muntner P, Hamm LL, Jones DW, Batuman V, Fonseca V, et al. The metabolic syndrome and chronic kidney disease in U.S. adults. Ann Intern Med. 2004;140(3):167–74. https://doi.org/10.7326/0003-4819-140-3-200402030-00007.

56. Zammit AR, Katz MJ, Derby C, Bitzer M, Lipton RB. Metabolic syndrome and smoking are associated with future development of advanced chronic kidney disease in older adults. Cardioren Med. 2016;6(2):108–15. https://doi.org/10.1159/000441624.

57. Yoon YE, Choi KH, Lee KS, Kim KH, Yang SC, Han WK. Impact of metabolic syndrome on postdonation renal function in living kidney donors. Transplant Proc. 2015;47(2):290–4. https://doi.org/10.1016/j.transproceed.2014.10.051.

58. Doucet B, Kostner K, Kaiser O, Hawley C, Isbel N. Live donor study - implications of kidney donation on cardiovascular risk with a focus on lipid parameters including lipoprotein A. Nephrology (Carlton). 2016;21(10):901–4. https://doi.org/10.1111/nep.12792.

59. Mejia-Vilet JM, Cordova-Sanchez BM, Arreola-Guerra JM, Alberu J, Morales-Buenrostro LE. Facing the metabolic syndrome epidemic in living kidney donor programs. Ann Transplant. 2016;21:456–62.

60. Marcusa DP, Schaubel DE, Woodside KJ, Sung RS. Impact of screening for metabolic syndrome on the evaluation of obese living kidney donors. Am J Surg. 2018;215(1):144–50. https://doi.org/10.1016/j.amjsurg.2017.08.019.

61. Glasser SP, Judd S, Basile J, Lackland D, Halanych J, Cushman M, et al. Prehypertension, racial prevalence and its association with risk factors: analysis of the REasons for Geographic And Racial Differences in Stroke (REGARDS) study. Am J Hypertens. 2011;24(2):194–9. https://doi.org/10.1038/ajh.2010.204.

62. Chu KH, Poon CK, Lam CM, Cheuk A, Yim KF, Lee W, et al. Long-term outcomes of living kidney donors: a single centre experience of 29 years. Nephrology (Carlton). 2012;17(1):85–8. https://doi.org/10.1111/j.1440-1797.2011.01524.x.

63. Klag MJ, Whelton PK, Randall BL, Neaton JD, Brancati FL, Ford CE, et al. Blood pressure and end-stage renal disease in men. N Engl J Med. 1996;334(1):13–8. https://doi.org/10.1056/nejm199601043340103.

64. Whelton PK, He J, Perneger TV, Klag MJ. Kidney damage in 'benign' essential hypertension. Curr Opin Nephrol Hypertens. 1997;6(2):177–83. https://doi.org/10.1097/00041552-199703000-00012.

65. Kannel WB, Gordon T, Schwartz MJ. Systolic versus diastolic blood pressure and risk of coronary heart disease. The Framingham study. Am J Cardiol. 1971;27(4):335–46. https://doi.org/10.1016/0002-9149(71)90428-0.

66. Castelli WP. Epidemiology of coronary heart disease: the Framingham study. Am J Med. 1984;76(2a):4–12. https://doi.org/10.1016/0002-9343(84)90952-5.

67. Al Ammary F, Luo X, Muzaale AD, Massie AB, Crews DC, Waldram MM, et al. Risk of ESKD in older live kidney donors with hypertension. Clin J Am Soc Nephrol. 2019;14(7):1048–55. https://doi.org/10.2215/cjn.14031118.

68. Organ Procurement and Transplantation Network (OPTN)/United Network for Organ Sharing (UNOS). Policy 14: Living Donation. Available at: https://optn.transplant.hrsa.gov/governance/policies/. Accessed: 7 Sept 2020.

69. Holscher CM, Bae S, Thomas AG, Henderson ML, Haugen CE, DiBrito SR, et al. Early hypertension and diabetes after living kidney donation: a national cohort study. Transplantation. 2019;103:1216. https://doi.org/10.1097/tp.0000000000002411.

70. Buhler FR, Vesanen K, Watters JT, Bolli P. Impact of smoking on heart attacks, strokes, blood pressure control, drug dose, and quality of life aspects in the International Prospective Primary Prevention Study in Hypertension. Am Heart J. 1988;115(1 Pt 2):282–8. https://doi.org/10.1016/0002-8703(88)90651-5.

71. Dikalov S, Itani HA, Richmond B, Vergeade A, Rahman SMJ, Boutaud O, et al. Tobacco smoking induces cardiovascular mitochondrial oxidative stress, promotes endothelial dysfunction and enhances hypertension. Am J Physiol Heart Circ Physiol. 2019;316:H639–46. https://doi.org/10.1152/ajpheart.00595.2018.

72. Orth SR, Hallan SI. Smoking: a risk factor for progression of chronic kidney disease and for cardiovascular morbidity and mortality in renal patients--absence of evidence or evidence of absence? Clin J Am Soc Nephrol. 2008;3(1):226–36. https://doi.org/10.2215/cjn.03740907.

73. Bleyer AJ, Shemanski LR, Burke GL, Hansen KJ, Appel RG. Tobacco, hypertension, and vascular disease: risk factors for renal functional decline in an older population. Kidney Int. 2000;57(5):2072–9. https://doi.org/10.1046/j.1523-1755.2000.00056.x.

74. Nolan MB, Martin DP, Thompson R, Schroeder DR, Hanson AC, Warner DO. Association between smoking status, preoperative exhaled carbon monoxide levels, and postoperative surgical site infection in patients undergoing elective surgery. JAMA Surg. 2017;152(5):476–83. https://doi.org/10.1001/jamasurg.2016.5704.

75. Yoon YE, Lee HH, Na JC, Huh KH, Kim MS, Kim SI, et al. Impact of cigarette smoking on living kidney donors. Transplant Proc. 2018;50(4):1029–33. https://doi.org/10.1016/j.transproceed.2018.02.050.

76. Heldt J, Torrey R, Han D, Baron P, Tenggardjaja C, McLarty J, et al. Donor smoking negatively affects donor and recipient renal function following living donor nephrectomy. Adv Urol. 2011;2011:929263. https://doi.org/10.1155/2011/929263.

77. Underwood PW, Sheetz KH, Cron DC, Terjimanian MN, Englesbe MJ, Waits SA. Cigarette smoking in living kidney donors: donor and recipient outcomes. Clin Transpl. 2014;28(4):419–22. https://doi.org/10.1111/ctr.12330.

78. Abecassis M, Adams M, Adams P, Arnold RM, Atkins CR, Barr ML, et al. Consensus statement on the live organ donor. JAMA. 2000;284(22):2919–26. https://doi.org/10.1001/jama.284.22.2919.

79. Garg AX, Meirambayeva A, Huang A, Kim J, Prasad GV, Knoll G, et al. Cardiovascular disease in kidney donors: matched cohort study. BMJ (Clinical research ed). 2012;344:e1203. https://doi.org/10.1136/bmj.e1203.

80. Reese PP, Bloom RD, Feldman HI, Rosenbaum P, Wang W, Saynisch P, et al. Mortality and cardiovascular disease among older live kidney donors. Am J Transplant. 2014;14(8):1853–61. https://doi.org/10.1111/ajt.12822.

81. Mjoen G, Hallan S, Hartmann A, Foss A, Midtvedt K, Oyen O, et al. Long-term risks for kidney donors. Kidney Int. 2014;86(1):162–7. https://doi.org/10.1038/ki.2013.460.

82. Fleisher LA, Fleischmann KE, Auerbach AD, Barnason SA, Beckman JA, Bozkurt B, et al. 2014 ACC/AHA guideline on perioperative cardiovascular evaluation and management of patients undergoing noncardiac surgery: a report of the American College of Cardiology/American Heart Association task force on practice guidelines. J Am Coll Cardiol. 2014;64(22):e77–137. https://doi.org/10.1016/j.jacc.2014.07.944.

83. Richardson R, Connelly M, Dipchand C, Garg AX, Ghanekar A, Houde I, et al. Kidney paired donation protocol for participating donors 2014. Transplantation. 2015;99(10 Suppl 1):S1–S88. https://doi.org/10.1097/tp.0000000000000918.

84. Newell KA, Formica RN, Gill JS, Schold JD, Allan JS, Covington SH, et al. Integrating APOL1 gene variants into renal transplantation: considerations arising from the American

Society of Transplantation Expert Conference. Am J Transplant. 2017;17(4):901–11. https://doi.org/10.1111/ajt.14173.

85. Locke JE, Sawinski D, Reed RD, Shelton B, MacLennan PA, Kumar V, et al. Apolipoprotein L1 and chronic kidney disease risk in young potential living kidney donors. Ann Surg. 2018;267(6):1161–8. https://doi.org/10.1097/sla.0000000000002174.

86. Freedman BI, Moxey-Mims MM, Alexander A, Astor BC, Birdwell KC, Bowden DW, et al. On behalf of APOLLO Steering Committee. APOL1 long-term kidney transplantation outcomes network (APOLLO): design and rationale. Kidney Int Rep. 2020;5:278–88. https://doi.org/10.1016/j.ekir.2019.11.022.

Infection and Cancer Screening in Living Donor Candidates

7

Mary Ann Lim, Eric Au, Blair Weikert, Germaine Wong, and Deirdre Sawinski

Evaluation and Management of the Living Donor Candidate to Prevent Infection Transmission

A crucial component of the living kidney donor evaluation includes the assessment of infectious risk through screening of donor candidates for infections that may affect their health and for infections with potential for inadvertent transmission to their transplant recipients. To facilitate this assessment, both the Organ Procurement and Transplantation Network (OPTN) and Kidney Disease: Improving Global Outcomes (KDIGO) have issued guidelines for infectious disease screening and evaluation of living donors [1, 2].

Donor-derived infections can be classified as "expected" or "unexpected" [2]. Scenarios such as that of cytomegalovirus (CMV) transmission from a CMV antibody-positive donor to a CMV antibody-negative recipient is considered "expected." These "expected" infections tend to occur not infrequently in recipients and are managed by surveillance and/or prophylactic strategies in the recipient post-transplant. "Unexpected" donor-derived infections are those that are transmitted despite screening because of false-negative serologic testing, such as transmission

M. A. Lim · D. Sawinski (✉)
Renal, Electrolyte and Hypertension Division, Department of Medicine, Perelman School of Medicine, Philadelphia, PA, USA
e-mail: Maryann.lim@uphs.upenn.edu; Deirdre.sawinski@uphs.upenn.edu

E. Au · G. Wong
Sydney School of Public Health, University of Sydney, Sydney, NSW, Australia
e-mail: e.au@sydney.edu.au; germaine.wong@health.nsw.gov.au

B. Weikert
Division of Infectious Diseases, Department of Medicine, Perelman School of Medicine, Philadelphia, PA, USA
e-mail: blair.weikert@uphs.upenn.edu

of human immunodeficiency virus (HIV) from a donor candidate after negative testing in the window period of infection.

A thorough medical history, physical examination, and laboratory testing are imperative to identify a history of prior infections and infectious disease risk factors in potential donors, thereby mitigating donor-derived disease transmissions. While routine screening for some transmissible infections is recommended universally, such as for CMV, Epstein-Barr (EBV), syphilis, HIV, hepatitis B virus (HBV), and hepatitis C virus (HCV), focused testing for other transmissible infections will depend on a particular donor candidate's risk factors.

In this section, we first review considerations to properly identify individuals at increased risk for certain infections. This is followed by a discussion of infections that are routinely screened for in all donor candidates as well as a review of seasonal and geographic infectious considerations. For each specific infection, we provide screening and confirmatory testing recommendations, optimum timing for testing, and implications of positive testing for proceeding with organ donation. A summary table (Table 7.1) is provided at the end of this chapter.

Identifying Risk Factors

The following factors should be considered and should be included in the medical history when evaluating a donor candidate's infectious risk:

- *Geographic risks:* place of birth, prolonged time of residence at certain locations, travel history, and military postings (if applicable)

- *Occupational risks:* healthcare work, veterinary care work, military service, landscaping, park ranger service, and any occupation that involves travel

- *Seasonal risks:* for mosquito or tick-borne diseases

- *Recreational risks:* hunting, camping, gardening, and other outdoor sports

- *Animal exposure:* pets, farm animals, lab/research animals, and occupational exposures

- *Sexual risks:* behaviors that confer an increased risk for transmission of HIV, HBV, or HCV infection as defined by the US Public Health Service (PHS) (Table 7.2) [3]

Donor candidates who have risk factors for, have a personal history of, or have been in close contact with/have family members with history of seasonal or geographic infections must see a transplant infectious disease expert as part of the evaluation process.

Table 7.1 Summary of recommended screening tests for living donor candidates. (Adapted from [1–11])

Disease	Who to screen	Screening test	Confirmatory test	Timing of testing	Implications for donation
CMV	All donor candidates	Anti-CMV IgG		At initial screening	Guide posttransplant care
EBV	All donor candidates	Anti-EBV IgG		At initial screening	Guide posttransplant care
Syphilis	All donor candidates	RPR, VDRL or TRUST	Anti-*T. pallidum* Ab	• At initial screening • If risk factors, repeat as close to donation as possible if risk factors	Donation after appropriate treatment of donor with latent disease may be considered with informed consent of recipient and monitoring posttransplant
HIV	All donor candidates	• Anti-HIV 1/2 Ab or Ag/Ab • If high risk: HIV NAT or Ag/Ab	HIV NAT or HIV Ag/Ab combination testing	• At initial screening and within 28 days of donation • If high risk, consider retesting 14 days before donation	Donation from HIV+ candidate contraindicated unless part of an approved research protocol
HBV	All donor candidates	• Anti-Hbc Ab and HBSAg	HBV NAT		Donation from HBsAg+ candidate contraindicated for non-immune recipient, but may be considered for recipients with protective immunity with informed consent of recipient, monitoring posttransplant, and possible recipient HBV treatment posttransplant
HCV	All donor candidates	Anti-HCV Ab and HCV NAT			Donation from HCV+ candidate contraindicated unless part of an approved research protocol
Histoplasmosis	Personal (residence or travel in high-risk geographical area), social (hobbies, employment), or medical risk factors (prior history)	• Chest radiograph • If symptoms of active disease: serum and urine antigen complement fixation, immunodiffusion			• Donation deferred until treatment of active disease (for least 3–6 months) and with negative serum antigen and urine antigen <2 ng/ml. • Close monitoring of recipient with clinical symptoms and serial urine and serum antigen testing

(continued)

Table 7.1 (continued)

Disease	Who to screen	Screening test	Confirmatory test	Timing of testing	Implications for donation
Coccidioidomycosis	Personal (residence or travel in high-risk geographical area), medical risk factors (prior history)	Chest radiograph, enzyme immunoassay	Complement fixation and immunodiffusion serologies		• Donation deferred for active disease until resolution of symptoms (if any), normalization of chest imaging, and at least a fourfold reduction in complement fixation titers. • Recipients should have pretransplant serologic testing. Close monitoring of recipient for clinical symptoms, and serologic testing if unexplained fever
Strongyloides	Personal (residence or travel in high risk geographical area), social (soil exposure from job/hobbies) or medical risk factors (prior history)	Strongyloides Ab testing (ELISA preferred) and/ or stool ova and parasites exam			• Donation may proceed after appropriate treatment • Consider treating donor for another round 2 weeks after initial treatment if risk for autoinfection
Chagas	Personal (residence or travel in high risk geographical area, children of mother from endemic area), medical (prior history, received transfusion in endemic area)	ELISA, indirect immunofluorescence, indirect hemagglutination	Confirmatory serologic testing		Donation considered on case by case basis

Tuberculosis	Personal (residence or travel in high-risk geographical area), social (employment, incarceration, homelessness, substance abuse), or medical risk factors (known untreated TB, prior history)	Chest radiograph, tuberculin skin testing, interferon gamma release assay	Acid-fast bacilli stain and culture for active infection	At initial testing, but repeat as close to donation as possible if with risk factors	• Donation contraindicated from candidates with active TB contraindicated. • Donation after complete treatment of active TB may be considered. • Donation after initiation of chemoprophylaxis of latent TB may be considered. • In both cases, informed consent of recipient and close follow-up posttransplant required. Consider chemoprophylaxis of recipient if donor did not complete latent TB treatment.
West Nile	Mosquito exposure, blood transfusion during high-risk season and at high-risk location	WNV NAT			Donation should be deferred
Zika	Mosquito exposure/ travel to endemic areas, sexually transmitted	NAT?			Donation should be deferred

Source: Adapted from [1–11]
Abbreviations: *CMV* Cytomegalovirus, *EBV* Epstein-Barr virus, *ELISA* Enzyme-linked immunosorbent assay, *HBV* Hepatitis B virus, *HCV* Hepatitis C virus, *HIV* Human immunodeficiency virus, *NAT* Nucleic acid test, *RPR* Rapid Plasma Reagin, *TRUST* Toluidine red unheated serum test, *TB* Tuberculosis, *VDRL* Venereal Disease Research Lab, *WNV* West Nile virus

Table 7.2 US Public Health Service (PHS) 2013 screening for factors associated with increased likelihood of recent HIV, HBV, or HCV infection. (From Seem et al. [3])

1. Have you had sex with a person known or suspected to have HIV, HBV, or HCV infection in the preceding 12 months?
2. For men – have you had sex with men (MSM) in the preceding 12 months?
3. For women – have you had sex with a man with a history of MSM behavior in the preceding 12 months?
4. Have you had sex in exchange for money or drugs in the preceding 12 months?
5. Have you had sex with a person who had sex in exchange for money or drugs in the preceding 12 months?
6. Have you had sex with a person who injected drugs by intravenous, intramuscular, or subcutaneous route for nonmedical reasons in the preceding 12 months?
7. Have you injected drugs by intravenous, intramuscular, or subcutaneous route for nonmedical reasons in the preceding 12 months?
8. Have you been in lockup, jail, or prison for more than 72 consecutive hours in the preceding 12 months?
9. Have you been newly diagnosed with, or have been treated for, syphilis, gonorrhea, *chlamydia,* or genital ulcers in the preceding 12 months?

Abbreviations: HIV human immunodeficiency virus, *HBV* hepatitis B virus, *HCV* hepatitis C virus

Routine Infectious Screening

Cytomegalovirus

CMV is a ubiquitous herpesvirus that infects most humans. It typically causes an asymptomatic or self-limited febrile illness in immunocompetent individuals and then establishes lifelong latent infection in various reservoir cells [12]. In kidney transplant recipients, CMV can manifest as asymptomatic viremia or as CMV disease, with symptoms such as fever, malaise, and diarrhea; CMV in the transplant recipient is associated with increased risk of allograft failure and death [12–14]. CMV disease in transplant recipients may result from reactivation of recipient's own latent infection or may be transmitted from a CMV-positive kidney donor. The American Society of Transplantation (AST) Infectious Disease Community of Practice (ID-COP) recommends that all donors and transplant candidates should be tested for anti-CMV antibodies (IgG) prior to transplantation to allow for risk stratification and guide prevention strategies and/or prophylaxis [2, 12].

While the highest risk scenario for development of CMV disease is with a CMV antibody-positive donor kidney transplanted into a CMV antibody-negative recipient [14–16], transplant recipients who have anti-CMV IgG are still at risk for CMV reactivation; their risk of developing CMV viremia is the same as those who are CMV +/R-, but they are less likely to develop symptomatic disease [17]. The presence of anti-CMV antibodies in the living donor candidate should not preclude organ donation; rather, this should inform necessary prevention and prophylactic strategies to prevent recipient CMV disease, along with anticipation, early recognition, and prompt treatment of recipient CMV infection or disease should it develop [2, 12, 14].

Epstein-Barr Virus (EBV)

Similar to other members of the herpesvirus family, EBV establishes latency in lymphocytes after initial acute infection, which presents as infectious mononucleosis in most cases; EBV also has the potential for reactivation in the setting of an immunocompromised state. In contrast to the immunocompetent host, EBV reactivation in transplant recipients is usually asymptomatic but increases the likelihood for development of posttransplant lymphoproliferative disorders (PTLD) [18, 19]. All donors and transplant candidates should be tested for anti-EBV antibodies (IgG) prior to transplantation [2]. The presence of anti-EBV IgG should not preclude organ donation but donor and recipient EBV status impacts posttransplant care – EBV-naïve recipients who receive organs from donors with latent EBV infection are more prone to develop EBV-positive PTLD [18, 19].

Syphilis

Syphilis has had a resurgence in the United States since the late 1990s, with a steady increase in the number of cases reported to the Centers for Disease Control and Prevention (CDC). In 2017, the CDC reported 9.5 cases of primary and secondary syphilis in the United States per 100,000 population [20]. Transmission of the spirochete *Treponema pallidum*, the organism responsible for syphilis, is typically via sexual contact; however, transmission through organ transplantation has been reported [21, 22]. The current recommendation is to screen all organ donors for syphilis using a Food and Drug Administration (FDA)-cleared screening or diagnostic test [23]. Screening for syphilis involves initial testing with a non-treponemal test (Rapid Plasma Reagin [RPR] or Venereal Disease Research Laboratory [VDRL] test) and confirmation of any positive result using a treponemal-specific test. Non-treponemal tests are positive in 70–100% of recently infected individuals, becoming undetectable 1–5 years after successful treatment; however, individuals with immunologic or inflammatory disorders can have false-positive non-treponemal tests [24]. In contrast, treponemal-specific tests remain positive after treatment and cannot distinguish between recent, remote, and previously treated infections, but are more specific [24].

Living donor candidates with confirmed syphilis infection must be treated with penicillin; in cases with penicillin allergy, doxycyline is an acceptable alternative. The question of donation from an individual with positive serologic testing is more nuanced. In one report, two recipients were infected with syphilis after receiving organs from a deceased donor with previously treated disease, prompting recommendation for treatment of any recipients from deceased donors with positive serologic testing [21]. The 2017 KDIGO guideline recommends living kidney donation from individuals with latent syphilis may be considered after (1) adequate treatment of syphilis prior to donation, (2) informed consent of the recipient, and (3) establishment of a plan for recipient monitoring [2].

Human Immunodeficiency Virus, Hepatitis B Virus, and Hepatitis C Virus

Transmission of HIV, HBV, and HCV via organ transplantation is a known occurrence [4, 5, 25, 26]. All donor candidate evaluations should include US PHS risk factor screening (Table 7.2) [3]. Any donor candidate with positive risk factor screening should receive individualized counseling on strategies to prevent exposure to HIV, HBV, and HCV during the period prior to donation surgery. The 2017 KDIGO guideline recommends testing all donor candidates for HIV, HBV, and HCV [2]. Testing should be done as close to donation as possible but should be performed within 28 days of donation [2]. It remains controversial whether retesting of high-risk donor candidates closer to the time of donation surgery is necessary or effective [6]. Among transplant programs that retest living donors within 14 days prior to donation, retesting resulted in rare delays, but no cancellation of organ transplants [27].

There are three available HIV testing options: (1) HIV 1 and 2 antibody test, (2) a combined HIV 1 and 2 antibody and p24 antigen test, and (3) viral detection through HIV RNA nucleic acid testing (NAT). The time from infection to the development of detectable antibody can range from 22 days to 6 months; thus, individuals with newly acquired HIV infection may not necessarily have a positive antibody test during the window period [7]. NAT testing detects the virus earlier and reduces the window period to between 5.6 and 10.2 days [28]. The 2017 KDIGO guideline and 2013 PHS guideline recommend that all donor candidates be tested for antibodies to HIV using anti-HIV 1/2 Ab testing or HIV Ag/Ab combination assay, while high-risk donor candidates be tested using HIV NAT testing or HIV Ag/Ab combination assay [2, 3].

HIV-positive individuals were excluded from living donation until recently. In 2013, the HIV Organ Policy Equity (HOPE) Act repealed aspects of the 1984 National Organ Transplant Act (NOTA) that prohibited the known procurement or transplantation of organs from HIV-positive donors. Currently, transplantation of organs from HIV-infected donors to HIV-infected recipients is allowed, but can only happen under the context of research approved by institutional review board [29]. In 2019, the first kidney transplantation in the United States from an HIV-infected living donor was reported [30].

The 2017 KDIGO guideline and 2013 PHS guideline recommend that all donor candidates be screened for HCV using both anti-HCV antibody testing and HCV RNA testing by NAT [2, 3]. Unlike HBV, antibodies against HCV are not protective and persist lifelong, even in individuals who spontaneously clear the virus; it is therefore crucial to know both the HCV antibody and HCV RNA (or NAT) status of any living donor candidate. Prior to the availability of direct acting antivirals (DAAs) for the treatment of HCV, active HCV infection was considered an absolute contraindication to living donation for two reasons: (1) the risk of HCV transmission to the recipient and (2) the risk for HCV-associated kidney disease in the donor. However, with the advent of DAAs, the status of HCV-positive individuals as donor candidates is evolving. It is generally accepted practice at most centers to transplant HCV antibody-positive but NAT-negative deceased donor kidneys into

HCV-negative recipients; no documented transmissions from kidneys in this setting have yet been reported [31]. Because transplantation of kidneys from HCV viremic deceased donors into HCV-negative patients has been performed with promising results, some transplant centers are now doing this under clinical practice protocols [32, 33]. It is plausible that living kidney donation from previously treated HCV-positive donors to HCV-negative recipients may be considered the norm in the future. Donor safety (e.g., donor renal and hepatic function) and recipient safety (ensuring a period of sustained viral response in the donor) should be carefully balanced with the health risks associated with the potential recipient remaining on dialysis.

All donor candidates should undergo HBV screening using anti-hepatitis B core IgG (anti-HBcAb) and hepatitis B surface antigen (HBsAg) testing [2, 3]. Donor candidates with positive anti-HBcAb should receive further testing with HBV NAT to define the risks of transmission. Donors with positive anti-HBcAb, but negative HBsAg and HBV NAT, appear to have low risk of transmission in non-liver organ donations; therefore, no further therapy is needed for kidney transplant recipients from these donors [33]. However, if the recipient has no protective immunity, one may consider antiviral therapy for 1 year following transplant [34]. Because of the potential risk of donor kidney disease, we do not recommend living donation from donors with positive HBsAg and/or HBV NAT, regardless of recipient's protective immunity.

Seasonal and Geographic Infections

Endemic Fungal Infections

Histoplasmosis *Histoplasma capsulatum* can be found worldwide, but is most common in North and Central America, specifically in the Ohio and Mississippi River valleys in the United States [35]. It is typically acquired from inhaling airborne *Histoplasma* spores. Hence, donor candidates who have occupations or hobbies that involve disturbance of and exposure to contaminated bird and bat droppings, such as spelunking, cave exploration, cleaning chicken coops, or construction, are at increased risk of histoplasmosis. Infection is typically asymptomatic, but when present, symptoms can include fever, night sweats, lymphadenopathy, cough, and pulmonary nodules.

However, even in endemic areas, only 0.5% of transplant recipients develop histoplasmosis [8]. Additionally, as 1–5% of healthy persons have positive antigen or antibodies, the AST-ID COP does not recommend routine antigen and antibody screening of all donors from endemic areas [8]. Donors at higher risk of disease transmission include those with a recent or current infection or with a history of active disease. Hence, donor candidates who have a prior history of histoplasmosis, undiagnosed pneumonia in the 2 years preceding donation, or any symptoms suggestive of active infection should have pulmonary imaging performed, along with serologic testing [1, 35]. A positive serum or urine antigen, complement fixation titers of $\geq 1:32$, and H precipitin band by agar gel immunodiffusion all suggest active infection. Organ donation should be deferred for any candidate who has active disease until they (1) are treated for at least 3–6 months (usually with itraconazole), (2) have a negative serum antigen, and (3) have a urine antigen that is <2 ng/ml. The risk of disease transmission following adequate therapy and resolution of antigenemia and antigenuria is low; therefore recipients of adequately treated donors do not require specific prophylaxis [1, 8, 9]. However, informed consent is advised, and close monitoring for clinical symptoms and serial (monthly to quarterly) urine and serum antigen testing of recipients for a year following transplant may be prudent [1].

Coccidioidomycosis *Coccidioides immitis* is found in the San Joaquin Valley in California, and *Coccidioides posadasii* is found in desert soil in the southwestern part of the United States (including Southwestern Arizona and West Texas), Northern Mexico, and parts of Central and South America [1, 8, 36]. The incidence of coccidioidomycosis in transplant recipients ranges from 1.5% to 8.7% in endemic areas [37]. Donor-derived transmissions have been reported and often result in significant morbidity and mortality [38].

Transmission rates of coccidioidomycosis, even by asymptomatic individuals, are high, and because donor-derived disease causes significant morbidity and mortality in transplant recipients, some experts recommend screening all donors who have lived or had a prolonged stay in endemic areas with serologic testing (enzyme-linked immunosorbent assays (ELISA) followed by confirmatory complement fixation and immunodiffusion assays) with or without chest imaging [1, 38]. Donor candidates who have fever, weight loss, and "pneumonia" that is poorly responsive to therapy or unexplained abnormal chest imaging should also be screened and may require sputum cultures or bronchoscopy with culture of bronchoalveolar lavage fluid [1]. Serologic testing should also be performed in donor candidates with known history of coccidioidomycosis as persistently positive serologies may indicate viable organisms [1].

Any potential donor whose initial evaluation suggests evidence of active coccidioidomycosis infection should be further evaluated to determine extent of disease, which will then inform type and length of therapy. Organ donation should be deferred in active coccidioidomycosis infection until treatment is complete and infection is controlled [1, 8]. This usually means resolution of symptoms, normalization of chest imaging, and at least a fourfold reduction in complement fixation titer [1]. Guidelines recommend lifelong prophylaxis for recipients of organs from coccidioidomycosis serology-positive donors, and thus recipient informed consent should be obtained before living donor transplantation [1, 8]. However, prophylaxis does not completely eliminate the risk of infection in recipients and posttransplant surveillance is recommended, ideally at 3–4-month intervals initially and then once or twice per year. A rising antibody titer indicates infection, which must be promptly treated. Any unexplained fever in a recipient of a transplant from a coccidioidomycosis serology-positive donor merits further serologic workup, as well as the necessary cultures to facilitate diagnosis and guide therapy [8].

Endemic Parasitic Infections

Strongyloides *Strongyloides stercoralis* is an intestinal nematode that is endemic in tropical and subtropical countries, but can also be found in the Appalachia and southeastern United States [38]. Initial *Strongyloides* infection occurs when the larvae enter the skin of individuals who walk barefoot in soil contaminated with feces. Infection is often asymptomatic in immunocompetent individuals, but can lead to hyperinfection and disseminated disease in immunocompromised persons [39–43]. Though rare, transmission via transplantation has been reported with significant mortality risks [39–41]. OPTN has mandated screening for *Strongyloides* in donor candidates from endemic areas [1].

The AST-ID COP recommends screening for *Strongyloides* in high-risk donor candidates, defined as (1) born or lived in endemic areas; (2) having occupations such as farming, coal mining, or occupations that involve direct contact with contaminated soil, human waste, or sewage; (3) having eosinophilia and a history of travel to endemic areas; and (4) prior history of *Strongyloides* infection [10].

Donor candidates should be screened by *Strongyloides* serology, and anyone with positive antibody testing should be evaluated by an infectious disease expert. ELISA have higher sensitivity (90%), specificity (99%), positive predictive (97%), and negative predictive (95%) values and are preferred over other methods [40]. The gold standard for diagnosis is stool exam; however, this is only reliable during active larval shedding and may be negative in asymptomatic chronic infection. Infected donors should be treated with a minimum of two consecutive daily doses of ivermectin 200 ug/kg prior to donation [10]. Because of the risk of autoinfection, some experts recommend repeating this in 2 weeks [10]. No follow-up testing is recommended posttreatment, such that the treated donor candidate considered cured and able to proceed with donation, unless re-exposure has occurred [10].

Chagas Disease *Trypanosoma cruzi*, the protozoan parasite responsible for Chagas disease, is estimated to be present in 6–7 million people worldwide, most of whom live in Central America [44]. Based on most recent estimates, approximately 300,000 individuals in the United States are infected with *T. Cruzi* [11, 45]. Infection is typically vector-borne via contact with feces of infected triatomine insects, although vertical transmissions from mother to infant and transmission through blood transfusions and organ transplantation have been reported [10, 46].

Although transmission via living kidney donation has not yet been reported in the United States, this has been described in Mexico and South America [10, 11, 46]. Deceased donor transmission has been reported in the United States [10, 11]. In a report describing the cumulative CDC experience from 2001 to 2011 of recipients who received organs from *T. Cruzi* seropositive donors, with a median follow-up of 29 weeks, transmission was confirmed in two of the 15 (13%) kidney recipients and in the single simultaneous pancreas kidney recipient (100%) [46]. The simultaneous pancreas kidney recipient was diagnosed after presenting with symptoms and eventually died from Chagas myocarditis, while the kidney recipients were both diagnosed by monitoring [46].

The Chagas in Transplant Working Group recommends screening all donor candidates who are born in Latin America for Chagas disease [11]. The AST-ID COP also recommends screening in the following high-risk groups: (1) candidates who were born or lived in endemic areas, (2) children of women who lived in endemic areas whose *T.cruzi* status is positive or unknown, (3) candidates who have received blood transfusions in endemic regions, and (4) candidates with prior history of Chagas disease [10]. Screening serologic testing to detect antibodies must be done in all of these high-risk groups with any of the three commercially available testing kits [10]. If the screening test is positive, a confirmatory test should be performed, and the candidates should be referred to an infectious disease physician. A living donor who is infected with Chagas should receive 30–60 days of trypanocidal treatment prior to the procedure [47]. Type of treatment should be determined with the help of an infectious disease specialist. It is unknown what the risk of transmission is from donor to recipient after they receive therapy [47]. Kidney donation from a candidate with positive serologic testing can be considered on a case-by-case basis after treatment of the donor candidate before donation, informed consent of the recipient, and recipient monitoring after transplant [2, 10]. The Chagas in Transplant Working Group does not recommend against kidney transplantation from this group of donors, as long as appropriate plans for long-term monitoring and follow-up are in place [11]. Posttransplant follow-up of any recipient of kidney from a *T.cruzi*-positive donor must be coordinated with local infectious disease support and should include blood polymerase chain reaction (PCR) testing (through the CDC) for *T. cruzi* DNA and review of peripheral blood smear weekly × 2 months, then every 2 weeks for 3–6 months, and monthly thereafter until 24 months or potentially indefinitely [9–11, 47]. Prophylactic therapy in the recipient is not recommended; however, prompt treatment should be given in the event of detection of any *T. cruzi* infection in the recipient, with benznidazole as first-line therapy or nifurtimox as second-line therapy [10, 11, 47].

Endemic Bacterial Infections

Tuberculosis *Mycobacterium tuberculosis* is one of the most common bacterial causes of donor-derived infections in solid organ transplantation [48]. Although only 4% of posttransplant tuberculosis (TB) is thought to be donor derived, an estimated 17% of recipients with donor-derived TB die as a consequence of the infection [49]. The risk of transmission from a donor with active TB is estimated to be approximately 30%, and while the actual risk of transmission from donors with untreated latent TB is unknown, transmission is thought to be possible [9]. TB transmission has been reported from both deceased and living donors [49].

Consensus-based recommendations for TB screening in living donor candidates include [2, 49]:

1. Risk stratification by:
   (a) Place of birth, residence, or travel to a high risk-geographic area
   (b) Social risk factors including employment (healthcare, prison, homeless shelter, military), incarceration, homelessness, substance abuse, and known TB contact
   (c) Medical risk factors including history of untreated TB, evidence of prior TB, or signs/symptoms consistent with active TB
2. Chest X-ray
3. Consideration for urinalysis, urine acid-fast bacilli smear and culture, and genitourinary imaging of donor candidates from areas with high TB prevalence
4. Immune-based diagnostic testing with tuberculin skin test (TST) or interferon gamma release assay (IGRA) of all donor candidates or those considered increased risk

Active TB is considered a contraindication to living donation [2, 49]. Living kidney donation after adequate therapy of active TB may be considered after (1) informed consent of the recipient and (2) establishing a plan to monitor the recipient and treat posttransplant if indicated. Administration of recipient prophylaxis after transplantation from a living donor with a history of treated active TB infection is controversial, and posttransplant monitoring by an infectious disease expert is advised.

Any donor candidate with latent TB should receive chemoprophylaxis before kidney donation [2, 49]. Kidney donation from individuals with latent TB may be considered under the guidance of an infectious disease expert with initiation of chemoprophylaxis in the donor candidate before donation, informed consent of the recipient, and recipient monitoring after transplant [2, 49]. Chemoprophylaxis of kidney recipients from donors with latent TB should be guided by infectious disease expertise and will depend on donors' length of therapy at the time of donation [2, 49].

Endemic Viral Infections

West Nile Virus *West Nile virus* (WNV) is a flavivirus that primarily infects birds and mosquitoes. Although transmission to humans is primarily through bites from infected *Culex* mosquitoes, transmission has been reported to occur via blood transfusions and organ donation [10, 50, 51]. Once infected, symptoms can range from asymptomatic disease to neuroinvasive disease; in fact, WNV is the most common cause of human neuroinvasive arboviral disease in the continental United States since the late 1990s [51]. In 2016, over 2000 cases of WNV infections were reported to the CDC, and more than 1300 of these were thought to be neuroinvasive [52, 53]. Immunocompromised individuals are more prone to developing neuroinvasive disease (one in 40 infections in immunocompromised individuals, compared to one in 150 immunocompetent individuals) [54]. Reports of transmission via organ transplantation have all been from deceased donation [10, 50, 51]. In a case report and literature review that included published US and Italian data from 2003 to 2011, nine deceased donors transmitted WNV to 24 of 27 recipients (89%), 17 of whom developed encephalitis [50].

Because of the seasonal nature of WNV transmission, year-round testing is not cost-effective. Current OPTN Ad Hoc Disease Transmission Advisory Committee (DTAC) guidance recommends serologic screening of all living donor candidates during periods of WNV activity in areas where they live, work, or have travelled [55]. Two options are given to establish WNV activity: (1) determine when local blood bank switch from year-round mini-pool testing to individual testing, or (2) assume WNV activity from May to November and test everyone during this time frame [10]. The latter may be less cost-effective and give higher false-positive rates, but is simpler, involves less coordination, and is easier for transplant programs to implement [10].

Living donor candidates should be advised on protective measures against mosquito exposures and should ideally be tested for WNV within 2 weeks of organ donation. Testing should include WNV NAT with any one of the two FDA-approved tests [10]. Antibody testing may also be considered since two of nine reported deceased donor transmissions had negative NAT testing but positive IgM antibodies; however, interpretation of positive tests may be complicated by the fact that (1) antibody testing for this purpose has not been evaluated and validated, (2) WMV IgM and IgG may persist for longer than what may be considered relevant (positive for >500 days and 5 years after resolution of viremia, respectively), and (3) WNV antibodies may cross-react with other viruses [10, 56]. There is no effective treatment for WNV; therefore, the AST ID-COP recommends that donation should be delayed for 28 days when WNV NAT screening is positive, followed by repeat NAT and WNV IgM Ab testing, with further decisions based on combined results in consultation with an infectious disease expert.

Zika Virus *Zika virus* (ZKV) is a flavivirus transmitted by *Aedes aegypti*. First recognized in Brazil in 2014, the CDC now lists many countries in Asia, Africa, Central and South America, the Pacific Islands, and the Caribbean as areas where Zika virus can be found [57]. Although 80% of individuals with ZKV are asymptomatic, 20% will have clinical symptoms including rash, arthralgias, conjunctivitis, and encephalitis. Data on Zika virus infection in immunosuppressed patients is limited [58]. Zika virus infection can be sexually transmitted, and congenitally acquired infection has been associated with significant morbidity and mortality; it is therefore a concern for both male and female transplant recipients [59–61]. The risk for transmission of Zika virus via organ donation is unknown but is, theoretically, possible because of the Zika virus transmission in blood transfusions [62]. The 2016 OPTN DTAC guidance recommends considering donor deferral if the living donor candidate (or his/her sexual partner) has a history of travel to endemic areas within 28 days, but donation likely can be considered after an appropriate wait time with consultation from an infectious disease expert [58]. In the case of potential living donors with confirmed Zika infection, donation should be deferred when possible.

Evaluation and Management of the Living Donor Candidate to Prevent Cancer Transmission

Cancer transmission from a kidney donor is a rare event, but can lead to significant morbidity and mortality in transplant recipients. The outcomes of a living donor who develops cancer after donation may also be compromised in the context of reduced kidney function from donation. Screening strategies should be in place to protect donor health and safety and limit the risk of disease transmission through living donation.

Donor-related malignancy can be due to either direct transmission of cancer (donor cancer transmission) or due to cancer arising in cells of donor origin (donor-derived). Donor transmission refers to cancers that develop in transplant recipients due to the transmission of tumors that existed in the donor at the time of transplantation. Donor-derived malignancies are cancers from donor cells where there is no prior clinical history of cancer.

In this section, we first review the current guidelines for cancer screening and evaluation of cancer risks in living kidney donor candidates. We also discuss the available approaches for preventing donor-related malignancy. The epidemiology of donor cancer transmission is described, particularly in the context of donors with a prior cancer history. Finally, we summarize published evidence on recipient outcomes when donor-derived cancer or donor transmission of cancer has occurred.

Cancer Screening in Living Donor Candidates

A thorough history and physical examination of all living kidney donor candidates should be undertaken to evaluate for evidence of past or current malignancy prior to donation and transplantation. The evaluation should include assessing for signs or symptoms of possible malignancy such as new lumps or masses, changes in bowel habit or blood in stool, unintentional weight loss, and details of any previous cancer diagnosis and associated treatment. Donors should be asked about risk factors for cancer such as smoking history and family cancer history. The 2017 Kidney Disease: Improving Global Outcomes (KDIGO) clinical practice guideline and various national and regional guidelines recommend that donor candidates undergo age-appropriate cancer screening tests as recommended for the general population in the donor candidate's place of residence [2, 63, 64]. For donor candidates of the appropriate age and sex, this testing will generally include colorectal cancer screening with fecal occult blood testing or colonoscopy, breast cancer screening with mammography, and cervical cancer screening with Papanicolaou (Pap) test and/or a human papillomavirus (HPV) DNA test [65, 66]. A list of common cancer screening tests is provided in Table 7.3.

Table 7.3 Cancer screening in the evaluation of living donor candidates. (Adapted from American Cancer Society recommendations for the general population [65])

Cancer type	Age	Screening tests
Breast	45 years or older	Mammography every year (age 45–54) or every 1–2 years (55 or older and expected to live 10 or more years)
Cervical	21–29 years	Cervical cytology (Papanicolaou test) every 3 years
	30–65 years	Cervical cytology every 3 years alone or high-risk human papillomavirus (HPV) DNA test every 5 years in combination with cytology (co-testing)
	Over 65 years	No screening if normal result on regular screening for past 10 years
Colorectal	45–75 years	Annual or biennial fecal occult blood testing or colonoscopy
Lung	55–74 years	Low-dose CT scan of lung annually for candidates with at least 30 pack-year smoking history who currently smoke or have quit within the past 15 years
Prostate	Based on risk profile	Individual decision on screening based on risks and benefits. Age criteria for those considering screening • Average risk: 50–69 years • African American or one first-degree relative with prostate cancer: 45 years or older • Multiple family members: 40 years or older

Risk of Cancer Transmission

Evidence on the risk of donor cancer transmission comes largely from observational studies such as case reports, case series, and registry studies. A systematic review of all published peer-reviewed case reports, case series, and registry studies of donor cancer transmission in kidney transplantation until November 2012 found a total of 104 cases of transmitted cancer, with the most common transmitted cancer types being kidney cancers (19%), melanoma (17%), lymphoma (14%), and lung cancers (14%) [67]. Recent analyses from various national registries (including both deceased and living donors) in Europe and the United States have shown an overall low donor cancer transmission risk of around 0.01–0.06% for transplants from all donors, i.e., both donors with and without a known history of cancer [68–71]. In two studies – one from the Italian Transplant Network and the National Transplant Centre (CNT) [69] (29,858 transplants from 11,271 donors) and one from the UK Transplant Registry (30,765 transplants from 14,986 donors) [68] – none of the donors for the reported cases of donor-transmitted cancer were known to have cancer at the time of donation. Reassuringly, in a separate study of all solid organ transplants performed between 1990 and 2008 using the UK Transplant Registry and matched cancer data from the National Cancer Data Repository examining the risk of cancer transmission from donors characterized as having high or unacceptable risk as defined by guidelines from the Council of Europe and the OPTN (Table 7.4), no instances of donor cancer transmission were found in the 133 recipients of organs from 61 donors [73].

The risk of donor cancer transmission is dependent on the type of donor cancer (Table 7.4). In the Israel Penn International Transplant Tumor Registry, a registry with voluntary reporting of outcomes from solid organ transplants from both deceased and living donors with a known history of malignancy, 124 cases of donor cancer transmission were recorded in 296 transplants between 1965 and 2003 [74]. The highest rates of donor cancer transmission occurred in choriocarcinoma (93%), melanoma (74%), and renal cell carcinomas (61%). For deceased donors with

Table 7.4 Summary of risk categories for donor cancer transmission. (From Nalesnik et al. [72])

Risk category	Transmission risk estimate	Cancer type	Recommended acceptance (recipient risk perspective)
No significant risk	0%	Benign tumors	Standard
Minimal	<0.1%	• Skin basal cell and squamous cell carcinoma • Non-melanoma skin cancer in situ • Cervical carcinoma in situ • Noninvasive papillary carcinoma • Resected solitary renal cell carcinoma ≤1 cm, Fuhrman grade I–II	Clinical judgment and informed consent
Low	0.1–1%	• Low-grade CNS tumor (WHO grade I or II) • Resected solitary renal cell carcinoma >1–4 cm, Fuhrman grade I-II • Treated non-CNS malignancy ≥5 years prior with >99% probability of cure	Use in recipients at significant risk without transplant, after informed consent
Intermediate	1–10%	• Breast carcinoma in situ • Colon carcinoma in situ • Resected solitary renal cell carcinoma 4–7 cm, Fuhrman grade I–II • Treated non-CNS malignancy ≥5 years prior with 90–99% probability of cure	Use generally not recommended
High	>10%	• Malignant melanoma • Breast, colon, lung cancer • Renal cell carcinoma >7 cm or Fuhrman grade II–IV • High-grade CNS tumor (WHO grade III or IV) • Leukemia, lymphoma, sarcoma	Not recommended

primary intracranial malignancies, a UK study of 448 donors between 1985 and 2001 found no recorded cases of cancer transmission [75].

However, there are limitations to these estimates of donor cancer transmission, including selective reporting and publication biases as well as incomplete and inaccurate recording in donor and transplant registries [76]. As such, the true incidence of donor cancer transmission could not be ascertained or determined with certainty. In order to better assess the risks of donor cancer transmission, several programs have been established to improve the reporting of donor cancer transmission events. In the United States, potential donor-derived disease transmission events for both deceased and living donor recipients, including suspected donor-transmitted tumors, should be reported to the OPTN [77]. In addition, the NOTIFY library is an online global vigilance and surveillance database which has been set up by the WHO (World Health Organization) and the Italian National Transplant Centre to monitor and collect information on adverse occurrences due to organ or tissue donation [78].

Donor Candidates with a History of Cancer

In donor candidates with a history of cancer, the evaluation process needs to protect the health of the potential donor and minimize the risk of cancer transmission to the transplant recipient. An assessment should be made in discussion with the donor's oncologist regarding the risk of cancer recurrence and the potential need for future treatments, particularly treatments which rely on sufficient kidney function or may cause kidney impairment and subsequently increase the donor's risk of chronic kidney disease or kidney failure. Consideration should also be given to the need for follow-up or restaging imaging which may require adequate kidney function such as computer tomography (CT) and magnetic resonance imaging (MRI) scans with contrast.

In general, active malignancy is an absolute contraindication to organ donation, except for low-grade non-melanoma skin cancers and select cases where a nephrectomy is performed for the treatment of renal cell carcinoma (addressed below). Donation is also contraindicated in donor candidates with a history of cancers with the potential for late recurrence, such as breast cancer and melanoma. In other situations, living kidney donation may be appropriate after successful treatment of cancer and an appropriate waiting period, based on observational studies on the risks of cancer transmission to the recipient [72]. The OPTN DTAC [72] and the European Directorate for the Quality of Medicines and Healthcare (EDQM) [79] have defined risk categories for donor transmission of certain cancer types and provided recommendations on the use of organs from both deceased and living donors. These recommendations are based on review of existing literature (comprising case reports, case series, and registry studies of cancer transmission risk) and expert consensus. A summary of risk categories for donor cancer transmission and recommendations by the OPTN DTAC is provided in Table 7.4 [72]. Recommendations are also provided for benign tumors confirmed by histopathological examination (Table 7.5) [72]. Certain benign tumors have the potential for malignant transformation, and

Table 7.5 Benign tumors and potential for malignancy. (From Nalesnik et al. [72])

Organ/site	Malignant potential	Benign tumor type (and associated malignancy)
Soft tissue, vessels, nerves, blood vessels	Potential for associated malignancy	Paraganglioma (malignant paraganglioma)
	Minimal malignant potential	• Chondroma • Dermatofibroma • Fibroma • Hemangioma • Leiomyoma • Lipoblastoma • Lipoma • Lymphangioma • Osteoma
Thyroid and parathyroid	Potential for associated malignancy	• Follicular adenoma (follicular carcinoma) • Pleomorphic adenoma (adenocarcinoma)
	Minimal malignant potential	Parathyroid adenoma
Salivary gland	Potential for associated malignancy	Pleomorphic adenoma (adenocarcinoma)
	Minimal malignant potential	• Basal cell adenoma • Cystadenoma • Myoepithelioma • Oncocytoma • Sebaceous adenoma • Warthin tumor
Nose, nasopharynx, oropharynx	Minimal malignant potential	• Craniopharyngioma • Nasopharyngeal angiofibroma • Pyogenic granuloma • Sinonasal (Schneiderian) papilloma • Squamous papilloma
Heart and pericardium	Potential for associated malignancy	• Atrial myxoma • Mesothelioma of AV node (malignant mesothelioma)
	Minimal malignant potential	• Fibroma • Papillary fibroelastoma • Rhabdomyoma
Lungs and pleura	Minimal malignant potential	Pulmonary hamartoma
Liver and biliary	Potential for associated malignancy	• Hepatocellular adenoma (hepatocellular carcinoma) • Von Meyenburg complex (VMC) (cholangiocarcinoma)
	Minimal malignant potential	• Adenomyoma • Bile duct adenoma • Cavernous hemangioma • Focal nodular hyperplasia

(continued)

Table 7.5 (continued)

Organ/site	Malignant potential	Benign tumor type (and associated malignancy)
Gastrointestinal tract	Potential for associated malignancy	Adenoma (adenocarcinoma)
	Minimal malignant potential	Fundic gland polyp
Kidney and urinary tract	Potential for associated malignancy	• Angiomyolipoma (may coexist with renal cell neoplasms) • Bladder paraganglioma (malignant paraganglioma) • Oncocytoma (may coexist with renal cell carcinoma)
	Minimal malignant potential	• Cystic nephroma • Fibroepithelial polyp • Metanephric adenoma • Renomedullary interstitial cell tumor
Adrenal	Potential for associated malignancy	Pheochromocytoma (malignant pheochromocytoma)
Ovary, fallopian tubes, uterus	Minimal malignant potential	• Adenofibroma • Adenomatoid tumor • Benign cystadenoma • Benign ovarian fibroma/thecoma • Cystadenofibroma • Dermoid cyst • Endometrial polyp • Luteoma of pregnancy • Ovarian surface papilloma • Uterine leiomyoma
Placenta	Minimal malignant potential	Placental chorangioma
Testes, prostate, seminal vesicles	Minimal malignant potential	• Nephrogenic adenoma • Leiomyoma • Adenomatoid tumor
Breast	Minimal malignant potential	Fibroadenoma

this needs to be considered in the assessment of living donor candidates; by comparison, other benign tumors have little malignant potential, and donation can occur without concern of donor cancer transmission. In all cases of potential organ donation from a donor with a previous history of cancer, the transplant candidate should be counseled about the risks of cancer transmission from the donor so that an informed decision in relation to transplantation options can be made.

Living Donation in the Setting of Known Cancer

It is generally recommended by most clinical practice guidelines that acceptance of donors with prior histories of solid organ and hematological cancers should be considered only in exceptional circumstances following discussion of the risk and benefits with the transplant candidate [2, 63, 64]. However, small renal cell carcinomas may provide a unique circumstance when tumor excision may be curative and mitigate transmission risk sufficiently to allow a kidney to be used for transplantation. Cases of transplantation of kidneys removed from donors with small renal cell carcinomas (TNM stage T1a), with back-table resection of the tumor prior to transplantation, have been reported. Case reports and case series totaling close to 100 living donor transplants have described good transplant outcomes and low rates of cancer recurrence/transmission [80–83]. The 2017 KDIGO living donor guideline recommends that donor candidates with high-grade Bosniak renal cysts (III or higher) or small (T1a) renal cell carcinoma curable by nephrectomy may be acceptable for donation on a case-by-case basis [2]. Procurement and transplantation of living donor kidneys with Bosniak (III or higher) renal cysts or small (T1a) renal cell carcinoma curable in the donor by nephrectomy and amenable to complete excision before implantation should proceed only after detailed informed consent of donor and recipient and donor and recipient understanding and acceptance of these risks. Similarly, the 2018 British Transplant Society-Renal Association Living Donor Kidney Transplantation Guidelines recommend that donor candidates with an incidental small renal mass (<4 cm) that appears to be renal cell carcinomas may be considered on a case-by-case basis with ex vivo resection of tumor, after multidisciplinary input from nephrology, urology, and oncology teams and appropriate informed consent from both donor and recipient [64].

It should be emphasized that decisions on the management of renal tumors should always be made in the best interest of the specific patient with consideration of the full range of possible treatment options including nephron-sparing surgery (partial nephrectomy), cryotherapy, and radio-ablation, rather than focused on the aim of organ donation [64]. Potential transplant recipients need to be counseled on the risks of cancer recurrence and the benefits of transplantation compared to waiting for a deceased donor organ. After transplantation, both the donor and recipient should receive surveillance monitoring for the possibility of cancer recurrence as per usual recommendations after nephron-sparing surgery for renal tumors [81].

Outcomes after Donor Cancer Transmission

While donor cancer transmission occurs rarely, the outcomes after donor cancer transmission are poor, with high rates of graft loss and mortality [48, 67, 74]. Treatment options for donor-transmitted cancers may include reduction in immunosuppression (with an associated risk of graft rejection and graft loss), removal of transmitted cancer in the transplanted kidney via graft nephrectomy, and other standard cancer therapies such as chemotherapy and radiotherapy [67]. In donor-derived

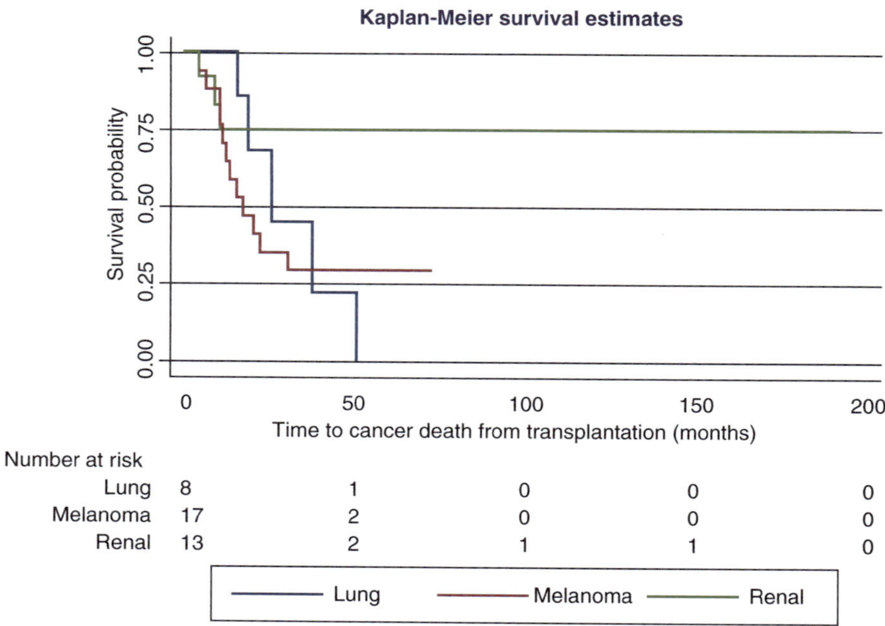

Fig. 7.1 Survival of recipients after diagnosis of donor-transmitted cancer. (From Xiao et al. [67])

malignancies reported to the OPTN, 50% for recipients (10 out of 20) were reported to have died from the transmitted malignancy [48]. High rates of mortality were also reported for certain cancer types in the Israel Penn International Transplant Tumor Registry, with 68% mortality for transmitted choriocarcinoma, 58% for malignant melanoma, and 15% for renal cell carcinoma [74]. In a systematic review of donor cancer transmission by Xiao et al. [67], high rates of cancer-related deaths were reported for donor-transmitted melanoma (median time from transplantation to death of 12.5 months) and donor-transmitted lung cancer (median time from transplantation to death of 25.0 months) (Fig. 7.1). A more favorable prognosis was reported for donor-transmitted renal cancers, with a 5-year survival rate of over 70% in this study.

Conclusion

Living donor candidates must undergo a comprehensive predonation assessment to ensure the health of the potential donor and minimize the risk of inadvertent transmission of infections and cancers to the intended recipient.

Donor-derived infections can be mitigated by obtaining a thorough medical history that includes detailed social history, comprehensive physical examination, and directed laboratory testing. Routine screening for CMV, EBV, syphilis, HIV, HBV, and HCV is universally recommended for all donors, while focused testing for other transmissible seasonal and geographic infections will depend on a particular donor candidate's risk profile. As new infections emerge and patterns of old infections change, standardized protocols for monitoring and reporting these infections will help inform future guidelines.

Age-appropriate cancer screening (such as breast, colorectal, and cervical cancer screening) is also mandatory prior to donation. Donor candidates with active malignancy are generally deemed unsuitable to be organ donors; however, donor candidates with non-melanoma skin cancers and donors with low-grade, small, and localized renal cell carcinoma may be acceptable for donation on a case-by-case basis. Current guidelines also suggest that those with prior solid organ and hematological malignancies including melanoma and lung and breast cancers should be considered ineligible to donate. Evidence-based guidelines are needed to inform the cancer-free time interval before a potential donor with history of cancer with low transmission risk could donate, if donation is deemed appropriate. On a global scale, there is an urgent need for accurate, current, and ongoing reporting of suspected and actual donor-transmitted cancers.

References

1. Organ Procurement and Transplantation Network (OPTN). Recognizing seasonal and geographically endemic infections in organ donors: considerations during living donor evaluation. Available at: https://optn.transplant.hrsa.gov/media/1138/seasonal_disease_guidance.pdf. Accessed: 7 Sept 2020.
2. Lentine KL, Kasiske BL, Levey AS, Adams PL, Alberú J, Bakr MA, et al. KDIGO clinical practice guideline on the evaluation and care of living kidney donors. Transplantation. 2017;101.(8S Suppl 1:S1–S109. https://doi.org/10.1097/tp.0000000000001769.
3. Seem DL, Lee I, Umscheid CA, Kuehnert MJ, United States Public Health Service. PHS guideline for reducing human immunodeficiency virus, hepatitis B virus, and hepatitis C virus transmission through organ transplantation. Public Health Rep. 2013;128(4):247–343. https://doi.org/10.1177/003335491312800403.
4. Natov SN, Pereira BJ. Transmission of viral hepatitis by kidney transplantation: donor evaluation and transplant policies (part 1: hepatitis B virus). Transpl Infect Dis. 2002;4(3):117–23. https://doi.org/10.1034/j.1399-3062.2002.t01-1-01002.x.
5. Natov SN. Transmission of viral hepatitis by kidney transplantation: donor evaluation and transplant policies (part 2: hepatitis C virus). Transpl Infect Dis. 2002;4(3):124–31. https://doi.org/10.1034/j.1399-3062.2002.t01-2-01002.x.
6. Blumberg EA, Ison MG, Pruett TL, Segev DL, Optimal Testing of the Live Organ Donor Consensus Conference Participants. Optimal testing of the live organ donor for blood-borne viral pathogens: the report of a consensus conference. Am J Transplant. 2013;13(6):1405–15. Epub 2013 Apr 19. https://doi.org/10.1111/ajt.12205.
7. Ison MG, Grossi P, AST Infectious Diseases Community of Practice. Donor-derived infections in solid organ transplantation. Am J Transplant. 2013;13(Suppl 4):22–30. https://doi.org/10.1111/ajt.12095.
8. Singh N, Huprikar S, Burdette SD, Morris MI, Blair JE, Wheat LJ, American Society of Transplantation, Infectious diseases Community of Practice, Donor-Derived Fungal Infection Working Group. Donor-derived fungal infections in organ transplant recipients: guidelines of the American Society of Transplantation, infectious diseases community of practice. Am J Transplant. 2012;12(9):2414–28. https://doi.org/10.1111/j.1600-6143.2012.04100.x.

9. Clemente WT, Pierrotti LC, Abdala E, Morris MI, Azevedo LS, López-Vélez R, Cuenca-Estrella M, et al. Recommendations for management of endemic diseases and travel medicine in solid-organ transplant recipients and donors: Latin America. Transplantation. 2018;102(2):193–208. https://doi.org/10.1097/tp.0000000000002027.

10. Levi ME, Kumar D, Green M, Ison MG, Kaul D, Michaels MG, et al. Considerations for screening live kidney donors for endemic infections: a viewpoint on the UNOS policy. Am J Transplant. 2014;14(5):1003–11. https://doi.org/10.1111/ajt.12666.

11. Chin-Hong PV, Schwartz BS, Bern C, Montgomery SP, Kontak S, Kubak B, et al. Screening and treatment of Chagas disease in organ transplant recipients in the United States: recommendations from the Chagas in transplant working group. Am J Transplant. 2011;11(4):672–80. https://doi.org/10.1111/j.1600-6143.2011.03444.x.

12. Razonable RR, Humar A, AST Infectious diseases Community of Practice. Cytomegalovirus in solid organ transplantation. Am J Transplant. 2013;13(Suppl 4):93–106. https://doi.org/10.1111/ajt.12103.

13. Razonable RR. Epidemiology of cytomegalovirus disease in solid organ and hematopoietic stem cell transplant recipients. Am J Health Syst Pharm. 2005;62(Suppl 1):S7–S13. https://doi.org/10.1093/ajhp/62.suppl_1.s7.

14. Kotton C, Kumar D, Caliendo AM, Åsberg A, Chou S, Danziger-Isakov L, et al. Updated international consensus guidelines on the management of cytomegalovirus in solid-organ transplantation. Transp J. 2013;96(4):333–60. https://doi.org/10.1097/tp.0b013e31829df29d.

15. Abbott KC, Hypolite IO, Viola R, Poropatich RK, Hshieh P, Cruess D, et al. Hospitalizations for cytomegalovirus disease after renal transplantation in the United States. Epidemiology. 2002;12(6):402–9. https://doi.org/10.1016/s1047-2797(01)00283-6.

16. Khoury JA, Storch GA, Bohl DL, Schuessler RM, Torrence SM, Lockwood M, et al. Prophylactic versus preemptive oral valganciclovir for the management of cytomegalovirus infection in adult renal transplant recipients. Am J Transplant. 2006;6(9):2134–43. https://doi.org/10.1111/j.1600-6143.2006.01413.x.

17. Hartmann A, Sagedal S, Hjelmesaeth J. The natural course of cytomegalovirus infection and disease in renal transplant recipients. Transplantation. 2006;82(2 Suppl):S15–7. https://doi.org/10.1097/01.tp.0000230460.42558.b0.

18. Walker RC, Marshall WF, Strickler JG, Wiesner RH, Velosa JA, Habermann TM, et al. Pretransplantation assessment of the risk of lymphoproliferative disorder. Clin Infect Dis. 1995;20(5):1346–53. https://doi.org/10.1093/clinids/20.5.1346.

19. McDonald RA, Smith JM, Ho M, Lindblad R, Ikle D, Grimm P, et al. Incidence of PTLD in pediatric renal transplant recipients receiving basiliximab, calcineurin inhibitor, sirolimus and steroids. Am J Transplant. 2008;8(5):984–9. https://doi.org/10.1111/j.1600-6143.2008.02167.x.

20. Centers for Disease Control and Prevention. Sexually transmitted diseases surveillance 2017: syphilis. Available at: https://www.cdc.gov/std/stats17/syphilis.htm. Accessed: 7 Sept 2020.

21. Cortes NJ, Afzali B, MacLean D, Goldsmith DJ, O'Sullivan H, Bingham J, et al. Transmission of syphilis by solid organ transplantation. Am J Transplant. 2006;6(10):2497–9. Epub 2006 Jul 6. https://doi.org/10.1111/j.1600-6143.2006.01461.x.

22. Tariciotti L, Das I, Dori L, Perera MT, Bramhall SR. Asymptomatic transmission of Treponema pallidum (syphilis) through deceased donor liver transplantation. Transpl Infect Dis. 2012;14:321–5. https://doi.org/10.1111/j.1399-3062.2012.00745.x.

23. Theodoropoulos N, Jaramillo A, Penugonda S, Wasik C, Brooks K, Ladner DP, et al. Improving syphilis screening in deceased organ donors. Transplantation. 2015;99(2):438–43. https://doi.org/10.1097/tp.0000000000000323.

24. Seña AC, White BL, Sparling PF. Novel Treponema pallidum serologic tests: a paradigm shift in syphilis screening for the 21st century. Clin Infect Dis. 2010;51(6):700–8. https://doi.org/10.1086/655832.

25. Ison MG, Llata E, Conover CS, Friedewald JJ, Gerber SI, Grigoryan A, et al. Transmission of human immunodeficiency virus and hepatitis C virus from an organ donor to four transplant recipients. Am J Transplant. 2011;11(6):1218–25. https://doi.org/10.1111/j.1600-6143.2011.03597.x.

26. Centers for Disease Control and Prevention (CDC). HIV transmitted from a living organ donor--New York City, 2009. MMWR Morb Mortal Wkly Rep. 2011;60(10):297–301. https://pubmed.ncbi.nlm.nih.gov/21412210/.

27. Echenique IA, Cohen D, Rudow DL, Ison MG. Impact of repeat testing of living kidney donors within 14 days of the transplant procedure: a multicenter retrospective survey. Transpl Infect Dis. 2014;16(3):403–11. https://doi.org/10.1111/tid.12219.

28. Busch MP, Glynn SA, Stramer SL, Strong DM, Caglioti S, Wright DJ, et al. A new strategy for estimating risks of transfusion-transmitted viral infections based on rates of detection of recently infected donors. Transfusion. 2005;45(2):254–64. https://doi.org/10.1111/j.1537-2995.2004.04215.x.

29. Health Resources and Services Administration (HRSA), Department of Health and Human Services (HHS). Organ procurement and transplantation: Implementation of the HIV Organ Policy Equity Act. Final rule. Fed Regist. 2015;80(89):26464–7. https://pubmed.ncbi.nlm.nih.gov/25985481/.

30. Bernstein L. First living HIV-positive donor provides kidney for transplant in medical breakthrough. The Washington Post 2019. Available at: https://www.washingtonpost.com/national/health-science/first-living-hiv-positive-donor-provides-kidney-for-transplant-in-medical-breakthrough/2019/03/28/29894312-50bc-11e9-88a1-ed346f0ec94f_story.html. Accessed: 7 Sept 2020.

31. de Vera ME, Volk ML, Ncube Z, Blais S, Robinson M, Allen N, et al. Transplantation of hepatitis C virus (HCV) antibody positive, nucleic acid test negative donor kidneys to HCV negative patients frequently results in seroconversion but not HCV viremia. Am J Transplant. 2018;18(10):2451–6. https://doi.org/10.1111/ajt.15031.

32. Reese PP, Abt PL, Blumberg EA, Van Deerlin VM, Bloom RD, Potluri VS, et al. Twelve-month outcomes after transplant of hepatitis C-infected kidneys into uninfected recipients: a single-group trial. Ann Intern Med. 2018;169(5):273–81. https://doi.org/10.7326/m18-0749.

33. Goldberg DS, Abt PL, Reese PP, THINKER Trial Investigators. Transplanting HCV-infected kidneys into uninfected recipients. N Engl J Med. 2017;377(11):1105. https://doi.org/10.1056/nejmc1709315.

34. Huprikar S, Danziger-Isakov L, Ahn J, Naugler S, Blumberg E, Avery RK, et al. Solid organ transplantation from hepatitis B virus-positive donors: consensus guidelines for recipient management. Am J Transplant. 2015;15(5):1162–72. https://doi.org/10.1111/ajt.13187.

35. Manos NE, Ferebee SH, Kerschbaum WF. Geographic variation in the prevalence of histoplasmin sensitivity. Dis Chest. 1956;29(6):649–68. https://doi.org/10.1378/chest.29.6.649.

36. Sunenshine RH, Anderson S, Erhart L, Vossbrink A, Kelly PC, Engelthaler D, et al. Public health surveillance for coccidioidomycosis in Arizona. Ann N Y Acad Sci. 2007;1111:96–102. https://doi.org/10.1196/annals.1406.045.

37. Blair JE, Logan JL. Coccidioidomycosis in solid organ transplantation. Clin Infect Dis. 2001;33(9):1536–44. https://doi.org/10.1086/323463.

38. Kusne S, Taranto S, Covington S, Kaul DR, Blumberg EA, Wolfe C, et al. Coccidioidomycosis transmission through organ transplantation: a report of the OPTN Ad Hoc Disease Transmission Advisory Committee. Am J Transplant. 2016;16(12):3562–7. https://doi.org/10.1111/ajt.13950.

39. Centers for Disease Control and Prevention (CDC). Transmission of Strongyloides stercoralis through transplantation of solid organs--Pennsylvania, 2012. MMWR Morb Mortal Wkly Rep. 2013;62(14):264–6. https://pubmed.ncbi.nlm.nih.gov/23575239/.

40. Le M, Ravin K, Hasan A, Clauss H, Muchant DG, Pasko JK, et al. Single donor-derived strongyloidiasis in three solid organ transplant recipients: case series and review of the literature. Am J Transplant. 2014;14(5):1199–206. https://doi.org/10.1111/ajt.12670.

41. Abanyie FA, Gray EB, Delli Carpini KW, Yanofsky A, McAuliffe I, Rana M, et al. Donor-derived Strongyloides stercoralis infection in solid organ transplant recipients in the United States, 2009–2013. Am J Transplant. 2015;15(5):1369–75. https://doi.org/10.1111/ajt.13137.

42. Coster LO. Parasitic infections in solid organ transplant recipients. Infect Dis Clin North Am. 2013;27(2):395–427. Epub 2013 Mar 29. https://doi.org/10.1016/j.idc.2013.02.008.

43. Abdalhamid BA, Al Abadi AN, Al Saghier MI, Joudeh AA, Shorman MA, Amr SS. Strongyloides stercoralis infection in kidney transplant recipients. Saudi J Kidney Dis Transpl. 2015;26(1):98–102. https://doi.org/10.4103/1319-2442.148752.
44. World Health Organization. Chagas disease. Available at: http://www.who.int/news-room/fact-sheets/detail/chagas-disease-(american-trypanosomiasis). Accessed: 7 Sept 2020.
45. Bern C, Montgomery SP. An estimate of the burden of Chagas disease in the United States. Clin Infect Dis. 2009;49(5):e52–4. https://doi.org/10.1086/605091.
46. Huprikar S, Bosserman E, Patel G, Moore A, Pinney S, Anyanwu A, et al. Donor-derived Trypanosoma cruzi infection in solid organ recipients in the United States, 2001–2011. Am J Transplant. 2013;13(9):2418–25. https://doi.org/10.1111/ajt.12340.
47. Pierrotti LC, Carvalho NB, Amorin JP, Pascual J, Kotton CN, Lopez-Velez R. Chagas disease recommendations for solid-organ transplant recipients and donors. Transplantation. 2018;102(2S Suppl2):S1–7. https://doi.org/10.1097/tp.0000000000002019.
48. Ison MG, Nalesnik MA. An update on donor-derived disease transmission in organ transplantation. Am J Transplant. 2011;11(6):1123–30. https://doi.org/10.1111/j.1600-6143.2011.03493.x.
49. Morris MI, Daly JS, Blumberg E, Kumar D, Sester M, Schluger N, et al. Diagnosis and management of tuberculosis in transplant donors: a donor-derived infections consensus conference report. Am J Transplant. 2012;12(9):2288–300. https://doi.org/10.1111/j.1600-6143.2012.04205.x.
50. Winston DJ, Vikram HR, Rabe IB, Dhillon G, Mulligan D, Hong JC, et al. Donor-derived West Nile virus infection in solid organ transplant recipients: report of four additional cases and review of clinical, diagnostic, and therapeutic features. Transplantation. 2014;97(9):881–9. https://doi.org/10.1097/tp.0000000000000024.
51. Iwamoto M, Jernigan DB, Guasch A, Trepka MJ, Blackmore CG, Hellinger WC, et al. Transmission of West Nile virus from an organ donor to four transplant recipients. N Engl J Med. 2003;348(22):2196–203. https://doi.org/10.1056/nejmoa022987.
52. Centers for Disease Control and Prevention. West Nile virus. Available at: https://www.cdc.gov/westnile/index.html. Accessed: 7 Sept 2020.
53. Burakoff A, Lehman J, Fischer M, Staples JE, Lindsey NP. West Nile virus and other nationally notifiable arboviral diseases - United States, 2016. MMWR Morb Mortal Wkly Rep. 2018;67(1):13–7. https://doi.org/10.15585/mmwr.mm6701a3.
54. Kumar D, Prasas GV, Zaltzman J, Levy GA, Humar A. Community-acquired West Nile virus infection in solid-organ transplant recipients. Transplantation. 2004;77:339–402. https://doi.org/10.1097/01.tp.0000101435.91619.31.
55. Organ Procurement and Transplantation Network (OPTN). Identifying risk factors for West Nile virus (WNV) during evaluation of potential living donors. Available at: https://optn.transplant.hrsa.gov/resources/guidance/identifying-risk-factors-for-west-nile-virus-wnv-during-evaluation-of-potential-living-donors/. Accessed: 7 Sept 2020.
56. Busch MP, Kleinman SH, Tobler LH, Kamel HT, Norris PJ, Walsh I, et al. Virus and antibody dynamics in acute West Nile virus infection. J Infect Dis. 2008;198(7):984–93. https://doi.org/10.1086/591467.
57. Centers for Disease Control and Prevention. Zika virus. https://www.cdc.gov/zika/index.html. Accessed: 7 Sept 2020.
58. Organ Procurement and Transplantation Network (OPTN). Guidance on Zika virus. Available at: https://optn.transplant.hrsa.gov/news/guidance-on-zika-virus/. Accessed: 7 Sept 2020.
59. Reynolds MR, Jones AM, Petersen EE, Lee EH, Rice ME, Bingham A, et al. Vital signs: update on Zika virus-associated birth defects and evaluation of all U.S. infants with congenital Zika virus exposure - U.S. Zika pregnancy registry, 2016. MMWR Morb Mortal Wkly Rep. 2017;66(13):366–73. https://doi.org/10.15585/mmwr.mm6613e1.
60. Satterfield-Nash A, Kotzky K, Allen J, Bertolli J, Moore CA, Pereira IO, et al. Health and development at age 19–24 months of 19 children who were born with microcephaly and laboratory evidence of congenital Zika virus infection during the 2015 Zika virus outbreak - Brazil, 2017. MMWR Morb Mortal Wkly Rep. 2017;66(49):1347–51. https://doi.org/10.15585/mmwr.mm6649a2.

61. Polen KD, Gilboa SM, Hills S, Oduyebo T, Kohl KS, Brooks JT, et al. Update: interim guidance for preconception counseling and prevention of sexual transmission of Zika virus for men with possible Zika virus exposure - United States, august 2018. MMWR Morb Mortal Wkly Rep. 2018;67(31):868–71. https://doi.org/10.15585/mmwr.mm6731e2.

62. Magnus MM, Espósito DLA, Costa VAD, Melo PS, Costa-Lima C, Fonseca BALD. Risk of Zika virus transmission by blood donations in Brazil. Hematol Transfus Cell Ther. 2018;40(3):250–4. https://doi.org/10.1016/j.htct.2018.01.011.

63. Tong A, Chapman JR, Wong G, de Bruijn J, Craig JC. Screening and follow-up of living kidney donors: a systematic review of clinical practice guidelines. Transplantation. 2011;92(9):962–72. https://doi.org/10.1097/tp.0b013e3182328276.

64. British Transplant Society (BTS). Guidelines for living donor kidney transplantation. 4th ed. 2018. Available at: https://bts.org.uk/wp-content/uploads/2018/07/FINAL_LDKT-guidelines_June-2018.pdf. Accessed: 7 Sept 2020.

65. American Cancer Society (ACS). Guidelines for the early detection of cancer. 2018. Available at: https://www.cancer.org/healthy/find-cancer-early/cancer-screening-guidelines/american-cancer-society-guidelines-for-the-early-detection-of-cancer.html. Accessed: 7 Sept 2020.

66. Australian Government Department of Health. Cancer screening. 2018. Available at: http://www.cancerscreening.gov.au/. Accessed: 7 Sept 2020.

67. Xiao D, Craig JC, Chapman JR, Dominguez-Gil B, Tong A, Wong G. Donor cancer transmission in kidney transplantation: a systematic review. Am J Transplant. 2013;13(10):2645–52. https://doi.org/10.1111/ajt.12430.

68. Desai R, Collett D, Watson CJ, Johnson P, Evans T, Neuberger J. Cancer transmission from organ donors-unavoidable but low risk. Transplantation. 2012;94(12):1200–7. https://doi.org/10.1097/tp.0b013e318272df41.

69. Eccher A, Lombardini L, Girolami I, Puoti F, Zaza G, Gambaro G, et al. How safe are organs from deceased donors with neoplasia? The results of the Italian Transplantation Network. J Nephrol. 2019;32(2):323–30. https://doi.org/10.1007/s40620-018-00573-z.

70. Kauffman HM, Cherikh WS, McBride MA, Cheng Y, Hanto DW. Deceased donors with a past history of malignancy: an organ procurement and transplantation network/united network for organ sharing update. Transplantation. 2007;84(2):272–4. https://doi.org/10.1097/01.tp.0000267919.93425.fb.

71. Kauffman HM, McBride MA, Cherikh WS, Spain PC, Marks WH, Roza AM. Transplant tumor registry: donor related malignancies. Transplantation. 2002;74(3):358–62. https://doi.org/10.1097/00007890-200208150-00011.

72. Nalesnik MA, Woodle ES, Dimaio JM, Vasudev B, Teperman LW, Covington S, et al. Donor-transmitted malignancies in organ transplantation: assessment of clinical risk. Am J Transplant. 2011;11(6):1140–7. https://doi.org/10.1111/j.1600-6143.2011.03565.x.

73. Desai R, Collett D, Watson CJE, Johnson P, Evans T, Neuberger J. Estimated risk of cancer transmission from organ donor to graft recipient in a national transplantation registry. Br J Surg. 2014;101(7):768–74. https://doi.org/10.1002/bjs.9460.

74. Buell JF, Beebe TM, Trofe J, Gross TG, Alloway RR, Hanaway MJ, et al. Donor transmitted malignancies. Ann Transplant. 2004;9(1):53–6. https://pubmed.ncbi.nlm.nih.gov/15478892/.

75. Watson CJE, Roberts R, Wright KA, Greenberg DC, Rous BA, Brown CH, et al. How safe is it to transplant organs from deceased donors with primary intracranial malignancy? An analysis of UK registry data. Am J Transplant. 2010;10(6):1437–44. https://doi.org/10.1111/j.1600-6143.2010.03130.x.

76. Engels EA, Castenson D, Pfeiffer RM, Kahn A, Pawlish K, Goodman MT, et al. Cancers among US organ donors: a comparison of transplant and cancer registry diagnoses. Am J Transplant. 2014;14(6):1376–82. https://doi.org/10.1111/ajt.12683.

77. Organ Procurement and Transplantation Network (OPTN) / United Network for Organ Sharing (UNOS). Policy 15: identification of transmissible diseases. Available at: https://optn.transplant.hrsa.gov/governance/policies/. Accessed: 7 Sept 2020.

78. Chapman J, D'Errico-Grigioni A, Matsanz R. The transmission of malignancies. NOTIFY: exploring vigilance notification for organs, tissues and cells. Bologna: Testi Centro Nazionale Trapianti; 2011. p. 78–97.
79. European Directorate for the Quality of Medicines & Healthcare. Guide to the quality and safety of organs for transplantation. 2018. Available at: https://www.edqm.eu/en/guide-quality-and-safety-organs-transplantation. Accessed: 7 Sept 2020.
80. Lugo-Baruqui JA, Guerra G, Chen L, Burke GW, Gaite JA, Ciancio G. Living donor renal transplantation with incidental renal cell carcinoma from donor allograft. Transpl Int. 2015;28(9):1126–30. https://doi.org/10.1111/tri.12594.
81. Lugo-Baruqui A, Guerra G, Arocha A, Burke GW, Ciancio G. Use of kidneys with small renal tumors for transplantation. Curr Urol Rep. 2016;17(1):3. https://doi.org/10.1007/s11934-015-0557-z.
82. Sener A, Uberoi V, Bartlett ST, Kramer AC, Phelan MW. Living-donor renal transplantation of grafts with incidental renal masses after ex-vivo partial nephrectomy. BJU Int. 2009;104(11):1655–60. https://doi.org/10.1111/j.1464-410x.2009.08681.x.
83. Nicol DL, Preston JM, Wall DR, Griffin AD, Campbell SB, Isbel NM, et al. Kidneys from patients with small renal tumours: a novel source of kidneys for transplantation. BJU Int. 2008;102(2):188–92. https://doi.org/10.1111/j.1464-410x.2008.07562.x.

Evaluation of Genetic Kidney Disease in Living Donor Candidates

8

Christie P. Thomas and Jasmin Divers

Introduction

The first successful kidney transplantation occurred in 1954 between two 23-year-old identical twins and was accomplished without the need for immunosuppression in the recipient. The twin donor is reported to have had no perioperative complications and lived for another 56 years without evident kidney disease despite genetic identity to his recipient twin brother [1, 2]. Since then living kidney donation has become common, with approximately 6000 living kidney donations performed in the United States each year, and is the preferred therapy for optimal outcomes in the kidney recipient. While outcomes in living donors are generally good, in recent years it has been recognized that living donors face a small but significant increase in the risk of kidney failure, compared to similar healthy persons who did not donate [3, 4]. One recently identified risk factor for long-term kidney failure risk in living donors is biological relatedness to their recipient, suggesting an impact of shared genetic risk factors that predispose to chronic kidney disease (CKD) [5–8]. Compared to unrelated living donors, first-degree relatives (i.e., siblings, parents, offspring) have a two- to fourfold increased risk of end-stage kidney disease (ESKD), and identical twins have a 3.5–22.5-fold increased risk of ESKD after a median follow-up of 11–12 years [6, 8]. Anecdotal reports of donors presenting

C. P. Thomas (✉)
Department of Internal Medicine and Pediatrics, Carver College of Medicine,
University of Iowa and Veterans Affairs Medical Center, Iowa City, IA, USA
e-mail: christie-thomas@uiowa.edu

J. Divers
Division of Health Services Research, Department of Foundations of Medicine,
New York University Long Island School of Medicine, New York, NY, USA

Winthrop Research Institute, Mineola, NY, USA
e-mail: Jasmin.Divers@nyulangone.org

K. L. Lentine et al. (eds.), *Living Kidney Donation*,
https://doi.org/10.1007/978-3-030-53618-3_8

years after donation with the same kidney diseases that also affected their family member illustrate the importance of screening presymptomatic living kidney donor candidates for genetic variants that are associated with kidney disease [5, 9]. Similarly, the presence of two *apolipoprotein L1 (APOL1)* renal risk variants has been associated with ESKD in living kidney donors [10, 11]. In this chapter we review selected monogenic renal diseases as well as two major renal disease susceptibility traits (*APOL1* renal risk variants, sickle cell trait) and provide guidelines for their evaluation in living kidney donor candidates.

ESKD and the Role of Kidney Transplantation

Options for management of ESKD include chronic dialysis and kidney transplantation. Kidney transplantation is the optimal treatment for patients with ESKD, as it offers superior survival and improves quality of life, at lower cost to the healthcare system [12]. There are not enough deceased-donor kidneys to meet the demand for kidney transplantation, which has led to recognition of the important role of living kidney donation to fill the gap. In some parts of the world, the only practical renal replacement therapy option is living donor transplantation. Furthermore, not only does living donor kidney transplantation reduce or avoid time on dialysis among patients with ESKD, but living donor transplants are almost always superior to deceased-donor kidneys, offering better long-term kidney allograft and patient survival. In the United States alone, the number of kidney transplants from living donors increased from 1,817 in 1988 to 6,857 in 2019 [13].

Scope of Risks to Living Kidney Donors

Living kidney donation is not without risks to the donor. These include the perioperative risks common to any abdominal surgery, psychosocial risks that arises from post-operative depression or distress from an adverse recipient or donor outcome, and financial risks from uncompensated expenses as well as potential loss of income associated with the donation process. Long-term risks of living kidney donation also include ESKD after donation. Reasons for this increased risk may include decreased reserve after donation of half of one's nephron mass, combined with other environmental or genetic hits. These may include the shared genetic risk variants that cause or contribute to the ESKD in the recipient, the presence of other renal disease susceptibility traits, and postdonation renal injury related to common causes of ESKD in the general population, such as diabetes and hypertension [7, 8, 14]. Although several genetic diseases and genetic variants may increase the perioperative risk of complications (e.g., Factor V Leiden increasing thrombosis risk, ryanodine receptor variants increasing malignant hyperthermia risk), this chapter discusses monogenic renal diseases and major genetic susceptibility traits that are associated with increased risk of ESKD among living kidney donors.

Risk of Kidney Disease after Living Donation

The long-term risk of ESKD among living donors was not appreciated until recently with initial studies reporting that the incidence of ESKD was much lower following living donation compared to the general population [15]. However, this has changed with the publication of two large retrospective studies using more appropriate comparison groups of healthy non-donors, rather than the unscreened general population, which includes many persons who with medical contraindications to donation. In one landmark paper from the United States, the risk of ESKD following donation increased about tenfold on average over a 15-year period compared to matched healthy controls who did not donate [3]. In another study from Norway, a similar increase in risk of ESKD was seen in donors compared with matched healthy non-donors [4]. In the US studies, the risk of ESKD in donors was higher in men compared to women, in obese vs non-obese persons, and in African Americans and Hispanics compared to non-Hispanic whites, with the highest risk seen in young African American men [3, 6, 7]. Importantly, compared to an unrelated donor, donors biologically related to their recipient appear to have an overall 1.7-fold increased risk of postdonation ESKD with higher risk based on degree of relatedness and ancestry [7]. For example, in updated analyses of similar US datasets, the adjusted hazard ratio for ESKD at 20 years for a full sibling or parent of a recipient was 1.87 and 2.01, respectively [6]. When analyzed further by ancestry, the adjusted hazard ratio (aHR) for ESKD in sibling donors was 2.0 among white persons and 4.1 among black persons; the aHR for identical twin donors suggested a 3.5-fold risk among white persons and 22.5-fold risk among black persons [8]. Although the cause of ESKD in the recipient or donor in these cases was not reported, there are anecdotal reports of living donors who later developed the same renal diseases that affected their relative, including focal segmental glomerulosclerosis (FSGS), hemolytic uremic syndrome, or Alport syndrome [5, 9].

Diagnostic Tools to Estimate Risk of CKD and ESKD in Living Donor Candidates

Living donor candidates are thoroughly evaluated with testing including measurement of blood pressure, body mass index (BMI), blood glucose, urine albumin excretion kidney function (e.g., measured glomerular filtration rate (GFR) or creatinine clearance), as well as urinalysis and imaging studies [16]. Candidates with well-established risk factors for ESKD such as albuminuria, proteinuria, low renal function, and diabetes and hypertension are usually excluded from living donation. There are however many additional risk factors for advanced CKD or ESKD in the general population that typically do not get the same attention during a living donor candidate evaluation. In a large cohort of individuals who had health checkups in the Kaiser Permanente System (177,570 people, 5,275,957 follow-up years), prehypertension (aHR 1.72), male sex (aHR 1.22), BMI 25–30 kg/m^2 (aHR 1.65), ancestry (Asian aHR 1.83; African aHR 3.02), and uric acid >6.0 mg/dL (aHR 2.14) were identified as significant risk factors for the development of ESKD over a 25+-year follow-up period [17]. In other studies of cohorts of non-donors with up to 24 years of follow-up, microscopic hematuria (aHR 18.5), history of kidney stones (aHR 2.09), low birth weight (aHR 1.60), and small for gestational age (aHR 1.51) were identified as significant risk factors for ESKD [18–20]. In living donors, in addition, both obesity and a family history of ESKD have been identified as risk factors for kidney failure after donation [7, 21].

In donor candidates with a family history of inherited kidney disease, a disease-focused evaluation may be sufficient to screen the donor candidate if the cause of genetic disease in the recipient is known. A perfect screening test for a living donor would have a 100% negative predictive value; that is, the test would always exclude disease in an asymptomatic living donor. These include a negative ultrasound in a person age 40 or older with a first-degree relative with autosomal dominant poly-cystic kidney disease (ADPKD) or a negative slit lamp exam and normal plasma alpha-galactosidase-A (α-Gal-A) in a man with a family history of Fabry disease. However, clinical screening tests to exclude the future development of most renal diseases are not available. The problem of determining risk of genetic disease in an asymptomatic living donor candidate is compounded when the cause of ESRD in a related recipient candidate or other family member with kidney disease is not known or not recognized as monogenic in nature, as screening for a specific dis-ease in the donor is contingent on accurate phenotyping of the affected family member. The 2017 Kidney Disease: Improving Global Outcomes "Guideline for the Evaluation and Care of Living Donors" recommends that when the intended recipient is genetically related to the donor candidate, the cause of the intended recipient's kidney failure should be determined whenever possible [16]. The intended recipient should consent to share this medical information with the donor evaluation team and with the donor candidate if it could affect the decision to donate [16].

Genetic Mechanisms of CKD

Genetic disorders are inherited in a simple (monogenic) or complex fashion. Monogenic disorders, also known as Mendelian disorders, are typically rare and characterized by change in a specific protein level or function due to variant(s) in a single gene. Monogenic diseases may be autosomal or X-linked and behave pre-dominantly as dominant or recessive diseases. In a dominant disease, a single copy of an abnormal gene causes disease, while two copies are needed for recessive dis-eases [22]. The mechanism of dominant disease is either a gain of function where the abnormal gene product has a new or enhanced function (e.g., Liddle syndrome) or cytotoxicity (e.g., autosomal dominant tubulointerstitial kidney disease due to UMOD mutations, ADTKD-*UMOD*) or a dominant negative effect where the abnormal gene product interferes with the function of the normal allele (e.g., autosomal dominant nephrogenic diabetes insipidus due to aquaporin 2 mutation, NDI-*AQP2*). In other cases, a germline pathogenic heterozygous gene variant must be followed by an acquired or somatic mutation in the second allele for disease to occur (e.g., ADPKD-*PKD1*). Dominant diseases can less commonly occur from a null variant that reduces the total gene product, indicating that haploinsufficiency is also a model of dominant disease (e.g., ADTKD due to hepatocyte nuclear factor 1β mutations, ADTKD-*HNF1*β). In a recessive disease, both copies of a gene are abnormal, and the mechanism of disease is usually from loss or substantial reduction of the amount or function of the total gene product. Rarely, genetic disorders arise from variants in two genes (digenic inheritance) as has been reported with Bardet-Biedl syndrome [23]. In an X-linked recessive disorder, the hemizygous male with a single X-chromosome manifests the disease, while women, with some exceptions, are asymptomatic heterozygous carriers (e.g., Dent disease). In an X-linked dominant disorder on the other hand, the abnormal gene product exhibits a gain of function or a dominant negative effect, and men and women may be equally effected (e.g., X-linked hypophosphatemic rickets). Changes in the genetic code that can lead to dominant or recessive genetic disease are usually single nucleotide variants (SNVs) or small insertions or deletions (indels) but may also be deletions or insertions of larger tracts of DNA called copy number variations (CNVs). CNVs are now increasingly recognized as causing monogenic renal disease [24, 25]. Common chronic diseases, including hypertension, diabetes, and CKD, are known to run in families, which suggests a genetic contribution to their etiology. Unlike Mendelian disorders, these diseases are thought to result from multifactorial causes involving complex interactions between multiple genetic and environmental factors (e.g., diet, physical activity, smoking, neighborhood characteristics, exposure to pollutants).

The kidney is a highly complex organ with many different cell types and a multitude of specific functions that singly or together maintain homeostasis. A defect within any compartment of the kidney can lead to the development of CKD. Many monogenic disorders can cause CKD, including developmental renal and urological abnormalities, cystic and non-cystic ciliopathies, tubulointerstitial diseases, and glomerular diseases. The renal and urological structural defects are known as congenital abnormalities of the kidney and urinary tract (CAKUT), which can range from renal agenesis to posterior urethral valves. These malformations account for 50% of CKD in children, but some CAKUTs may not become clinically apparent until adulthood [26]. A CAKUT may present as an isolated renal disease or be part of a syndrome with extrarenal features. The cystic and non-cystic ciliopathies arise from genetic defects in structure or function of the cilia with ADPKD as the most common example. The ciliopathies also include other monogenic cystic kidney diseases and nephronophthisis, which can present as an isolated renal disease or as the renal manifestation of multisystem disorders such as Bardet-Biedl, COACH, Jeune, Joubert, Meckel-Gruber, and Sensenbrenner syndromes [27, 28]. Tubulointerstitial genetic diseases usually are associated with bland urine, minimal to absent proteinuria, and, generally, normal imaging findings, although a few medullary or corticomedullary cysts may be seen. Glomerular diseases present with hematuria and/or proteinuria, with anatomically normal-appearing kidneys.

Assigning Pathogenicity to Identified Genetic Variants

Single nucleotide variants (SNVs) are alterations of single nucleotide (adenine (A), cytosine (C), guanine (G), or thymine (T)) in the DNA sequence. The biologic impact of SNVs in coding regions depends on their type (synonymous versus missense), and in noncoding regions, their impact depends on their effect on RNA processing or gene regulation [29]. The output from sequencing large tracts of DNA by exome/genome sequencing or by targeted capture and resequencing requires sophisticated bioinformatic algorithms to sort through the thousands of variants to determine which variants to exclude because of poor sequencing quality and which to exclude based on allele frequency. Selection pressure reduces the overall frequency of deleterious single base pair substitutions in coding DNA and in associated regulatory sequences. The sequence data is compared with large population databases to exclude SNVs with high allele frequency and the remaining evaluated for potential pathogenic effects using software tools that examine nucleotide conservation, presumed or reported functional impact, and the correlation with a presenting phenotype. The pathogenicity of a variant is typically classified using American College of Medical Genetics (ACMG) criteria as benign, likely benign, variant of unknown significance (VUS), likely pathogenic, or pathogenic [30]. Variants that disrupt expression and/or function, such as gene deletions, frameshift, and splice site or truncation variants, are highly likely to be pathogenic. On the other hand, synonymous variants or common nonsynonymous variants are highly likely to be benign, while missense variants may be pathogenic, benign, or of unknown significance. The absence of a pathogenic or likely pathogenic variant does not automatically exclude a genetic disease. Some cases of genetic kidney disease may be caused by a genetic variant elsewhere in the gene that was not sequenced (e.g., intronic and upstream regulatory regions), a variant within the gene that was erroneously filtered out computationally, or variants in a new, yet unidentified, gene.

Methods of Genetic Testing

Gene-Focused Testing by PCR

When the specific genetic cause of ESKD is known to be a single nucleotide variant or a small indel, screening for the familial genetic disease or the specific variant is accomplished by polymerase chain reaction (PCR)-based sequencing to evaluate the entire coding region or the specific exon where the causal variant is located. However, with few single gene exceptions (e.g., *GLA* gene for Fabry, *CTNS* gene for cystinosis), most types of inherited kidney disease in a patient with ESKD are caused by one of many genes (e.g., inherited FSGS).

Broad-Based or Comprehensive Screening by Next-Generation Sequencing

In most cases where genetic testing may have a role, the cause of ESKD in the related recipient candidate is not known, or the specific renal disease can be caused by several genes (e.g., atypical hemolytic uremic syndrome (aHUS), FSGS) necessitating a broader approach to screening for genetic causes of kidney disease. Advances in rapid, large-scale, inexpensive sequencing of hundreds and thousands of genes or the entire genetic code, through techniques called next-generation sequencing (NGS) or massively parallel sequencing (MPS), provide the ability to interrogate any patient's DNA in an unbiased fashion to find pathogenic or likely pathogenic genetic variants that explain the patient's phenotype. The options for testing include screening the ~3 billion base pairs of the entire genome (genome sequencing), limiting sequencing to the protein coding exons (exome sequencing), or using a targeted approach to sequence all or a subset of renal gene exons [31–35]. NGS technology is however prone to error in presence of gene duplications and long repeat sequences [36] which potentially reduce its sensitivity in detecting variants in the proximal portion of polycystic kidney disease 1 (*PKD1*) *gene* (one of the genetic causes of ADPKD) and in detecting the insertion within the cytosine repeat of mucin 1 (*MUC1*) *gene* (one of the genetic causes of ADTKD). Additional techniques like long-range PCR for PKD1 and capillary sequencing for *MUC1* may be required [33, 36, 37].

Copy Number Variant Analysis

Many NGS-based testing services incorporate CNV analysis into their bioinformatic pipeline, and this should be part of the genetic screening of patients with uncharacterized renal disease and for selected diseases such as hepatocyte nuclear factor 1 beta (*HNF1β*)-mediated nephropathy where a microdeletion in chromosome 17q12, containing *HNF1β*, is a common mechanism for disease [33]. Orthogonal techniques such as array chromosomal gene hybridization (aCGH) and multiplex ligation-dependent probe amplification (*MLPA*) can also be used to identify CNVs and complement NGS-based approaches [38, 39].

Screening Living Donor Candidates for Individual Diseases

There are many monogenic renal diseases that cause ESKD, and it is not possible to describe a screening strategy for each of them. In the following section, we discuss the approach to screening living donor candidates for a few common diseases that are known to lead to ESKD in an affected family member. Table 8.1 also includes a few more diseases but the list is not intended to be comprehensive. Figure 8.1 outlines a simplified approach to testing for monogenic disease and renal disease susceptibility traits. The 2017 KDIGO guideline recommends that in cases where it

Table 8.1 Testing a donor candidate with family history of genetic disease (requires genotyping affected relative first). (From Kuppachi et al. [58])

Genetic disease	Affected gene	Phenotype	Genetic phenocopy	Donation from a relative?
Autosomal dominant disorders				
ADPKD	*PKD 1, PKD2, GANAB*	Bilateral cystic kidneys	*DNAJB11, HNF1B, NOTCH2, OFD1, PKHD1, TSC2*	Yes, if disease excluded[a]
ADTKD	*UMOD, MUC1 HNF1B, REN*	Normal to small kidneys, bland urine +/− few cysts	*DNAJB11*, all genetic causes of JN	Yes, if genetic screening negative[a]
Alport syndrome	*COL4A3, COL4A4*	GBM abnormality with focal or global GS	*MYH9*	Yes, if genetic screening negative[a]
TBMN	*COL4A3, COL4A4*	Thin GBM with hematuria		Caution in donor candidate with microscopic hematuria even if genetic screen negative
FSGS/SRNS	*ACTN4, ANLN, ARHGAP24, CD2AP, CFI, COL4A3, COL4A4, E2F3, INF2, LMX1B, TRPC6, WT1*	Focal and segmental GS and/ or steroid-resistant nephrotic syndrome	*CLCN5, FN1, PAX2*	Yes, if disease excluded[a]
Atypical HUS	*CFH, CFB, CFI, C3, MCP, PLG, THBD*	Thrombotic microangiopathy, +/− MAHA	*ADAMTS13*	Caution even if genetic screening negative
Autosomal recessive disorders				
ARPKD	*PKHD1*	Large kidneys, early renal failure	*PKD1, PKD2*	Yes, if negative or heterozygous carrier[b]
Juvenile nephronophthisis	*AHI1, ATXN10, IQCB1, CEP290, GLIS2, INVS, NEK8, NPHP1, NPHP3, NPHP4, RPGRIP1L, TMEM67, TTC21B, WDR19, XPNPEP3*	Normal to small kidneys, bland urine	*UMOD, MUC1 HNF1B, REN*	Yes, if negative or heterozygous carrier[b]
Alport syndrome	*COL4A3, COL4A4*	GBM abnormality with focal or global GS	*MYH9*	• Yes, if negative or heterozygous carrier[b] • Caution in donor candidate with microscopic hematuria

FSGS/SRNS	*ADCK4, ALG1, ANKFY1, ARHGDIA, COQ6, CRB2, CUBN, DGKE, DHTKD1, DLC1, EMP2, FAT1, GAPVD1, ITGB4, LAMA5, LAMB2, MYO1E, NPHS2, NUP133, NUP160, NUP85, NUP107, NUP205, NUP93, PLCE1, PDSS2, PMM2, PTPRO, SCARB2, SGPL1, XPO5, ZMPSTE24*	Focal segmental GS and/or steroid-resistant nephrotic syndrome	*CLCN5, FN1, PAX2*	• Yes, if negative or heterozygous carrier[b] • Caution with NPHS2 R229Q variant
Atypical HUS	*DGKE*	Thrombotic microangiopathy or MPGN	*CFH, CFB, CFI, C3, MCP, PLG, THBD*	Yes, if negative or heterozygous carrier[b]
X-linked diseases				
Alport syndrome	*COL4A5*	GBM abnormality with focal or global GS	*MYH9*	• Yes, if negative[a] • No if positive, except with caution in older heterozygous woman (>50) if no or minimal phenotype
Fabry disease	*GLA*	Zebra bodies on kidney biopsy, neuropathy, cardiac involvement		• Yes, if negative[a] • No if positive, except with caution in older heterozygous woman (>50) if no or minimal phenotype

Abbreviations: FSGS focal segmental glomerulosclerosis, *GS* glomerulosclerosis, *JN* juvenile nephronophthisis, *MAHA* microangiopathic hemolytic anemia, *SRNS* steroid-resistant nephrotic syndrome

[a]Requires identification of causal variant in affected individual

[b]Requires identification of both causal variants in affected individual

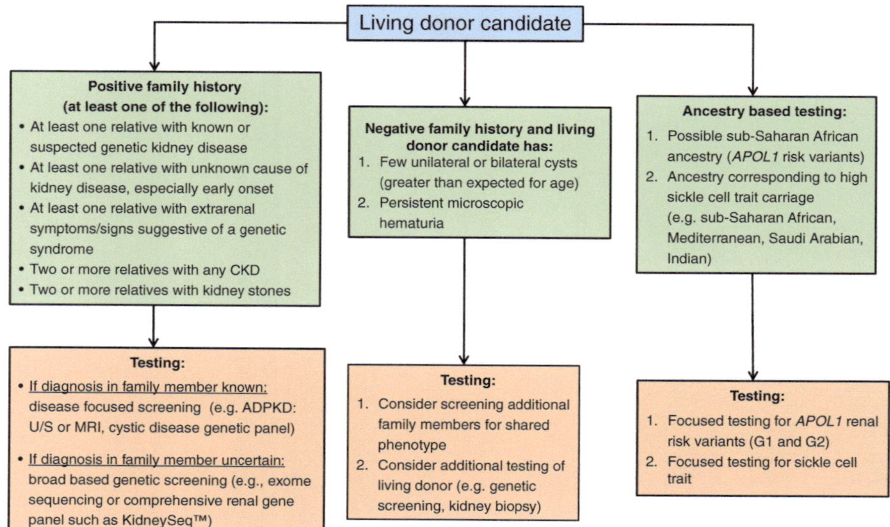

Fig. 8.1 Approach to testing for monogenic disease and renal disease susceptibility traits in living donor candidates. *Abbreviations: ADPKD* autosomal dominant polycystic kidney disease, *APOL1* apolipoprotein L1, *CKD* chronic kidney disease, *U/S* ultrasound, *MRI* magnetic resonance imaging

remains uncertain whether the donor candidate has a genetic kidney disease and whether the disease can cause kidney failure, donation should proceed only after informing the donor candidate of the risks of donation if the disease manifests later in life [16].

Autosomal Dominant Polycystic Kidney Disease

Causal genes PKD1, PKD2, GANAB

Clinical diagnosis ADPKD is the most common monogenic cause of ESKD. ADPKD presents with innumerable cysts of varying sizes in bilaterally enlarged kidneys. Together with a positive family history in a multigenerational context, the diagnosis can be established using ultrasound, computed tomography (CT), or magnetic resonance imaging (MRI).

Phenocopy Almost all patients with ADPKD who develop ESKD have heterozygous variants in *PKD1* or *PKD2*. In approximately 10% of cases, family history is absent which is generally thought to indicate the emergence of a de novo pathogenic variant in *PKD1* or *PKD2* or the presence of another cause of cystic kidney disease with much higher rates of de novo variants such as renal cysts with diabetes (*HNF1B*). Other conditions that phenocopy ADPKD include tuberous sclerosis (*TSC2*), orofacial digital syndrome (*OFD1*), Hajdu-Cheney syndrome (*NOTCH2*), autosomal recessive polycystic kidney disease (*PKHD1*), and acquired cystic kidney disease [28, 40]. Variants in *DNAJB11* are a recently described cause of autosomal dominant cystic kidney disease where the kidneys atrophy as kidney function declines [41]. If the imaging appearance is atypical especially with a negative family history, then phenocopies of polycystic kidney disease may need to be considered, and, in the absence of distinct syndromic features, genetic testing may be the only way to confirm a diagnosis.

Testing living donor candidates Normal kidney function or normal imaging studies do not exclude disease. In living donor candidates with a first-degree relative who has ADPKD, the modified Ravine criteria have been used to verify the absence of ADPKD [42]. Since ADPKD has age-dependent penetrance, the negative predicted value (NPV) of a normal renal ultrasound increases with age. Thus, the absence of cysts on ultrasound in at-risk individuals between the ages of 15–29, 30–39, and >40 years has a NPV of 90.8%, 98.3%, and 100%, respectively. Recently, MRI has been used as a screening tool for ADPKD. Compared with high-resolution ultrasound, in a single-center study, using MRI criteria of 5 cysts or less in both kidneys combined demonstrated 100% sensitivity and 100% negative predictive value in identifying and excluding ADPKD in a cohort aged between 16 and 40 years [43]. The limitations of imaging-based criteria for excluding ADPKD can be complemented or overcome by the use of predictive genetic testing, first to verify a genetic diagnosis in the affected family member followed by focused genetic screening to exclude ADPKD in the donor candidate [34, 44]. Genetic testing is particularly useful with younger living donor candidates, in the context of atypical disease, or when there is only one affected individual with the disease.

Autosomal Dominant Tubulointerstitial Disease

Causal genes *UMOD, MUC1, HNF1B*, and *REN*

Clinical diagnosis ADTKD is characterized by progressive decline in kidney function with bland urinalysis, minimal proteinuria, and a tendency for normal blood pressure. Ultrasound imaging is usually normal although a few cortical or corticomedullary cysts can be seen, the basis for its original name of medullary cystic kidney disease. A kidney biopsy will show non-specific interstitial fibrosis and tubular atrophy. Family history is likely to be positive, and some patients may present with juvenile onset gout. Immunohistochemical studies can show retention of mucin 1 within renal tubules, establishing a diagnosis of ADTKD-*MUC1* [45]. However, in practice, a definitive diagnosis is established by genetic testing.

Phenocopy Nephronophthisis is a clinical disease that is very similar to ADTKD in its clinical features and imaging findings. Nephronophthisis is autosomal recessive, and another sibling may be the only other affected individual. Based on the age of onset of advanced CKD/ESKD, nephronophthisis has been divided into the infantile, juvenile, and adult subtypes. In later stages of disease, *DNAJB11*-mediated disease may show a tubulointerstitial disease phenotype with normal or small kidneys and few or no cysts [41].

Testing living donor candidates Normal kidney function, urinalysis, and imaging studies do not exclude disease in a living donor candidate. Genetic testing in the affected family member to verify the basis for disease followed by focused testing of the living donor candidate is the only way to determine if a living donor candidate is not at risk for ADTKD. While testing for *UMOD*, *HNF1B*, and *REN* is widely available, testing for *MUC1* is only available through the Broad Institute [37].

Alport Nephropathy

Causal genes *COL4A3*, *COL4A4*, and *COL4A5*

Clinical diagnosis Alport syndrome is a disorder that begins with microscopic hematuria (and occasionally intermittent gross hematuria) with the subsequent development of progressive chronic kidney disease with or without increasing proteinuria, sensorineural hearing loss, and ocular findings of pigmentary retinal flecks and/or lenticonus [46]. The collagen 4 alpha chain abnormality results in characteristic abnormalities in the glomerular basement membrane such as thinning, abnormal lamellation, or splitting on electron microscopy. Light microscopic findings are variable and include focal segmental or global glomerulosclerosis. With increasing broad-based genetic screening of FSGS and/or steroid-resistant nephrotic syndrome, *COL4* variants are being identified in apparently sporadic and renal-limited cases of proteinuria. *COL4* variants are now considered to be the commonest cause of genetic FSGS in adults [47, 48], and affected patients are better labeled as having (non-syndromic) Alport nephropathy or collagen type 4 nephropathy. X-linked diseases from variants in *COL4A5* are the most commonly seen cases, with men most often affected and developing progressive CKD/ESKD, while most heterozygous women only develop hematuria although about 15% develop ESKD by age 60. The nature of the genetic variant impacts disease progression with null variants in *COL4A5* usually resulting in ESKD before the age of 30 in hemizygous men. Autosomal recessive disease from homozygous or compound heterozygous variants in *COL4A3* or *COL4* is seen in about 10% of Alport syndrome and usually presents with advanced CKD or ESKD at a young age. Heterozygous carriers of autosomal

Alport variants are generally asymptomatic and may present with microscopic hematuria and with thinned glomerular basement membranes on kidney biopsy [49]. This condition termed thin basement membrane disease is generally thought to be benign, but there appears to be variability in presentation even within families, with some individuals progressing to more advanced CKD and ESKD consistent with an autosomal dominant form of Alport nephropathy.

Phenocopy The commonest phenocopy for Alport nephropathy is IgA nephropathy, which characteristically presents with microscopic or intermittent macroscopic hematuria with some patients progressing to CKD and ESKD. It is important to note that some patients with IgA nephropathy may also carry pathogenic or likely pathogenic variants in *COL4A3*, *COL4A4*, or *COL4A5*, and it may be difficult to distinguish the contribution of the IgA deposition from the effect of *COL4* risk variants to the extent of kidney disease without clinical screening of other family members combined with segregation analysis [50]. *MYH9*-related disease, sometimes called Epstein or Fechtner syndromes, presents with nephritis, hearing loss, thrombocytopenia, and neutrophil inclusion granules and should also be considered in patients with kidney disease and thrombocytopenia [51].

Testing living donor candidates The only way to confirm the diagnosis of Alport nephropathy is by the identification of pathogenic or likely pathogenic variants in *COL4A3*, *A4*, or *A5* in patients with an appropriate clinical presentation. Establishing the genetic basis of Alport syndrome or Alport nephropathy is necessary to appropriately screen at-risk living donor candidates for the familial Alport gene variant. In the X-linked form of disease, the mother of an affected male is an obligate "carrier" unless the genetic variant arose de novo. All daughters of an affected male are carriers, and no sons will carry the abnormal genetic variant. All "carriers" of the X-linked variant are at risk for developing kidney disease beyond microscopic hematuria. In autosomal recessive Alport syndrome, both parents will be carriers, while siblings may inherit 0, 1, or 2 pathogenic variants. Autosomal dominant cases of Alport syndrome (about 5% of cases) have one mutation in either *COL4A3* or *COL4A4*. At-risk family members can be screened with urine microscopy, urine albumin excretion, estimated GFR, as well as hearing tests and ophthalmological examination. However, interpretation of a normal examination is difficult in the absence of genetic confirmation in the affected individual. In genetically confirmed autosomal recessive Alport syndrome, heterozygous carriers with no clinical or laboratory evidence of disease including microscopic hematuria may be allowed to donate after counseling. In X-linked disease, an older heterozygous female with no phenotype (e.g., mother) may also be allowed to donate after counseling. In autosomal dominant Alport or thin basement membrane disease, a single *COL4A3* or *A4* variant is enough for disease, and at-risk relatives carrying the familial variant should be counseled against donation.

Genetic FSGS (Including Diffuse Mesangial Sclerosis and Steroid-Resistant Nephrotic Syndrome)

Causal genes
- *Primary* (glomerular genes):
- Autosomal dominant: *ACTN4, ANLN, ARHGAP24, CD2AP, CFI, COL4A3, COL4A4, E2F3, INF2, LMX1B, TRPC6, WT1*
- Autosomal recessive: *ADCK4, ALG1, ANKFY1, ARHGDIA, COQ6, CRB2, CUBN, DGKE, DHTKD1, DLC1, EMP2, FAT1, GAPVD1, ITGB4, LAMA5, LAMB2, MYO1E, NPHS2, NUP133, NUP160, NUP85, NUP107, NUP205, NUP93, PLCE1, PDSS2, PMM2, PTPRO, SCARB2, SGPL1, XPO5, ZMPSTE24*
- X-linked: *COL4A5*
- Secondary (other renal genes): *CLCN5, NPHP4, PAX2, TTCB12*

Clinical diagnosis FSGS is a histological form of glomerular kidney disease, so named because one or more glomeruli (i.e., focal) show sclerosis typically, but not always involving a portion (i.e., segmental) of the glomerular tuft. FSGS can manifest clinically with varying degrees of proteinuria from asymptomatic sub-nephrotic proteinuria to frank nephrotic syndrome, and some will variably progress to advanced CKD and ESRD. Diffuse mesangial sclerosis (DMS) has a genetic origin and occurs primarily in children. It is another histological disorder that can overlap with FSGS and presents with proteinuria, including nephrotic syndrome. In DMS there is increased mesangial matrix initially with podocyte hypertrophy progressing to glomerulosclerosis. Children that present with nephrotic syndrome are often first treated with high-dose steroids, and only those that are steroid resistant are further evaluated by kidney biopsy or by genetic testing. Some patients with steroid-resistant nephrotic syndrome (SRNS) have diffuse mesangial sclerosis, while others have FSGS. The younger the patient, the higher the likelihood of a genetic basis for DMS, FSGS, and SRNS [52]. A positive family history or the presence of syndromic features also increases the likelihood of a monogenic cause of FSGS. FSGS may be primary (intrinsic to the podocyte) or secondary to viral infections, medications, or a response to any form of reduction in nephron number (congenital or acquired). Thus, FSGS may be a monogenic disease arising from pathogenic variants in one of several podocyte genes or from variants that affect the integrity of the glomerular basement membrane (GBM). Genetic FSGS may also result from variants that cause renal developmental defects or tubulointerstitial disease where the FSGS is likely an adaptive response to reduced functional nephrons. Specific genetic variants in the *APOL1* gene can substantially increase risk of FSGS and ESKD in patients with hypertension, HIV, sickle cell disease, or lupus nephritis and are discussed later in the chapter under renal disease risk variants.

Phenocopy There is little distinction between genetic forms of FSGS and non-genetic forms of FSGS. All primary and secondary forms of FSGS are thus phenocopies of genetic FSGS. In some patients with FSGS, a non-genetic cause for FSGS can be readily ascertained (e.g., HIV or bisphosphonate therapy), but in most cases, genetic screening is necessary to separate inherited from acquired causes of FSGS. On occasion, autosomal dominant fibronectin glomerulopathy can be misdiagnosed as FSGS because the fibronectin deposits can resemble the sclerosing lesions of FSGS [53].

Testing living donor candidates Like other genetic disorders, to appropriately screen the living donor candidate, the cause of FSGS in the affected family member must first be established. Except for a minority with distinct clinical or biopsy features of an acquired disease, patients with FSGS will need screening with a comprehensive gene panel to determine if it is a monogenic disease. A positive genetic diagnosis in the index patient then facilitates focused screening for the familial variant in the related living donor candidate. Negative result on genetic screening does not exclude disease but substantially reduces its likelihood, and the living donor candidate can use this information to weigh the long-term risks of donation [34].

Atypical HUS

Causal genes CFH, FI, FB, C3, MCP, THBD, PLG, DGKE

Clinical diagnosis The classic manifestation of aHUS is acute kidney injury from thrombotic microangiopathy (TMA) together with peripheral evidence of a microangiopathic hemolytic anemia (MAHA) characterized by schistocytes, thrombocytopenia, and sometimes a low complement C3 level [54, 55]. Some patients with aHUS may present with advanced CKD or ESRD with or without modest thrombocytopenia or other features of a MAHA, and diagnosis may only be suspected with the demonstration of chronic TMA features on a kidney biopsy. aHUS is known to be caused in the majority of cases by excessive activation of the alternate complement pathway, and variants in the complement C3 and its regulatory genes complement factor H (*CFH*), membrane cofactor protein (*MCP*), factor I (*CFI*), and factor B (*CFB*) have been identified in a significant fraction of patients with aHUS [56]. In other patients, aHUS is secondary to an autoantibody to CFH that inhibits CFH function, and in a smaller number, variants in genes that impact coagulation such as thrombomodulin (*THBD*), phospholipase G (*PLG*), and diacylglycerol kinase epsilon (*DGKE*) have also been identified [55, 57].

Phenocopy There are many other causes of TMA that can resemble aHUS, at least superficially. These include thrombotic thrombocytopenic purpura (TTP), lupus vasculitis, antiphospholipid antibody syndrome, malignant hypertension, and scleroderma renal crisis. These need to be differentiated from aHUS if necessary, by appropriate serological, histopathological, and/or genetic testing.

Testing living donor candidates Transplant candidates with suggestive clinical presentations should be screened for genetic variants in aHUS genes and for CFH autoantibodies to confirm the cause of ESKD, to determine need for terminal complement blockade to prevent recurrent disease, and to permit appropriate screening of their related living donor candidates. Most, but not all, patients with genetic variants in aHUS genes present with disease after a triggering event such as surgery, certain drugs, pregnancy/peripartum, or certain infections, suggesting that a second hit is required for disease [54]. The role a second hit explains the negative family history typically seen. aHUS from DGKe nephropathy is autosomal recessive and presents in infancy or early childhood, while all other forms are autosomal dominant with limited penetrance and can present at any age. In some familial cases, a normal examination and routine laboratory testing of a related living donor candidate do not exclude susceptibility to aHUS. Screening of the transplant candidate and identification of contributing gene variants allow the appropriate screening and acceptance of related living donor candidates. Some have argued that since the pathogenesis of aHUS is not fully understood and because not all affected patients have identifiable variants, it may be prudent to counsel any related donor candidate about the unknown risk of aHUS despite negative screening [58].

Fabry Disease

Causal genes *GLA*

Clinical diagnosis Fabry disease is a lysosomal storage disease arising from loss of function variants in the X-linked gene *GLA* encoding α-GAL A. In this disorder, abnormal glycosphingolipids accumulate in the lysosomes of podocytes and in vascular endothelial cells of the kidney and many other organ systems including the skin, the heart, and the peripheral and central nervous system. Classically affected patients present with acroparesthesias, neuropathic pain in the extremities, nonspecific gastrointestinal symptoms, and/or intolerance to hot weather, and the diagnosis is usually delayed for years. While males always have disease, some heterozygous females also manifest varying degrees of pathology, and the disease may be considered to be X-linked with variable expressivity in heterozygosity [59]. Males with suggestive symptoms or clinical findings such as angiokeratomata in the periumbilical area or the scrotum, cornea verticillata by slit lamp exam, or evidence of CKD or ESKD who also have low or absent plasma or leucocyte α-GAL A enzyme activity have confirmed Fabry disease. A kidney biopsy with lamellated inclusion bodies (myeloid or zebra bodies) in the podocytes and sometimes in vascular endothelial cells is strongly suggestive of Fabry disease. The disease is confirmed by measured α-GAL A enzyme level or screening the GLA gene for causal variants. In women, a normal α-GALA level does not exclude disease, and genetic testing in a patient with positive symptoms, signs, or laboratory evidence of disease is required.

Phenocopy Chloroquine, hydroxychloroquine, and amiodarone can cause proteinuric kidney disease with lysosomal zebra bodies indistinguishable from Fabry disease [60]. The diagnosis of a pseudo-lipidoses should be considered in patients presenting with a history of an appropriate drug exposure and a normal plasma α-GAL A level.

Testing living donor candidates Once the diagnosis is established in the affected family member and the α-GALA level is informative, an at-risk male donor candidate can be screened with kidney function testing and an α-GAL A level or focused screening of the familial GLA gene variant. In related asymptomatic females, a normal α-GAL A level does not exclude disease, and genetic screening is necessary to more accurately determine risk of Fabry disease.

Uncharacterized Renal Disease in Transplant Candidates

Although some genetic renal diseases such as ADPKD are rarely missed in patients with CKD, many other genetic renal disorders may not be recognized by the time the patient has developed ESKD and is being evaluated for a kidney transplant. There are many likely reasons for underestimation of monogenic kidney disease, especially in adults. These include the lack of a family history, unavailable or apparently normal imaging studies, absence or non-recognition of extrarenal syndromic features, and a non-diagnostic renal biopsy, especially if done late in advanced disease where non-specific glomerulosclerosis and interstitial fibrosis will likely obscure the original pattern of disease. In one large cohort of ESKD patients older than 45 years of age, exome sequencing identified a genetic cause in 9% of those with unknown cause of ESKD, 10% of those with a glomerulopathy, and 60% of those with a congenital or cystic renal disease, demonstrating that a significant number of monogenic diseases are undiagnosed [31]. Furthermore, unbiased testing with exome sequencing or targeted comprehensive renal gene panel testing such as KidneySeq™ demonstrates that even when genetic disease is suspected, the identified causal gene does not always correspond to the phenotype of the affected patient [31, 33]. In fact, more than half the patients with UMOD-mediated kidney disease did not have a tubulointerstitial phenotype [31]. When a first-degree relative of a transplant candidate is being evaluated as a living donor, unless the transplant candidate has a clear non-genetic cause of kidney disease, genetic testing with a broad-based genetic testing strategy of the transplant candidate and the related living donor candidate should be strongly considered [34].

Renal Disease Risk Variants: *APOL1* Renal Risk Variants and Sickle Cell Trait

In addition to the monogenic kidney diseases, at least two genetic traits are known to increase the risk of CKD. Two copies of *APOL1* renal risk variants (G1 or G2) are present in approximately 13% of African Americans and have been shown to substantially increase the risk of ESKD in African Americans with hypertension, HIV infection, systemic lupus erythematosus, and sickle cell disease [61–63]. In a large population-based cohort study of African Americans (REasons for Geographic and Racial Differences in Stroke (REGARDS)), the presence of two *APOL1* renal risk variants increased the risk of ESKD about 1.8-fold [64]. In one recent small study of living donors, the presence of two APOL1 renal risk variants was associated with a faster annual decline in eGFR postdonation at a median time of 12 years; two donors developed ESKD, both of whom carried an *APOL1* high-risk genotype [10]. Sickle cell trait (SCT), defined as the presence of one copy of sickle hemoglobin gene variant, exists among 8% of African Americans and was associated with increased risk of ESRD in the large REGARDS cohort, with a aHR of 2 [64].

Identification of the *APOL1* Gene

People of recent African ancestry (PRAA) including African Americans have an increased risk of ESRD [3, 65–68]. Efforts to find genetic variants that explain this disparity led to the identification of the *APOL1 gene* in the 22q12 region, and further gene-mapping efforts identified the G1 and G2 genotypes as the variants that are strongly associated with ESKD [61, 69]. These risk variants are located on the 3′ end of the *APOL1* gene; G1 refers to the rs73885319 nonsynonymous coding variants in linkage disequilibrium (Ser342Gly and Ile384Met), and G2, to the rs71785313 two amino-acid deletion delAsn388/Tyr389. Approximately 13% of PRAAs possess high-risk genotypes (G1/G1, G1/G2, or G2/G2), and these risk variants are enriched (23%) among first-degree relatives of ESKD cases [70].

Distribution of the *APOL1* Risk Variants

Environmental factors acting via natural selection in sub-Saharan African populations likely underlie the rise in frequency of the G1 and G2 variants. These variants appear to confer protection against African *Trypanosoma* parasites, which are transmitted by the tsetse fly (endemic to sub-Saharan African) and responsible for African sleeping sickness or trypanosomiasis [71]. Consequently, the *APOL1* renal risk variants have only been seen in PRAA, including individuals from Africa and recently admixed individuals in the New World such as African Americans, Afro-Caribbeans, and Afro-Latinos [72, 73].

Association Between *APOL1* Renal Risk Variants, ESKD, and CKD

The genetic association between *APOL1* renal risk variants and CKD/ESRD has been independently replicated in multiple studies. Initial studies reported strong association between the *APOL1* renal risk variants and the *MYH9* haplotype with ESKD; however, the association between ESKD and *MYH9* was no longer significant after accounting for *APOL1* [61]. Two copies of *APOL1* renal risk variants are strongly associated with FSGS and hypertension-attributed ESKD, with odds ratios of 10.5 (95% CI 6.0–18.4) and 7.3 (95% CI 5.6–9.5), respectively [61]. Subsequent studies showed that the *APOL1* renal risk variants, in addition to being enriched among first-degree relatives of patients with ESKD, were also associated with CKD, which was defined as eGFR <60 ml/min per 1.73 m^2 or albumin-to-creatinine ratio >30 mg/g [70]. Associations of *APOL1* high-risk genotypes with increased incidence of kidney disease, its faster progression, and younger age at dialysis initiation have also been described in longitudinal cohorts [62, 74–78]. In several studies, recipients of kidneys from deceased-donors with the two *APOL1* risk variants experienced shorter renal allograft survival, compared to those who received kidneys carrying none or one risk variant [79–82].

APOL1 and the Second Hit Hypothesis

The frequency of *APOL1* high-risk genotypes (G1/G1, G1/G2, or G2/G2) in the US African American population is approximately 13%. However, not all individuals who carry a high-risk genotype (2 risk variants) develop CKD or ESKD. Although some of the strongest effect sizes in the history of genetic association studies with a complex trait are observed with *APOL1*, these associations are often detected in presence of an environmental factor, i.e., a second hit. For example, an odds ratio of 29 (95% confidence interval: 13–68) was noted for the association between *APOL1* and HIV-associated nephropathy (HIVAN) [83]. Reported odds ratios for the association between *APOL1*, *ESKD*, and severe lupus nephritis range between 5.4 (95% CI: 2.4–14.1) and 2.72 (95% CI: 1.76–4.19) [84, 85]. Several potential second hits have been proposed, including viruses. There is accumulating evidence suggesting that therapeutic interferon may contribute to the development of FSGS among individuals who carry two *APOL1* risk variants [86]. Studies showed that the *APOL1* risk variants activate protein kinase R, which may provide a mechanism by which these variants damage podocytes [87]. We have reported that the JC polyoma virus appears to confer protection against CKD among individuals who carry the two *APOL1* risk variants [88–91].

Sickle Cell Trait

SCT is one of the most frequent hereditary hematologic conditions in the world. Like *APOL1*, the rise in the frequency of the SCT is due to positive selection under environmental pressure. An inverse relationship between the presence of the SCT and malaria has been observed [92–94]. SCT is seen in a wider range of populations; in addition to PRAA, these variants are observed in higher frequencies among individuals from South America, the Caribbean, Central America, Saudi Arabia, India, Turkey, Greece, and Italy [95]. Although homozygosity for the sickle hemoglobin gene variant (sickle cell anemia) can have severe renal manifestations ranging from albuminuria to ESKD and renal medullary carcinoma, renal effects are comparatively mild in those having the heterozygous trait (SCT) [96–100]. Pooled data from five large NHLBI cohorts (Atherosclerosis Risk in Communities Study [ARIC], Jackson Heart Study [JHS], Coronary Artery Risk Development in Young Adults [CARDIA], Multi-Ethnic Study of Atherosclerosis [MESA], and the

Women's Health Initiative [WHI]) demonstrated that the presence of SCT was associated with an increased risk of CKD, a greater decline in eGFR, and higher incidence of albuminuria [101]. In another study from a single healthcare system, the risk for incident CKD stage 3 (aHR 1.25; 95% CI 1.05:1.51) was increased in African Americans by the presence of SCT [102]. Lower eGFR levels were also seen among Hispanics with SCT [103].

Role of Sickle Cell Trait in Living Donation and Living Donor Kidney Transplantation

SCT trait is more prevalent in populations with limited access to transplantation, and data on transplantation outcomes are scant. One study from the 1970s, reporting on the experience of a few recipients with SCT from of a survey of transplant centers, suggested that the patient and graft survival was equivalent to those who did not have SCT [104]. There are no data on the renal outcomes following donor nephrectomy in living donors, and it is not clear whether nephrectomy changes incidence or progression of CKD postdonation. Practices in screening for SCT among living donor candidates vary between centers. In a survey conducted among 137 centers, 113 (83%) had no policy to screen donor candidates for the sickle trait, and only 39 out of 105 centers reported excluding donor candidates with SCT [105].

Role of *APOL1* in Living Donation and Living Donor Kidney Transplantation

There is considerable uncertainty about the role of *APOL1* genotyping in the evaluation and selection of living kidney donors of recent African ancestry. Case reports demonstrate that transplantation of a kidney from a living donor with two *APOL1* risk variants can lead to FSGS with early allograft failure in the recipient, along with postdonation ESKD in previously healthy donors [11, 106]. Doshi et al. reported an association of high-risk *APOL1* genotypes with faster eGFR decline among a small cohort of 136 living donors (19 with two *APOL1* risk variants). After a median of 11.3-year postdonation follow-up, advanced CKD (eGFR <45 ml/min/1.73m^2) was found in 15.2% of those with *APOL1* high-risk genotypes compared to 3.5% of those with low-risk genotypes (0 or 1 risk allele). Two of the 19 (11%) previously healthy living donors with *APOL1* high-risk genotypes developed ESKD [10]. The small, retrospective nature of the study leaves the field with an ongoing controversy [89, 107]. Some transplant programs routinely perform *APOL1* genotyping in the evaluation of living donor candidates of recent African ancestry and use this information in donor selection and counseling processes [108]. The 2017 KDIGO living donor guideline recommends that *APOL1* genotyping may be offered to living donor candidates with sub-Saharan African ancestors and that donor candidates should be informed that having two *APOL1* risk variants increases the lifetime risk of kidney failure but that the precise kidney failure risk for an affected individual after donation cannot currently be quantified [16]. Determining whether *APOL1* renal risk variants or SCT clearly increase the risk of ESKD after donation will need to await larger prospective collaborative multicenter studies, such as the national US *APOL1* Long-term Kidney Transplantation Outcomes Network (APOLLO, NCT03615235) and Living Donor Extended Time (LETO) study [109].

Interaction Between Sickle Cell and *APOL1*

There have been several efforts to evaluate the contribution of the *APOL1* risk variants to the nephropathy in sickle cell disease; however, results have been mixed. While one study found no association and in another the association did not reach statistical significance after correction for multiple testing, a third study [110, 111] reported a significant association of *APOL1* in 152 patients with sickle cell disease, with an odds ratio of 32.3 with a very wide C.I. (3.320 to 1005.7) [110–112]. A similar analysis in the REGARDS cohort found no interaction between SCT and *APOL1* on the risk of ESKD, although co-inheritance of the hemoglobin C trait and *APOL1* high renal genotype appear to increase the risk of prevalent CKD [64]. This is clearly an area where more research is needed [64].

Recommendation for Testing Living Donor Candidates for *APOL1* and the Sickle Cell Trait

The inheritance of a single copy of the sickle gene (SCT) and two copies of the *APOL1* risk variants are both recognized as risk factors for CKD/ESKD, and living donor candidates of the appropriate ancestry should be informed of the impact of these genetic variants on future kidney disease (Fig. 8.1). For the last several decades, SCT screening has been part of the routine newborn evaluation in the United States, and many affected donor candidates may already be aware of their diagnosis. For others, diagnosing SCT is most easily accomplished by hemoglobin electrophoresis, by isoelectric focusing, or by genetic testing. Screening for *APOL1* risk variants is performed by PCR and Sanger sequencing, and CLIA-approved testing is currently available at several laboratories. If the living donor candidate makes it through the initial screening tests and continues to be interested in donating, then those potentially at risk should be offered testing for both genetic traits. If the candidate has two *APOL1* risk variants, the presence or absence of other risk factors should be incorporated into overall risk stratification, and the final determination on donor candidacy should ideally be a shared decision respectful of donor autonomy.

Role of a Renal Genetics Clinic

We estimate that a significant number of transplant candidates have not had a careful evaluation for the cause of their kidney disease prior to their referral to a transplant center. About a third of diabetic patients with presumed diabetic kidney disease and a similar number with hypertension-attributed kidney disease appear to have a different cause of kidney disease [113–115]. Furthermore, it is well established that the Centers for Medicare & Medicaid Services (CMS) ESKD Reporting Form 2728, used by dialysis centers to certify the need for ESKD care, does not have the cause of ESKD listed in 57% of patients and the cause is misclassified in a significant fraction of others [116, 117]. Once a patient gets to a transplant center, reassessing the cause of ESKD can be a challenge but becomes especially important when considering biologically related living donor candidates. If locally available, a renal genetics clinic staffed with genetic counselors and physicians who have expertise in renal genetic disorders can determine need for additional testing, improve diagnosis of a variety of the renal disorders, and provide genetic counseling and screening of the at-risk related living donor candidate [118–120].

Summary

While current screening practices for living donor evaluation include criteria for excluding certain monogenic diseases such as ADPKD in those at risk, for many other genetic renal diseases, there are no clearly validated screening criteria to exclude familial disease in donor candidates except by confirming the diagnosis in an affected family member by genetic screening followed by focused genetic evaluation of the related living donor candidate. When there is considerable locus heterogeneity in the genetic basis for certain phenotypes or when the cause of ESKD is unknown, broad-based unbiased screening techniques such as exome sequencing or comprehensive renal gene panels (e.g., KidneySeq™) offer the potential for increased diagnostic precision, although the inevitable increased identification of variants of unknown significance increases the possibility of donor exclusion due to uncertainty. Prudence however dictates that consideration of genetic screening should be entertained for any donor candidate biologically related to another individual with a known monogenic kidney disease or where the cause of ESKD in the affected family member is unknown, especially if more than one family member are affected. In addition, two major genetic traits for advanced CKD are now known (SCT and *APOL1* renal risk variants), and living donor candidates from susceptible ancestry groups should be offered the option of testing for these traits to better estimate their risk of future kidney disease.

References

1. Merrill JP, Murray JE, Harrison JH, Guild WR. Successful homotransplantation of the human kidney between identical twins. JAMA. 1956;160(4):277–82. https://doi.org/10.1001/jama.1956.02960390027008.
2. In memoriam: Ronald Lee Herrick. Available at: https://www.findagrave.com/memorial/63560713. Accessed: 7 Sept 2020.
3. Muzaale AD, Massie AB, Wang M, et al. Risk of end-stage renal disease following live kidney donation. JAMA. 2014;311(6):579–86. https://doi.org/10.1001/jama.2013.285141.

4. Mjøen G, Hallan S, Hartmann A, Foss A, Midtvedt K, Øyen O, et al. Long-term risks for kidney donors. Kidney Int. 2014;86(1):162–7. https://doi.org/10.1038/ki.2013.460.
5. Matas AJ, Berglund DM, Vock DM, Ibrahim HN. Causes and timing of end-stage renal disease after living kidney donation. Am J Transplant. 2018;18(5):1140–50. https://doi.org/10.1111/ajt.14671.
6. Wainright JL, Robinson AM, Wilk AR, Klassen DK, Cherikh WS, Stewart DE. Risk of ESRD in prior living kidney donors. Am J Transplant. 2018;18(5):1129–39. https://doi.org/10.1111/ajt.14678.
7. Massie AB, Muzaale AD, Luo X, Chow EKH, Locke JE, Nguyen AQ, et al. Quantifying postdonation risk of ESRD in living kidney donors. J Am Soc Nephrol. 2017;28(9):2749–55. https://doi.org/10.1681/asn.2016101084.
8. Muzaale AD, Massie AB, Al Ammary F, Henderson ML, Purnell TS, Holscher CM, et al. Donor-recipient relationship and risk of ESKD in live kidney donors of varied racial groups. Am J Kidney Dis. 2020;75:333–41. https://doi.org/10.1053/j.ajkd.2019.08.020.
9. Winn MP, Alkhunaizi AM, Bennett WM, Garber RL, Howell DN, Butterly DW, et al. Focal segmental glomerulosclerosis: a need for caution in live-related renal transplantation. Am J Kidney Dis. 1999;33(5):970–4. https://doi.org/10.1016/S0272-6386(99)70435-X.
10. Doshi MD, Ortigosa-Goggins M, Garg AX, Li L, Poggio ED, Winkler CA, et al. APOL1 genotype and renal function of black living donors. J Am Soc Nephrol. 2018;29(4):1309–16. https://doi.org/10.1681/asn.2017060658.
11. Lentine KL, Mannon RB. Apolipoprotein L1: role in the evaluation of kidney transplant donors. Curr Opin Nephrol Hypertens. 2020;29(6):645–55. https://doi.org/10.1097/MNH.0000000000000653.
12. Axelrod DA, Schnitzler MA, Xiao H, Irish W, Tuttle-Newhall E, Chang SH, et al. An economic assessment of contemporary kidney transplant practice. Am J Transplant. 2018;18(5):1168–76. https://doi.org/10.1111/ajt.14702.
13. Organ Procurement and Transplantation Network (OPTN) National Data. Available at: https://optn.transplant.hrsa.gov/data/view-data-reports/national-data/#. Accessed: 7 Sept 2020.
14. Muzaale AD, Massie AB, Kucirka LM, Luo X, Kumar K, Brown RS, et al. Outcomes of live kidney donors who develop end-stage renal disease. Transplantation. 2016;100(6):1306–12. https://doi.org/10.1097/TP.0000000000000920.
15. Grams ME, Chow EK, Segev DL, Coresh J. Lifetime incidence of CKD stages 3–5 in the United States. Am J Kidney Dis. 2013;62(2):245–52. https://doi.org/10.1053/j.ajkd.2013.03.009.
16. Lentine KL, Kasiske BL, Levey AS, Adams PL, Alberu J, Bakr MA, et al. KDIGO clinical practice guideline on the evaluation and care of living kidney donors. Transplantation. 2017;101(8S Suppl 1):S1–S109. https://doi.org/10.1097/TP.0000000000001769.
17. Hsu CY, Iribarren C, McCulloch CE, Darbinian J, Go AS. Risk factors for end-stage renal disease: 25-year follow-up. Arch Intern Med. 2009;169(4):342–50. https://doi.org/10.1001/archinternmed.2008.605.
18. Vivante A, Afek A, Frenkel-Nir Y, Tzur D, Farfel A, Golan E, et al. Persistent asymptomatic isolated microscopic hematuria in Israeli adolescents and young adults and risk for end-stage renal disease. JAMA. 2011;306(7):729–36. https://doi.org/10.1001/jama.2011.1141.
19. El-Zoghby ZM, Lieske JC, Foley RN, Bergstralh EJ, Li X, Melton LJ, et al. Urolithiasis and the risk of ESRD. Clin J Am Soc Nephrol. 2012;7(9):1409–15. https://doi.org/10.2215/cjn.03210312.
20. Ruggajo P, Skrunes R, Svarstad E, Skjaerven R, Reisaether AV, Vikse BE. Familial factors, low birth weight, and development of ESRD: a nationwide registry study. Am J Kidney Dis. 2016;67(4):601–8. https://doi.org/10.1053/j.ajkd.2015.11.015.
21. Locke JE, Reed RD, Massie A, MacLennan PA, Sawinski D, Kumar V, et al. Obesity increases the risk of end-stage renal disease among living kidney donors. Kidney Int. 2017;91(3):699–703. https://doi.org/10.1016/j.kint.2016.10.014.

22. Veitia RA, Caburet S, Birchler JA. Mechanisms of Mendelian dominance. Clin Genet. 2018;93(3):419–28. https://doi.org/10.1111/cge.13107.

23. Katsanis N, Ansley SJ, Badano JL, Eichers ER, Lewis RA, Hoskins BE, et al. Triallelic inheritance in Bardet-Biedl syndrome, a Mendelian recessive disorder. Science. 2001;293(5538):2256–9. https://doi.org/10.1126/science.1063525.

24. Sanna-Cherchi S, Kiryluk K, Burgess Katelyn E, Bodria M, Sampson Matthew G, Hadley D, et al. Copy-number disorders are a common cause of congenital kidney malformations. Am J Hum Genet. 2012;91(6):987–97. https://doi.org/10.1016/j.ajhg.2012.10.007.

25. Snoek R, van Setten J, Keating BJ, Israni AK, Jacobson PA, Oetting WS, et al. NPHP1 (Nephrocystin-1) gene deletions cause adult-onset ESRD. J Am Soc Nephrol. 2018;29(6):1772–9. https://doi.org/10.1681/asn.2017111200.

26. Hildebrandt F. Genetic kidney diseases. Lancet. 2010;375(9722):1287–95. https://doi.org/10.1016/S0140-6736(10)60236-X.

27. Stokman M, Lilien M, Knoers N. Nephronophthisis. In: GeneReviews [internet]. Seattle: University of Washington; 2016, 1993–2017. Available at: https://www.ncbi.nlm.nih.gov/books/NBK368475/.

28. Armstrong ME, Thomas CP. Diagnosis of monogenic chronic kidney diseases. Curr Opin Nephrol Hypertens. 2019;28(2):183–94. https://doi.org/10.1097/MNH.0000000000000486.

29. Spencer DH, Zhang B, Pfeifer J. Chapter 8 - Single nucleotide variant detection using next generation sequencing. In: Kulkarni S, Pfeifer J, editors. Clinical genomics. Boston: Academic Press; 2015. p. 109–27.

30. Richards S, Aziz N, Bale S, Bick D, Das S, Gastier-Foster J, et al. Standards and guidelines for the interpretation of sequence variants: a joint consensus recommendation of the American College of Medical Genetics and Genomics and the Association for Molecular Pathology. Genet Med. 2015;17(5):405–23. https://doi.org/10.1038/gim.2015.30.

31. Groopman EE, Marasa M, Cameron-Christie S, Petrovski S, Aggarwal VS, Milo-Rasouly H, et al. Diagnostic utility of exome sequencing for kidney disease. N Engl J Med. 2019;380(2):142–51. https://doi.org/10.1056/NEJMoa1806891.

32. Mallett AJ, McCarthy HJ, Ho G, Holman K, Farnsworth E, Patel C, et al. Massively parallel sequencing and targeted exomes in familial kidney disease can diagnose underlying genetic disorders. Kidney Int. 2017;92(6):1493–506. https://doi.org/10.1016/j.kint.2017.06.013.

33. Mansilla M, Sompallae R, Nishimura C, Kwitek A, Kimble M, Freese M, et al. Targeted broad-based genetic testing by next generation sequencing informs diagnosis and facilitates management in patients with kidney diseases. Nephrol Dial Transplant. 2019;34. https://doi.org/10.1093/ndt/gfz173.

34. Thomas CP, Mansilla MA, Sompallae R, Mason SO, Nishimura CJ, Kimble MJ, et al. Screening of living kidney donors for genetic diseases using a comprehensive genetic testing strategy. Am J Transplant. 2017;17(2):401–10. https://doi.org/10.1111/ajt.13970.

35. Mallawaarachchi AC, Hort Y, Cowley MJ, McCabe MJ, Minoche A, Dinger ME, et al. Whole-genome sequencing overcomes pseudogene homology to diagnose autosomal dominant polycystic kidney disease. Eur J Hum Genet. 2016;24(11):1584–90. https://doi.org/10.1111/ajt.13970.

36. Alkan C, Sajjadian S, Eichler EE. Limitations of next-generation genome sequence assembly. Nat Methods. 2011;8(1):61–5. https://doi.org/10.1038/nmeth.1527.

37. Kirby A, Gnirke A, Jaffe DB, Baresova V, Pochet N, Blumenstiel B, et al. Mutations causing medullary cystic kidney disease type 1 lie in a large VNTR in MUC1 missed by massively parallel sequencing. Nat Genet. 2013;45(3):299–303. https://doi.org/10.1038/ng.2543.

38. Zhang C, Cerveira E, Romanovitch M, Zhu Q. Array-based comparative genomic hybridization (aCGH). Methods Mol Biol. 2017;1541:167–79. https://doi.org/10.1007/978-1-4939-6703-2_15.

39. Perne A, Zhang X, Lehmann L, Groth M, Stuber F, Book M. Comparison of multiplex ligation-dependent probe amplification and real-time PCR accuracy for gene copy number quantification using the beta-defensin locus. Biotechniques. 2009;47(6):1023–8. https://doi.org/10.2144/000113300.

40. Alves M, Fonseca T, de Almeida EAF. Differential diagnosis of autosomal dominant polycystic kidney disease. Brisbane: Codon Publications; 2015.
41. Cornec-Le Gall E, Olson RJ, Besse W, Heyer CM, Gainullin VG, Smith JM, et al. Monoallelic mutations to DNAJB11 cause atypical autosomal-dominant polycystic kidney disease. Am J Hum Genet. 2018;102(5):832–44. https://doi.org/10.1016/j.ajhg.2018.03.013.
42. Pei Y, Obaji J, Dupuis A, Paterson AD, Magistroni R, Dicks E, et al. Unified criteria for ultrasonographic diagnosis of ADPKD. J Am Soc Nephrol. 2009;20(1):205–12. https://doi.org/10.1681/asn.2008050507.
43. Pei Y, Hwang Y-H, Conklin J, Sundsbak JL, Heyer CM, Chan W, et al. Imaging-based diagnosis of autosomal dominant polycystic kidney disease. J Am Soc Nephrol. 2015;26(3):746–53. https://doi.org/10.1681/asn.2014030297.
44. Simms RJ, Travis DL, Durkie M, Wilson G, Dalton A, Ong AC. Genetic testing in the assessment of living related kidney donors at risk of autosomal dominant polycystic kidney disease. Transplantation. 2015;99(5):1023–9. https://doi.org/10.1097/tp.0000000000000466.
45. Živná M, Kidd K, Přistoupilová A, Barešová V, DeFelice M, Blumenstiel B, et al. Noninvasive immunohistochemical diagnosis and novel *MUC1* mutations causing autosomal dominant tubulointerstitial kidney disease. J Am Soc Nephrol. 2018;29(9):2418–31. https://doi.org/10.1681/asn.2018020180.
46. Savige J, Ariani F, Mari F, Bruttini M, Renieri A, Gross O, et al. Expert consensus guidelines for the genetic diagnosis of Alport syndrome. Pediatr Nephrol. 2019;34:1175–89. https://doi.org/10.1681/asn.2018020180.
47. Gast C, Pengelly RJ, Lyon M, Bunyan DJ, Seaby EG, Graham N, et al. Collagen (COL4A) mutations are the most frequent mutations underlying adult focal segmental glomerulosclerosis. Nephrol Dial Transplant. 2016;31:961–70. https://doi.org/10.1093/ndt/gfv325.
48. Malone AF, Phelan PJ, Hall G, Cetincelik U, Homstad A, Alonso AS, et al. Rare hereditary COL4A3/COL4A4 variants may be mistaken for familial focal segmental glomerulosclerosis. Kidney Int. 2014;86(6):1253–9. https://doi.org/10.1038/ki.2014.305.
49. Kashtan CE. Alport syndrome and thin basement membrane nephropathy. In: Adam MP, Ardinger HH, Pagon RA, Wallace SE, Bean LJH, Stephens K, et al., editors. GeneReviews((R)). Seattle: University of Washington; 1993.
50. Stapleton CP, Kennedy C, Fennelly NK, Murray SL, Connaughton DM, Dorman AM, et al. An exome sequencing study of 10 families with IgA nephropathy. Nephron. 2020;144(2):72–83. https://doi.org/10.1159/000503564.
51. Tabibzadeh N, Fleury D, Labatut D, Bridoux F, Lionet A, Jourde-Chiche N, et al. MYH9-related disorders display heterogeneous kidney involvement and outcome. Clin Kidney J. 2019;12(4):494–502. https://doi.org/10.1093/ckj/sfy117.
52. Sadowski CE, Lovric S, Ashraf S, Pabst WL, Gee HY, Kohl S, et al. A single-gene cause in 29.5% of cases of steroid-resistant nephrotic syndrome. J Am Soc Nephrol. 2015;26(6):1279–89. https://doi.org/10.1681/asn.2014050489.
53. Strom EH, Banfi G, Krapf R, Abt AB, Mazzucco G, Monga G, et al. Glomerulopathy associated with predominant fibronectin deposits: a newly recognized hereditary disease. Kidney Int. 1995;48(1):163–70. https://doi.org/10.1038/ki.1995.280.
54. Nester CM, Thomas CP. Atypical hemolytic uremic syndrome: what is it, how is it diagnosed, and how is it treated? Hematology Am Soc Hematol Educ Program. 2012;2012:617–25. https://doi.org/10.1182/asheducation-2012.1.617.
55. Goodship THJ, Cook HT, Fakhouri F, Fervenza FC, Frémeaux-Bacchi V, Kavanagh D, et al. Atypical hemolytic uremic syndrome and C3 glomerulopathy: conclusions from a "Kidney Disease: Improving Global Outcomes" (KDIGO) controversies conference. Kidney Int. 2017;91(3):539–51. https://doi.org/10.1016/j.kint.2016.10.005.
56. Nester CM, Barbour T, de Cordoba SR, Dragon-Durey MA, Fremeaux-Bacchi V, Goodship THJ, et al. Atypical aHUS: state of the art. Mol Immunol. 2015;67(1):31–42. https://doi.org/10.1016/j.molimm.2015.03.246.
57. Bu F, Zhang Y, Wang K, Borsa NG, Jones MB, Taylor AO, et al. Genetic analysis of 400 patients refines understanding and implicates a new gene in atypical hemolytic uremic syndrome. J Am Soc Nephrol. 2018;29:2809–19. https://doi.org/10.1681/asn.2018070759.

58. Kuppachi S, Smith RJH, Thomas CP. Evaluation of genetic renal diseases in potential living kidney donors. Curr Transplant Rep. 2015;2(1):1–14. https://doi.org/10.1007/s40472-014-0042-5.

59. Germain DP. In: Mehta A, Beck M, Sunder-Plassmann G, editors. General aspects of X-linked diseases. Oxford: Oxford PharmaGenesis; 2006.

60. Bracamonte ER, Kowalewska J, Starr J, Gitomer J, Alpers CE. Iatrogenic phospholipidosis mimicking Fabry disease. Am J Kidney Dis. 2006;48(5):844–50. https://doi.org/10.1053/j.ajkd.2006.05.034.

61. Genovese G, Friedman DJ, Ross MD, Lecordier L, Uzureau P, Freedman BI, et al. Association of trypanolytic ApoL1 variants with kidney disease in African-Americans. Science (New York, NY). 2010;329(5993):841–5. https://doi.org/10.1126/science.1193032.

62. Parsa A, Kao WH, Xie D, Astor BC, Li M, Hsu CY, et al. APOL1 risk variants, race, and progression of chronic kidney disease. N Engl J Med. 2013;369(23):2183–96. https://doi.org/10.1056/NEJMoa1310345.

63. Kruzel-Davila E, Wasser WG, Aviram S, Skorecki K. APOL1 nephropathy: from gene to mechanisms of kidney injury. Nephrol Dial Transplant. 2016;31(3):349–58. https://doi.org/10.1093/ndt/gfu391.

64. Naik RP, Irvin MR, Judd S, Gutiérrez OM, Zakai NA, Derebail VK, et al. Sickle cell trait and the risk of ESRD in blacks. J Am Soc Nephrol. 2017;28(7):2180–7. https://doi.org/10.1681/ASN.2016101086.

65. Lentine KL, Schnitzler MA, Xiao H, Saab G, Salvalaggio PR, Axelrod D, et al. Racial variation in medical outcomes among living kidney donors. N Engl J Med. 2010;363(8):724–32. https://doi.org/10.1056/NEJMoa1000950.

66. Lentine KL, Segev DL. Health outcomes among non-Caucasian living kidney donors: knowns and unknowns. Transpl Int. 2013;26(9):853–64. https://doi.org/10.1111/tri.12088.

67. Lentine KL, Schnitzler MA, Garg AX, Xiao H, Axelrod D, Tuttle-Newhall JE, et al. Race, relationship and renal diagnoses after living kidney donation. Transplantation. 2015;99(8):1723–9. https://doi.org/10.1097/TP.0000000000000733.

68. Taber DJ, Egede LE, Baliga PK. Outcome disparities between African Americans and Caucasians in contemporary kidney transplant recipients. Am J Surg. 2017;213(4):666–72. https://doi.org/10.1016/j.amjsurg.2016.11.024.

69. Tzur S, Rosset S, Shemer R, Yudkovsky G, Selig S, Tarekegn A, et al. Missense mutations in the APOL1 gene are highly associated with end stage kidney disease risk previously attributed to the MYH9 gene. Hum Genet. 2010;128(3):345–50. https://doi.org/10.1007/s00439-010-0861-0.

70. Freedman BI, Langefeld CD, Turner J, Nunez M, High KP, Spainhour M, et al. Association of APOL1 variants with mild kidney disease in the first-degree relatives of African American patients with non-diabetic end-stage renal disease. Kidney Int. 2012;82(7):805–11. https://doi.org/10.1038/ki.2012.217.

71. Cooper A, Ilboudo H, Alibu VP, Ravel S, Enyaru J, Weir W, et al. APOL1 renal risk variants have contrasting resistance and susceptibility associations with African trypanosomiasis. Elife. 2017;6:e25461. https://doi.org/10.7554/eLife.25461.

72. Limou S, Nelson GW, Kopp JB, Winkler CA. APOL1 kidney risk alleles: population genetics and disease associations. Adv Chronic Kidney Dis. 2014;21(5):426–33. https://doi.org/10.1053/j.ackd.2014.06.005.

73. Nadkarni GN, Gignoux CR, Sorokin EP, Daya M, Rahman R, Barnes KC, et al. Worldwide frequencies of APOL1 renal risk variants. N Engl J Med. 2018;379(26):2571–2. https://doi.org/10.1056/NEJMc1800748.

74. Grams ME, Rebholz CM, Chen Y, Rawlings AM, Estrella MM, Selvin E, et al. Race, APOL1 risk, and eGFR decline in the general population. J Am Soc Nephrol. 2016;27(9):2842–50. https://doi.org/10.1681/Asn.2015070763.

75. Peralta CA, Bibbins-Domingo K, Vittinghoff E, Lin F, Fornage M, Kopp JB, et al. APOL1 genotype and race differences in incident albuminuria and renal function decline. J Am Soc Nephrol. 2016;27(3):887–93. https://doi.org/10.1681/Asn.2015020124.

76. Lipkowitz MS, Freedman BI, Langefeld CD, Comeau ME, Bowden DW, Kao WH, et al. Apolipoprotein L1 gene variants associate with hypertension-attributed nephropathy and the rate of kidney function decline in African Americans. Kidney Int. 2013;83(1) 114–20. https://doi.org/10.1038/ki.2012.263.

77. O'Toole JF, Bruggeman LA, Sedor JR. APOL1 and proteinuria in the AASK: unraveling the pathobiology of APOL1. Clin J Am Soc Nephrol. 2017;12(11):1723–5. https://doi.org/10.2215/CJN.10680917.

78. Kanji Z, Powe CE, Wenger JB, Huang C, Ankers E, Sullivan DA, et al. Genetic variation in APOL1 associates with younger age at hemodialysis initiation. J Am Soc Nephrol. 2011;22(11):2091–7. https://doi.org/10.1681/ASN.2010121234.

79. Israni AK, Salkowski N, Gustafson S, Snyder JJ, Friedewald JJ, Formica RN, et al. New national allocation policy for deceased donor kidneys in the United States and possible effect on patient outcomes. J Am Soc Nephrol. 2014;25(8):1842–8. https://doi.org/10.1681/ASN.2013070784.

80. Reeves-Daniel AM, DePalma JA, Bleyer AJ, Rocco MV, Murea M, Adams PL, et al. The APOL1 gene and allograft survival after kidney transplantation. Am J Transplant. 2011;11(5):1025–30. https://doi.org/10.1111/j.1600-6143.2011.03513.x.

81. Freedman BI, Julian BA. Should kidney donors be genotyped for APOL1 risk alleles? Kidney Int. 2015;87(4):671–3. https://doi.org/10.1038/ki.2015.16.

82. Freedman BI, Pastan SO, Israni AK, Schladt D, Julian BA, Gautreaux MD, et al. APOL1 genotype and kidney transplantation outcomes from deceased African American donors. Transplantation. 2016;100(1):194–202. https://doi.org/10.1097/tp.0000000000000969.

83. Kopp JB, Nelson GW, Sampath K, Johnson RC, Genovese G, An P, et al. APOL1 genetic variants in focal segmental glomerulosclerosis and HIV-associated nephropathy. J Am Soc Nephrol. 2011;22(11):2129–37. https://doi.org/10.1681/ASN.2011040388.

84. Freedman BI, Langefeld CD, Andringa KK, Croker JA, Williams AH, Garner NE, et al. End-stage renal disease in African Americans with lupus nephritis is associated with APOL1. Arthritis Rheumatol. 2014;66(2):390–6. https://doi.org/10.1002/art.38220.

85. Larsen CP, Beggs ML, Saeed M, Walker PD. Apolipoprotein L1 risk variants associate with systemic lupus erythematosus-associated collapsing glomerulopathy. J Am Soc Nephrol. 2013;24(5):722–5. https://doi.org/10.1681/ASN.2012121180.

86. Nichols B, Jog P, Lee JH, Blackler D, Wilmot M, D'Agati V, et al. Innate immunity pathways regulate the nephropathy gene Apolipoprotein L1. Kidney Int. 2015;87(2):332–42. https://doi.org/10.1038/ki.2014.270.

87. Okamoto K, Rausch JW, Wakashin H, Fu Y, Chung J-Y, Dummer PD, et al. APOL1 risk allele RNA contributes to renal toxicity by activating protein kinase R. Commun Biol. 2018;1:188. https://doi.org/10.1038/s42003-018-0188-2.

88. Divers J, Núñez M, High KP, Murea M, Rocco MV, Ma L, et al. JC polyoma virus interacts with APOL1 in African Americans with nondiabetic nephropathy. Kidney Int. 2013;84(6):1207–13. https://doi.org/10.1038/ki.2013.173.

89. Freedman BI, Julian BA. Evaluation of potential living kidney donors in the APOL1 era. J Am Soc Nephrol. 2018;29:1079–81. https://doi.org/10.1681/ASN.2018020137.

90. Kruzel-Davila E, Divers J, Russell GB, Kra-Oz Z, Cohen MS, Langefeld CD, et al. JC Viruria is associated with reduced risk of diabetic kidney disease. J Clin Endocrinol Metab. 2019;104(6):2286–94. https://doi.org/10.1210/jc.2018-02482.

91. Freedman BI, Kistler AL, Skewes-Cox P, Ganem D, Spainhour M, Turner J, et al. JC polyoma viruria associates with protection from chronic kidney disease independently from apolipoprotein L1 genotype in African Americans. Nephrol Dial Transplant. 2018;33(11):1960–7. https://doi.org/10.1093/ndt/gfx368.

92. Williams TN, Mwangi TW, Wambua S, Alexander ND, Kortok M, Snow RW, et al. Sickle cell trait and the risk of Plasmodium falciparum malaria and other childhood diseases. J Infect Dis. 2005;192(1):178–86. https://doi.org/10.1086/430744.

93. Aidoo M, Terlouw DJ, Kolczak MS, McElroy PD, ter Kuile FO, Kariuki S, et al. Protective effects of the sickle cell gene against malaria morbidity and mortality. Lancet (London, England). 2002;359(9314):1311–2. https://doi.org/10.1016/S0140-6736(02)08273-9.

94. Allison AC. Protection afforded by sickle-cell trait against subtertian malarial infection. Br Med J. 1954;1(4857):290–4. https://doi.org/10.1136/bmj.1.4857.290.

95. Piel FB, Patil AP, Howes RE, Nyangiri OA, Gething PW, Williams TN, et al. Global distribution of the sickle cell gene and geographical confirmation of the malaria hypothesis. Nat Commun. 2010;1:104. https://doi.org/10.1038/ncomms1104.

96. Ataga KI, Derebail VK, Archer DR. The glomerulopathy of sickle cell disease. Am J Hematol. 2014;89(9):907–14. https://doi.org/10.1002/ajh.23762.

97. Stuart MJ, Nagel RL. Sickle-cell disease. Lancet (London, England). 2004;364(9442):1343–60. https://doi.org/10.1016/S0140-6736(04)17192-4.

98. Derebail VK, Nachman PH, Key NS, Ansede H, Falk RJ, Kshirsagar AV. High prevalence of sickle cell trait in African Americans with ESRD. J Am Soc Nephrol. 2010;21(3):413–7. https://doi.org/10.1681/asn.2009070705.

99. Nath KA, Hebbel RP. Sickle cell disease: renal manifestations and mechanisms. Nat Rev Nephrol. 2015;11(3):161–71. https://doi.org/10.1038/nrneph.2015.8.

100. Cazenave M, Koehl B, Nochy D, Tharaux P-L, Audard V. Spectrum of renal manifestations in sickle cell disease. Nephrol Ther. 2014;10(1):10–6. https://doi.org/10.1016/j.nephro.2013.07.366.

101. Naik RP, Derebail VK, Grams ME, Franceschini N, Auer PL, Peloso GM, et al. Association of sickle cell trait with chronic kidney disease and albuminuria in African Americans. JAMA. 2014;312(20):2115–25. https://doi.org/10.1001/jama.2014.15063.

102. Olaniran KO, Allegretti AS, Zhao SH, Achebe MM, Eneanya ND, Thadhani RI, et al. Kidney function decline among black patients with sickle cell trait and sickle cell disease: an observational cohort study. J Am Soc Nephrol. 2020;31(2):393–404. https://doi.org/10.1681/asn.2019050502.

103. Dueker ND, Della-Morte D, Rundek T, Sacco RL, Blanton SH. Sickle cell trait and renal function in hispanics in the United States: the Northern Manhattan study. Ethn Dis. 2017;27(1):11–4. https://doi.org/10.18865/ed.27.1.11.

104. Chatterjee SN. National study on natural history of renal allografts in sickle cell disease or trait. Nephron. 1980;25(4):199–201. https://doi.org/10.1159/000181781.

105. Reese PP, Hoo AC, Magee CC. Screening for sickle trait among potential live kidney donors: policies and practices in US transplant centers. Transpl Int. 2008;21(4):328–31. https://doi.org/10.1111/j.1432-2277.2007.00611.x.

106. Kofman T, Audard V, Narjoz C, Gribouval O, Matignon M, Leibler C, et al. APOL1 polymorphisms and development of CKD in an identical twin donor and recipient pair. Am J Kidney Dis. 2014;63(5):816–9. https://doi.org/10.1053/j.ajkd.2013.12.014.

107. Ross LF, Thistlethwaite JR Jr. Introducing genetic tests with uncertain implications in living donor kidney transplantation: ApoL1 as a case study. Prog Transplant. 2016;26(3):203–6. https://doi.org/10.1177/1526924816654608.

108. Cohen DM, Mittalhenkle A, Scott DL, Young CJ, Norman DJ. African American living-kidney donors should be screened for APOL1 risk alleles. Transplantation. 2011;92(7):722–5. https://doi.org/10.1097/TP.0b013e31822eec39.

109. Freedman BI, Moxey-Mims MM, Alexander AA, Astor BC, Birdwell KA, Bowden DW, et al. APOL1 long-term kidney transplantation outcomes network (APOLLO): design and rationale. Kidney Int Rep. 2020;5(3):278–88. https://doi.org/10.1016/j.ekir.2019.11.022.

110. Ashley-Koch AE, Okocha EC, Garrett ME, Soldano K, De Castro LM, Jonassaint JC, et al. MYH9 and APOL1 are both associated with sickle cell disease nephropathy. Br J Haematol. 2011;155(3):386–94. https://doi.org/10.1111/j.1365-2141.2011.08832.x.

111. Hicks PJ, Langefeld CD, Lu L, Bleyer AJ, Divers J, Nachman PH, et al. Sickle cell trait is not independently associated with susceptibility to end-stage renal disease in African Americans. Kidney Int. 2011;80(12):1339–43. https://doi.org/10.1038/ki.2011.286.

112. Kormann R, Jannot A-S, Narjoz C, Ribeil J-A, Manceau S, Delville M, et al. Roles of APOL1 G1 and G2 variants in sickle cell disease patients: kidney is the main target. Br J Haematol. 2017;179(2):323–35. https://doi.org/10.1111/bjh.14842.

113. Sharma SG, Bomback AS, Radhakrishnan J, Herlitz LC, Stokes MB, Markowitz GS, et al. The modern spectrum of renal biopsy findings in patients with diabetes. Clin J Am Soc Nephrol. 2013;8(10):1718–24. https://doi.org/10.2215/cjn.02510213.
114. Christensen PK, Larsen S, Horn T, Olsen S, Parving HH. Causes of albuminuria in patients with type 2 diabetes without diabetic retinopathy. Kidney Int. 2000;58(4):1719–31. https://doi.org/10.1046/j.1523-1755.2000.00333.x.
115. Caetano ER, Zatz R, Saldanha LB, Praxedes JN. Hypertensive nephrosclerosis as a relevant cause of chronic renal failure. Hypertension. 2001;38(2):171–6. https://doi.org/10.1161/01.hyp.38.2.171.
116. Layton JB, Hogan SL, Jennette CE, Kenderes B, Krisher J, Jennette JC, et al. Discrepancy between medical evidence form 2728 and renal biopsy for glomerular diseases. Clin J Am Soc Nephrol. 2010;5(11):2046–52. https://doi.org/10.2215/cjn.03550410.
117. Tucker BM, Freedman BI. Need to reclassify etiologies of ESRD on the CMS 2728 medical evidence report. Clin J Am Soc Nephrol. 2018;13(3):477–9. https://doi.org/10.2215/cjn.08310817.
118. Thomas CP, Freese ME, Ounda A, Jetton JG, Holida M, Noureddine L, et al. Initial experience from a renal genetics clinic demonstrates a distinct role in patient management. Genet Med. 2020;22:1025–35. https://doi.org/10.1038/s41436-020-0772-y.
119. Mallett A, Fowles LF, McGaughran J, Healy H, Patel C. A multidisciplinary renal genetics clinic improves patient diagnosis. Med J Aust. 2016;204(2):58–9. https://doi.org/10.5694/mja15.01157.
120. Alkanderi S, Yates LM, Johnson SA, Sayer JA. Lessons learned from a multidisciplinary renal genetics clinic. QJM. 2017;110(7):453–7. https://doi.org/10.1093/qjmed/hcx030.

Perioperative Evaluation and Management of Living Donor Candidates

9

Gretchen Edwards, Beatrice P. Concepcion, and Rachel C. Forbes

Overview of Preoperative Evaluation of the Living Kidney Donor and Frequency of Complications

While most living kidney donors experience good outcomes and quality of life after donation, kidney donation is associated with risks of potential short- and long-term surgical, medical, psychosocial, and financial complications [1]. The goals of the preoperative evaluation of the living kidney donor candidate include assessing a donor candidate's risk of perioperative complications to determine if they are suitable to proceed, stratifying perioperative risk, performing suitable preoperative testing, counseling patients on their perioperative risks, and optimizing patients for surgery to minimize complications. Careful medical history, physical exam, and appropriate preoperative testing are required to assess a donor candidate's risk to determine if it is acceptable to proceed with donation and to identify conditions that may require additional management to optimize the safety of surgery and kidney donation. The 2017 Kidney Disease: Improving Global Outcomes (KDIGO) Clinical Practice Guideline on the Evaluation and Care of Living Kidney Donors includes recommendations for the preoperative evaluation and management for donors and recognizes there are few evidence-based recommendations for this aspect of living donor care. For this reason, perioperative considerations for living

G. Edwards
Division of General Surgery, Department of Surgery, Vanderbilt University Medical Center, Nashville, TN, USA

B. P. Concepcion
Division of Nephrology and Hypertension, Department of Medicine, Vanderbilt University Medical Center, Nashville, TN, USA

R. C. Forbes (✉)
Division of Kidney and Pancreas Transplantation, Department of Surgery, Vanderbilt University Medical Center, Nashville, TN, USA
e-mail: rachel.forbes@vumc.org

© Springer Nature Switzerland AG 2021
K. L. Lentine et al. (eds.), *Living Kidney Donation*,
https://doi.org/10.1007/978-3-030-53618-3_9

kidney donors are often extrapolated from populations not specific to living donors [2]. In the United States, the Organ Procurement and Transplantation Network (OPTN) policy mandates minimum requirements for the evaluation of living donor candidates.

Living donor nephrectomy has been safely performed since the 1950s and carries a low risk of complications. In a US study of integrated donor registry data and national death records for 80,347 donors (1994–2009), 90-day all-cause mortality was 0.03% based on 25 deaths [3]. Prior studies including a survey of US programs and a UK registry reported similar all-cause mortality rates [4, 5]. Based on US administrative data, Schold et al. reported an overall incidence of perioperative complications after donor nephrectomy of 7.9% and identified digestive (32%), respiratory (14%), procedural (13%), urinary (11%), hemorrhage (11%), infectious (9%), and cardiac (4%) complications. Limitations of this study included lack of data linkages to donor status and assumptions regarding acute care hospitalizations [6]. Lentine et al. evaluated US donor registry data to examine 14,964 donors (2008–2012) and identified postoperative complications in 16.8%, most commonly gastrointestinal (4.4%), bleeding (3.0%), respiratory (2.5%), and surgical/anesthesia-related injuries (2.4%); however, the incidence of major complications (Clavien grading system 4 or 5 [7]) was 2.5% [8]. Similar findings were also reported by a Norwegian registry study of 1022 living kidney donations from 1997 to 2008 showing a rate of 2.9% for major and 18% for minor complications by Clavien grading [9]. In a study of 1042 living donors from 12 Canadian and five Australian centers (2004–2014), 13% experienced 142 perioperative complications (55 intraoperative; 87 postoperative); 90% of complications were minor, and the incidence of major complications in the cohort was 1% [10].

Readmission rates after living donor nephrectomy have been examined in a study of integrated US registry data, administrative academic hospital consortium data, and pharmacy claims warehouse data [11]. Among 14,959 donors (2008–2012), 2.9% were readmitted within 90 days post-donation. Those donors with the highest predonation opioid use were more than twice as likely to experience a readmission (6.8 vs. 2.6%). Other groups with a statistically significant increased risk for readmission postoperatively include women, African Americans, spouses, exchange participants, uninsured donors, donors with predonation eGFR <60 mL/min per 1.73 m^2, donors with predonation pulmonary disease, and those who underwent robotic nephrectomy.

Thus, perioperative management, preoperatively, intraoperatively, and postoperatively, is important for reducing the risk of complications and facilitating optimal postsurgical recovery and return to predonation function.

History and Physical Exam

A thorough history and physical exam is necessary to evaluate a potential living kidney donor for not only perioperative risk but also long-term risk of renal dysfunction and other complications. OPTN policy requires documentation of the following components prior to living donation: personal history of significant medical conditions (including kidney-specific personal history), surgical history, active and past medications, family medical history, and social history (Table 9.1) [12].

Assessment of personal history of significant medical conditions should include discussion and documentation of the presence of hypertension, lung disease, prior history of coronary artery disease (CAD), prior evaluation for CAD, other heart disease, autoimmune disease, bleeding or clotting disorders, hematologic disorders, prior malignancy, and history of infections. Special attention should be dedicated to

Table 9.1 OPTN requirements for living donor medical evaluations. (From [12])

This evaluation must be completed	Including evaluation for and assessment of this information
General donor history	1. A personal history of significant medical conditions which include but are not limited to: (a) Hypertension (b) Diabetes (c) Lung disease (d) Heart disease (e) Gastrointestinal disease (f) Autoimmune disease (g) Neurologic disease (h) Genitourinary disease (i) Hematologic disorders (j) Bleeding or clotting disorders (k) History of cancer including melanoma 2. History of infections 3. Active and past medications with special consideration for known nephrotoxic and hepatotoxic medications or chronic use of pain medication 4. Allergies 5. An evaluation for coronary artery disease
General family history	• Coronary artery disease • Cancer
Social history	• Occupation • Employment status • Health insurance status • Living arrangements • Social support • Smoking, alcohol, and drug use and abuse • Psychiatric illness, depression, suicide attempts • Increased risk behavior as defined by the US Public Health Services (PHS) Guideline
Physical exam	• Height • Weight • BMI • Vital signs • Examination of all major organ systems

kidney-specific personal history including episodes of kidney injury or dysfunction, diabetes (including gestational diabetes), nephrolithiasis, recurrent urinary tract infections, genetic renal diseases, and known prior episodes of proteinuria or hematuria [12]. Women should be asked about prior hypertensive disorders of pregnancy including preeclampsia, as well as future childbearing plans [2]. Providers should also inquire about active and past medications, including nephrotoxic medications (particularly nonsteroidal anti-inflammatory agents) as well as chronic pain medications [11–12].

Assessment of prior surgical history is particularly important given that laparoscopic nephrectomy approaches (e.g., hand-assisted, "mini open," or pure laparoscopic) by trained surgeons are currently preferred, as laparoscopic nephrectomy is associated with significantly less pain, shorter hospitalization time, and shorter time to recovery compared to open nephrectomy [13]. Previous or complex prior surgical history or anatomical considerations may increase the risks of laparoscopic nephrectomy and may warrant an open technique for procurement [2]. When assessing family medical history of kidney disease, it is important to delineate the type of disease, age of onset, and extrarenal signs and symptoms. Family history of genetic kidney disease including autosomal dominant polycystic kidney disease (ADPKD) should be assessed. Additionally, the clinician should assess family history of cancer (including renal cell carcinoma), CAD, diabetes, and hypertension. Screening for behaviors that confer increased risk of transmissible infections including human immunodeficiency virus, hepatitis B, or hepatitis C should be performed. Physical exam should include vital signs, measurement of height and weight for assessment of body mass index (BMI), and examination of all major organ systems. Blood pressure should be measured on at least two occasions or by 24-hour or overnight ambulatory blood pressure monitoring.

Preoperative Laboratory and Imaging Tests

The following laboratory and imaging tests are usually obtained as part of the donor candidate evaluation: complete blood count (CBC) including platelet count, blood type, prothrombin time (PT) or international normalized ratio (INR), partial thromboplastin time (PTT), complete metabolic panel, and fasting lipid panel (including total, high-density lipoprotein [HDL], low-density lipoprotein [LDL], triglycerides) (Table 9.2). Glucose tolerance test or glycosylated hemoglobin (HbA1C) is recommended for those with family history of diabetes or otherwise at high risk of diabetes. Urinalysis with microscopy, measurement of urinary protein and albumin excretion, and measurement of glomerular filtration rate (GFR) by isotopic methods or creatinine clearance calculated from 24-hour urine collection are all also indicated [3]. Donor candidates with family history of ADPKD should be assessed by imaging and possibly genetic testing to reliably exclude ADPKD in the potential donor, as is discussed in Chap. 8. The assessment of donor candidates with a history of nephrolithiasis includes review of clinical history, imaging, and 24-hour urine stone profile, as discussed in Chap. 4. Among premenopausal women, quantitative

Table 9.2 OPTN requirements for living donor laboratory and imaging testing. (From [12])

This evaluation must be completed	Including evaluation for and assessment of this information
General laboratory and imaging tests	• Complete blood count (CBC) with platelet count • Blood type and subtype as specified in *14.5: Living Donor Blood Type Determination and Reporting* and its subsections • Prothrombin time (PT) or international normalized ratio (INR) • Partial thromboplastin time (PTT) • Metabolic testing (to include electrolytes, BUN, creatinine, transaminase levels, albumin, calcium, phosphorus, alkaline phosphatase, bilirubin) • HCG quantitative pregnancy test for premenopausal women without surgical sterilization • Chest X-ray • Electrocardiogram (ECG)
Transmissible disease screening transmissible	Infectious disease testing must be performed in a CLIA-certified laboratory or in a laboratory meeting equivalent requirements as determined by Centers for Medicare and Medicaid Services (CMS) using FDA-licensed, approved, or cleared tests. Testing must include *all* the following: 1. CMV (*Cytomegalovirus*) antibody 2. EBV (Epstein-Barr virus) antibody 3. HIV antibody (anti-HIV) testing or HIV antigen/antibody (Ag/Ab) combination test as close as possible, but within 28 days prior to organ recovery 4. Hepatitis B surface antigen (HBsAg) testing as close as possible, but within 28 days prior to organ recovery 5. Hepatitis B core antibody (anti-HBc) testing as close as possible, but within 28 days prior to organ recovery 6. Hepatitis C antibody (anti-HCV) testing as close as possible, but within 28 days prior to organ recovery 7. HCV ribonucleic acid (RNA) by nucleic acid test (NAT) as close as possible, but within 28 days prior to organ recovery 8. Syphilis testing If a living donor is identified as being at increased risk for HIV, HBV, and HCV transmission according to the US Public Health Services (PHS) Guideline, testing must also include HIV ribonucleic acid (RNA) by NAT or HIV antigen/antibody (Ag/Ab) combination test. This does not apply to donors whose only increased risk factor is receiving hemodialysis within the preceding 12 months, as they are at risk only for HCV according to the US Public Health Services (PHS) Guideline. For tuberculosis (TB), living donor recovery hospitals must determine if the donor is at increased risk for this infection. If TB risk is suspected, testing must include screening for latent infection using either: • Intradermal PPD • Interferon gamma release assay (IGRA)

HCG pregnancy test is required to confirm the absences of pregnancy at the time of donation surgery. Electrocardiogram, chest radiograph, and anatomic assessment of the kidneys are obtained preoperatively, as discussed in Chap. 4.

Preoperative Evaluation for Risk Stratification and to Minimize Complications

Cardiac

Comprehensive guidelines regarding perioperative cardiac risk stratification and the appropriate testing needed prior to undergoing noncardiac surgery are published periodically by the American College of Cardiology and the American Heart Association Task Force [14]. A preoperative electrocardiogram (ECG) is required by OPTN policy in the United States and is useful to establish a baseline and to evaluate for abnormalities. Some transplant programs routinely perform preoperative noninvasive cardiac testing in older living kidney donor candidates (e.g., stress electrocardiogram or nuclear stress test in candidates age >=50); there is no evidence to support use of noninvasive testing in those without symptoms or reduced functional capacity [15]. For individuals without active cardiac symptoms with exercise tolerance defined as the ability to achieve at least four metabolic energy equivalents (e.g., an ability to walk two blocks on ground level or carry two bags of groceries up one flight of stairs without symptoms), no additional cardiac testing is typically warranted.

Bleeding

Bleeding risk guidelines for presurgical evaluation from the British Committee for Standards in Hematology recommend performing a detailed bleeding history including family history of bleeding, previous personal excessive bleeding history, or use of antithrombotic drugs [16]. If any of these are positive, then additional coagulation testing should be performed; otherwise it is not needed. Although there is minimal evidence related to donor nephrectomy, OPTN policy requires both an assessment of bleeding history in the medical history and the performance of coagulation testing [12]. Regarding antiplatelet use in the context of surgical risk, a recent multicenter randomized trial of perioperative aspirin use before noncardiac surgery that included 10,010 patients found that perioperative aspirin increased the risk of major bleeding but had no effect of the risk of death or nonfatal myocardial infarction [17]. The American College of Surgeons recommends that aspirin, prasugrel, and ticagrelor should be suspended for 5–7 days before low/high bleeding risk surgery [18].

Venous Thromboembolism (VTE)

Recent guidelines are available regarding perioperative venous thromboembolism risk and risk stratification. Options for prophylaxis include early ambulation, mechanical prophylaxis, and unfractionated or low-molecular-weight heparin. Older age, obesity, and use of oral contraceptives (particularly estrogen-based) or hormone replacement are risk factors for VTE [19]. In our practice, patients receive heparin 5000 units subcutaneously prior to induction along with sequential compression devices (SCDs). Postoperatively, patients are administered heparin 5000 units subcutaneously every 8 hours, sequential compression devices are placed while they are not ambulating, and ambulation is encouraged as soon as possible including the night of surgery.

The risk of using estrogen-based oral contraceptive (OCP) medications before surgery should be balanced against the harms of pro-coagulation. Barrier birth control can be an appropriate option in the weeks before surgery; however, practices vary in requirements for cessation of OCP or estrogen-containing hormonal agents in the weeks prior to donation surgery.

Pulmonary

Assessing preoperative risk for pulmonary complications includes identifying conditions such as chronic obstructive pulmonary disease or congestive heart failure [20]. Preoperative spirometry and chest radiography are not recommended to predict pulmonary risk; however, chest radiography is required by OPTN policy for living donors [12]. Donor candidates should be counseled on the risks of perioperative complications and long-term health risks related to use of tobacco products, including the risk of damage to the remaining kidney. Candidates should be advised to abstain from use of tobacco products and referred to a tobacco cessation support program if possible [2]. A meta-analysis reviewing six randomized controlled trials found that smoking cessation decreased the risk of postoperative complications [21]. We recommend that donor candidates should abstain from use of tobacco products at least 4 weeks prior to donation surgery, and we encourage them to maintain lifelong abstinence. After surgery, postoperative deep breathing, incentive spirometry, and early ambulation are encouraged to reduce the risk of pulmonary complications.

Intraoperative Donor Nephrectomy Considerations

While Chap. 13 provides full discussion of nephrectomy approaches, here we will discuss intraoperative anesthetic considerations. Donors are at moderate risk for the development of VTE events in the perioperative period after nephrectomy, and, as above, in our practice, we administer perioperative prophylactic low-molecular-weight heparin. Based on the 2017 Centers for Disease Control and Prevention Guideline for the Prevention of Surgical Site Infection, we recommend administration of prophylactic antibiotics (e.g., 2 g of cefazolin) to reduce the risk for surgical site infections [22]. As bleeding is a rare but possible complication, two large-bore intravascular catheters should be inserted. Invasive monitoring such as arterial blood pressure and central venous pressure is not indicated during or after routine donor nephrectomy surgery. General anesthesia with endotracheal intubation is necessary due to the need for muscle relaxation to reduce intra-abdominal pressure and to achieve the desired degree of abdominal distention, as well as to control ventilation during pneumoperitoneum. Many centers utilize regional neuraxial pain control such as transversus abdominis plane blocks and minimize perioperative narcotics while using intraoperative ketamine and perioperative lidocaine [23].

The major risk to the kidney that is being transplanted is ischemia, which can manifest as delayed graft function in the recipient. Therefore, it is critical to prevent decreased renal perfusion by maintaining adequate intravascular volume and mean arterial pressure (MAP). Specific measures include intravascular volume expansion, avoidance of vasopressors, and tolerance of mild hypercapnia [24].

Intravascular Volume Expansion

Intravascular volume should be expanded with crystalloid solution throughout the nephrectomy procedure to maintain optimal renal perfusion with urine output greater than 0.5 mL/kg/hr throughout the operation. This is particularly important among patients undergoing laparoscopic nephrectomy (as compared to open) to counteract the effect of pneumoperitoneum. However, an upper limit to fluid administration (e.g., intraoperative fluid restriction of 3 mL/kg/hr while maintaining a target urine output) had also been suggested to prevent bowel edema and the incidence of ileus [25]. It is recommended that pneumoperitoneum created with insufflation of carbon dioxide should be maintained at 15 mm Hg or less to preserve renal perfusion. Additionally, many centers administer 12.5–25 g of mannitol IV or 5 mg doses of furosemide at times intraoperatively when blood supply to the kidney may be jeopardized, such as during insufflation for laparoscopy [26].

Avoidance of Vasopressors

Vasopressors are avoided if possible, as these agents interfere with renal perfusion. However, because maintenance of MAP is extremely important for graft function, ephedrine may be administered in bolus doses of 5–25 mg (combined alpha and beta agonism) to treat fluid-resistant hypotension. Pure alpha agonists should be avoided [27].

Tolerance of Mild Hypercapnia

Mild hypercapnia typically develops during laparoscopy with carbon dioxide insufflation. To address this hypercapnia in non-donor nephrectomy laparoscopy, minute ventilation is generally increased by 20–30% by increasing the respiratory rate while maintaining a constant tidal volume. However, among patients undergoing laparoscopic donor nephrectomy, it is recommended that mild hypercapnia be tolerated as it may improve perfusion due to vasodilation and increased cardiac output and may increase tissue oxygenation due to rightward shift of the oxyhemoglobin dissociation curve [28].

Postoperative Management of the Living Kidney Donor

The laparoscopic approach to donor nephrectomy has transformed the practice of living kidney donation. A meta-analysis by Nanidis et al. in 2008 evaluated 73 studies that included 3751 and 2843 living kidney donors who had undergone laparoscopic or open nephrectomy, respectively [29]. Compared with open nephrectomy, those who underwent laparoscopic nephrectomy had a significantly shorter hospital length of stay and quicker return to work (by 1.48 days and 2.58 weeks, respectively). Transplant recipients from donors in both groups had similar rates of delayed allograft function and allograft loss. A more recent systematic review of 190 studies (over 32,000 living donor nephrectomies) evaluated perioperative complications after minimally invasive donor nephrectomy, documenting 0.01% mortality [30]. Enhanced recovery protocols (ERP) are also increasingly recognized as an important component of decreasing disincentives to donation. Initially developed to improve postoperative length of stay after colectomy, ERP has now been applied to living kidney donation at many centers. ERP measures are typically described in three phases: preoperative, intraoperative, and postoperative (Fig. 9.1) [31].

Enhanced Recovery Protocols

The preoperative phase of ERP focuses on the donor's physiologic readiness to undergo nephrectomy. Donors who smoke or use other tobacco products are strongly encouraged to abstain from tobacco use. At many centers in accordance with American Society of Anesthesiologists guidelines [32], patients are instructed to consume clear, nonprotein-containing beverages up to 2 hours before the scheduled operative time. Patients may be given acetaminophen and 300 mg gabapentin as preoperative pain control adjuncts to allow narcotic minimization. Utilization of regional neuraxial blocks, including transversus abdominis plane (TAP) blocks with bupivicaine, can also be performed preoperatively. Intraoperative ketamine and lidocaine are often utilized to minimize narcotic use. As above, restricted use of

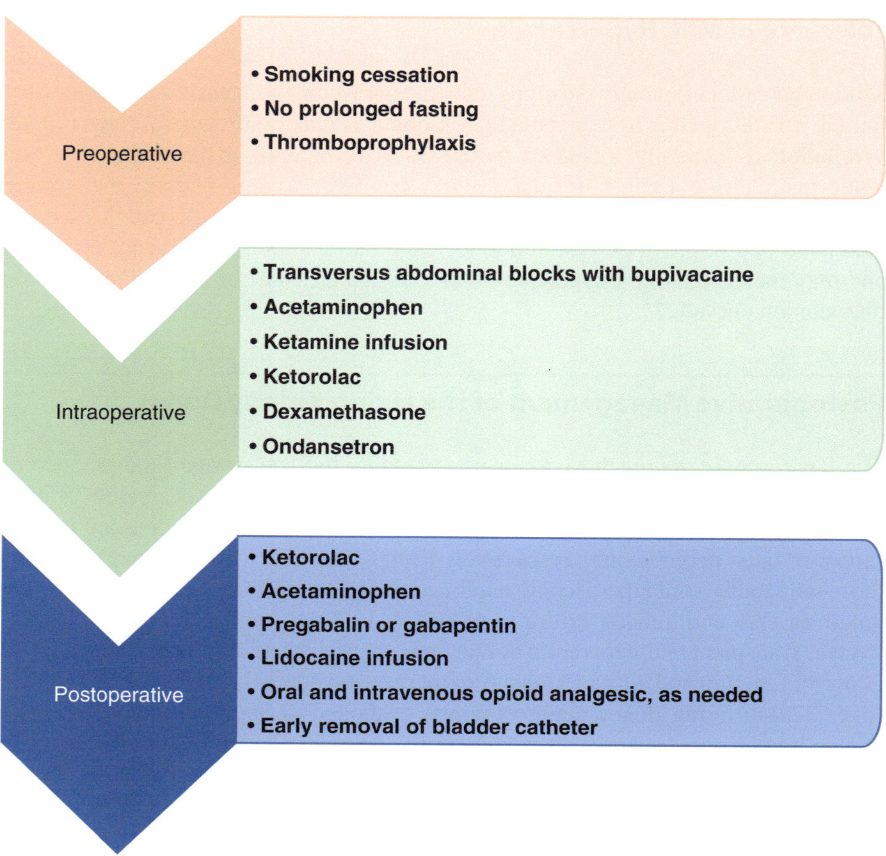

Fig. 9.1 Considerations for living donor nephrectomy enhanced recovery protocols

intraoperative fluids, while maintaining a target urine output of 0.5 mL/kg/hr [26], may prevent bowel edema and subsequently decrease the incidence of ileus. Furthermore, perioperative ketolorac is used by many centers without adverse effects, as a means to decrease total narcotic use [31, 33].

Postoperatively after living donor nephrectomy, patients are given clear liquids immediately and advanced to a regular diet as soon as tolerated. Postoperative multimodal therapies are employed to allow for narcotic minimization including lidocaine infusion, ketorolac, gabapentinoids, cyclobenzaprine, and scheduled acetaminophen. Many centers have employed ERPs in the care of living donors. A single-center study evaluated the effect of ERP by analyzing groups pre-and post-implementation. Findings showed a reduction in median length of stay from 2.0 to 1.0 days after donor nephrectomy ($p < 0.01$) and overall narcotic use decreased by nearly 50% (45.6 vs. 21.3; $p < 0.01$), whereas pain scores remained similar [31]. No significant increase in readmissions or outpatient opioid analgesic utilization needs was seen in the ERP group. Other centers have had similar results of postoperative reduction in length of stay and narcotic use [5]. Expected length of stay after living donor nephrectomy is typically 1–2 days [25, 31]. Optimization of the patient experience via a multimodal approach to pain control as well as enhanced recovery with expedited discharge to home helps to reduce barriers to living kidney donation.

After discharge from the hospital, living donors are usually seen in the surgical clinic for an exam within the first month. Laboratory testing may be obtained at this postoperative visit. In the United States, OPTN policy requires laboratory testing (serum creatinine, urine protein) and assessment of medical health at 6 months, 1 year, and 2 years post-donation [34]. One single-center study that evaluated living kidney donor quality of life, pain, and activity level using SF-36, EQ-5D, and the visual analog pain scale found that post-donation quality of life was worse after 2 weeks post-donation but returned to baseline between months 1 and 3 [35]. Pain scales were also worse after donation but returned to baseline after 3 months. Patients may be counseled and encouraged that they should approach their predonation function by around 3–6 months.

In summary, a thoughtful and systematic approach to the perioperative experience of living kidney donors supports successful surgical outcomes for both the living donor and their transplant recipient. Overall, while postoperative complications are experienced by up to 20% of donors, major complications occur in less than 3%, and death is rare at an incidence of less than 0.03%. Postoperative return to predonation function for donors may take as long as 3–6 months. Ensuring that a living kidney donor is optimized for donor nephrectomy includes assessing for medical and surgical risk factors, bleeding mitigation by holding antiplatelet agents such as aspirin for at least 5–7 days, administering appropriate VTE prophylaxis, and encouraging smoking cessation for at least 4 weeks. Preoperative administration of non-narcotic analgesics or neuraxial anesthesia reduces the need for perioperative narcotics. Intraoperative attention to fluid administration and blood pressure is important to support allograft function; balancing this consideration with restrictive fluid resuscitation may improve postoperative donor outcomes by decreasing ileus. Postoperative ERP further guides multimodal agent utilization to decrease narcotic consumption, pain, and hospital length of stay. Future work should seek to optimize risk stratification and approaches to minimizing the risk of perioperative complications in all living donors.

References

1. Lentine KL, Patel A. Risks and outcomes of living donation. Adv Chronic Kidney Dis. 2012;19(4):220–8. https://doi.org/10.1053/j.ackd.2011.09.005.
2. Lentine KL, Kasiske BL, Levey AS, Adams PL, Alberú J, Bakr MA, et al. KDIGO clinical practice guideline on the evaluation and care of living kidney donors Transplantation. 2017;101(Suppl 8S):S1–S109. https://doi.org/10.1097/TP.0000000000001769.
3. Segev DL, Muzaale AD, Caffo BS, Mehta SH, Singer AL, Taranto SE, et al. Perioperative mortality and long-term survival following live kidney donation. JAMA. 2010;303(10):959–66. https://doi.org/10.1001/jama.2010.237.

4. Matas AJ, Bartlett ST, Leichtman AB, Delmonico FL. Morbidity and mortality after living kidney donation, 1999–2001: a survey of United States transplant centers. Am J Transplant. 2003;3(7):830–4. https://pubmed.ncbi.nlm.nih.gov/12814474/.

5. Hadjianastassiou VG, Johnson RJ, Rudge CJ, Mamode N. 2509 living donor nephrectomies, morbidity and mortality, including the UK introduction of laparoscopic donor surgery. Am J Transplant. 2007;7(11):2532–7. https://doi.org/10.1111/j.1600-6143.2007.01975.x.

6. Schold JD, Goldfarb DA, Buccini LD, Rodrigue JR, Mandelbrot DA, Heaphy EL, et al. Comorbidity burden and perioperative complications for living kidney donors in the United States. Clin J Am Soc Nephrol. 2013;8(10):1773–82. https://doi.org/10.2215/CJN.12311212.

7. Clavien PA, Barkun J, de Oliveira ML, Vauthey JN, Dindo D, Schulick RD, et al. The Clavien-Dindo classification of surgical complications: five-year experience. Ann Surg. 2009;250(2):187–96. https://doi.org/10.1097/SLA.0b013e3181b13ca2.

8. Lentine KL, Lam NN, Axelrod D, Schnitzler MA, Garg AX, Xiao H, et al. Perioperative complications after living kidney donation: a national study. Am J Transplant. 2016;16(6):1848–57. https://doi.org/10.1111/ajt.13687.

9. Mjoen G, Oyen O, Holdaas H, Line P. Morbidity and mortality in 1022 consecutive living donor nephrectomies: benefits of a living donor registry. Transplantation. 2009;88(11):1273–9. https://doi.org/10.1097/TP.0b013e3181bb44fd.

10. Garcia-Ochoa C, Feldman LS, Nguan C, Monroy-Cuadros M, Arnold J, Boudville N, et al. Perioperative complications during living donor nephrectomy: results from a multicenter cohort study. Can J Kidney Health Dis. 2019;6:2054358119857718. https://doi.org/10.1177/2054358119857718.

11. Lentine KL, Lam NN, Schnitzler MA, Hess GP, Kasiske BL, Xiao H, et al. Predonation prescription opioid use: a novel risk factor for readmission after living kidney donation. Am J Transplant. 2017;17(3):744–53. https://doi.org/10.1111/ajt.14033.

12. Organ Procurement and Transplantation Network (OPTN/United Network for Organ Sharing). Policy 14: Living Donation. Available at: https://optn.transplant.hrsa.gov/governance/policies/. Accessed: 7 Sept 2020.

13. Wilson CH, Sanni A, Rix DA, Soomro NA. Laparoscopic versus open nephrectomy for live kidney donors. Cochrane Database Syst Rev. 2011;(11):CD006124. https://doi.org/10.1002/14651858.CD006124.pub2.

14. Fleisher LA, Beckman JA, Brown KA, Calkins H, Chaikof EL, Fleischmann KE, et al. ACC/AHA 2007 guidelines on perioperative cardiovascular evaluation and care for noncardiac surgery: a report of the American College of Cardiology/American Heart Association task force on practice guidelines. Circulation. 2007;116:e418–99. https://doi.org/10.1161/CIRCULATIONAHA.107.185699.

15. Ferket BS, Genders TS, Colkesen EB, Visser JJ, Spronk S, Steyerberg EW, et al. Systemic review of guidelines on imaging of asymptomatic coronary artery disease. J Am Coll Cardiol. 2011;57(15):1591–600. https://doi.org/10.1016/j.jacc.2010.10.055.

16. Chee YL, Crawford JC, Watson HG, Greaves M. Guidelines on the assessment of bleeding risk prior to surgery or invasive procedures. British Committee for Standards in Haematology. Br J Haematol. 2008;140(5):496–504. https://doi.org/10.1111/j.1365-2141.2007.06968.x.

17. Devereaux PJ, Mrkobrada M, Sessler DI, Leslie K, Alonso-Coello P, Kurz A, et al. Aspirin in patients undergoing noncardiac surgery. N Engl J Med. 2014;370(16):1494–503. https://doi.org/10.1056/NEJMoa1401105.

18. Hornor MA, Duane TM, Ehlers AP, Jensen EH, Brown PS, Pohl D, et al. American College of Surgeons' guidelines for the perioperative management of antithrombotic medication. J Am Coll Surg. 2018;227(5):521–36.e1. https://doi.org/10.1016/j.jamcollsurg.2018.08.183.

19. Guyatt GH, Akl EA, Crowther M, Gutterman DD, Schuunemann HJ. Executive summary: antithrombotic therapy and prevention of thrombosis, 9th ed: https://doi.org/American College of Chest Physicians evidence-based clinical practice guidelines. Chest. 2012;141(2 Suppl) v:7S–47S.

20. Qaseem A, Snow V, Fitterman N, Hornbake ER, Lawrence VA, Smetana GW, et al. Risk assessment for and strategies to reduce perioperative pulmonary complications for patients undergoing

noncardiothoracic surgery: a guideline from the American College of Physicians. Ann Intern Med. 2006;144(8):575–80. https://doi.org/10.7326/0003-4819-144-8-200604180-00008.

21. Mills E, Eyawo O, Lockhart I, Kelly S, Wu P, Ebbert JO. Smoking cessation reduces postoperative complications: a systematic review and meta-analysis. Am J Med. 2011;124(2):144–154e.148. https://doi.org/10.1016/j.amjmed.2010.09.013.

22. Berrios-Torres SI, Umscheid CA, Leas B, Stone EC, Kelz RR, et al. Centers for Disease Control and Prevention guideline for the prevention of surgical site infection, 2017. JAMA Surg. 2017;152(8):784–91. https://doi.org/10.1001/jamasurg.2017.0904.

23. Forbes RC, King AK, McGrane T, Hale D, Sandberg W, Wanderer J, et al. Enhanced recovery after surgery pathway for living donor nephrectomy patients decreases length of stay and narcotic utilization. [abstract]. Am J Transplant. 2017;17(suppl 3):788–9.

24. Lemmens HJM. Anesthesia for living kidney donors. Avidan M, Brennan DC, editors. UpToDate. Waltham, MA: UpToDate Inc. Available at: https://www.uptodate.com. Accessed: 7 Sept 2020.

25. Rege A, Leraas H, Vikraman D, Ravindra K, Brennan T, Miller T, et al. Could the use of an enhanced recovery protocol in laparoscopic donor nephrectomy be an incentive for live kidney donation? Cureus. 2016;8(11):e889. https://doi.org/10.7759/cureus.889.

26. Tiggeler RG, Berden JH, Oitsma AJ, Koene RA. Prevention of acute tubular necrosis in cadaveric kidney transplantation by the combined use of mannitol and moderate hydration. Ann Surg. 1985;201(2):246–51. https://doi.org/10.1097/00000658-198502000-00020.

27. Albanèse J, Leone M, Garnier F, Bourgoin A, Antonini F, Martin C. Renal effects of norepinephrine in septic and nonseptic patients. Chest. 2004;126(2):534–9. https://doi.org/10.1378/chest.126.2.534.

28. Joshi GP, Cunningham A. In: Clinical Anesthesia, Barash PG, editors. Anesthesia for laparoscopic and robotic surgeries, vol. 7. Philadelphia: Lippincott Williams Wilkins; 2013. p. 1257–73.

29. Nanidis TG, Antcliffe D, Kokkinos C, Borysiewicz CA, Darzi AW, Tekkis PP, et al. Laparoscopic versus open live donor nephrectomy in renal transplantation: a meta-analysis. Ann Surg. 2008;247(1):58–70. https://doi.org/10.1097/SLA.0b013e318153fc13.

30. Kortram K, Ijzermans JN, Frank JM. Perioperative events and complications in minimally invasive live donor nephrectomy: a systematic review and meta-analysis. Transplantation. 2016;100(11):2264–75. https://doi.org/10.1097/TP.0000000000001327.

31. Waits SA, Hilliard P, Sheetz KH, Sung RS, Englesbe MJ. Building the case for enhanced recovery protocols in living kidney donors. Transplantation. 2015;99:405–8. https://doi.org/10.1097/TP.0000000000000328.

32. Practice Guidelines for Preoperative Fasting and the Use of Pharmacologic Agents to Reduce the Risk of Pulmonary Aspiration. Application to healthy patients undergoing elective procedures: an updated report by the American Society of Anesthesiologists task force on preoperative fasting and the use of pharmacologic agents to reduce the risk of pulmonary aspiration. Anesthesiology. 2017;126(3):376–93. https://doi.org/10.1097/ALN.0000000000001452.

33. Campsen J, Call T, Allen CM, Presson AP, Martinez E, Rofaiel G, et al. Prospective, double-blind, randomized clinical trial comparing an ERAS pathway with ketorolac and pregabalin versus standard of care plus placebo during live donor nephrectomy for kidney transplant. 2019;19(6):1777–81. https://doi.org/10.1111/ajt.15242.

34. Organ Procurement and Transplantation Network (OPTN) / United Network for Organ Sharing (UNOS). Policy 18: Data Submission Requirements. Available at: http://optn.transplant.hrsa.gov/ContentDocuments/OPTN_Policies.pdf. Accessed: 7 Sept 2020.

35. Dageforde LA, Feurer ID, Moore DE. Longitudinal health-related quality of life, pain, and activity in kidney donors [abstract]. Am J Transplant. 2014;14(suppl 2):68–9.

Compatibility, Kidney Paired Donation, and Incompatible Living Donor Transplants

10

Neetika Garg, Jagbir Gill, and Didier A. Mandelbrot

In this chapter, we review the major types of biologic incompatibility, ABO and HLA, that transplant candidates face, along with the various crossmatch techniques used to assess incompatibility. Subsequently, we discuss in detail the two main approaches used to overcome incompatibility and facilitate living donor transplantation: kidney paired donation and desensitization.

Compatibility

Assessment of compatibility in a potential recipient with respect to their potential donor is essential to ensure successful transplantation. From an immunologic standpoint, a transplant recipient candidate is considered compatible with their donor candidate if the pair can proceed with transplantation without crossing any of the two major antibody-mediated barriers to transplantation: (1) ABO incompatibility from anti-ABO antibodies and (2) HLA incompatibility from preformed donor-specific antibodies.

N. Garg (✉) · D. A. Mandelbrot
Division of Nephrology, Department of Medicine, University of Wisconsin-Madison, Madison, WI, USA
e-mail: ngarg@medicine.wisc.edu; damandel@medicine.wisc.edu

J. Gill
Division of Nephrology, Department of Medicine, The University of British Columbia, Vancouver, BC, Canada
e-mail: JAGill@providencehealth.bc.ca

© Springer Nature Switzerland AG 2021
K. L. Lentine et al. (eds.), *Living Kidney Donation*,
https://doi.org/10.1007/978-3-030-53618-3_10

ABO Incompatibility

ABO antigens are glycoproteins that were discovered in the context of red blood cells and blood transfusion by Karl Landsteiner in 1901. They are also expressed on endothelial cells and epithelial cells. As a result, ABO antigens expressed on donor kidneys may be targets for an antibody-mediated immune response due to ABO antibodies in recipients and thereby mediate allograft rejection and loss.

ABO blood type consists of four common types: A, B, AB, and O. ABO compatibility between donor kidneys and recipients follows the same rules as in blood transfusion. Blood type O donors are universal donors, and transplant candidates with blood type AB are universal recipients. Transplants outside of blood type compatibility rules are considered ABO-incompatible, with the exception of A_2 or A2B to B transplants and A_2 to O transplants in selected recipients. Blood type A consists of two main subtypes: A_1 and non-A_1, with nearly 20%of individuals with blood type A being non-A_1 [1]. Most non-A_1 individuals are subtype A_2, and A_2 is often used as a shorthand for non-A_1, but several other non-A_1 subtypes exist. Among non-A_1 individuals, the A antigenic expression is both quantitatively and qualitatively lower. As a result, kidneys from A_2 donors can be successfully transplanted into blood type B or O recipients using the same immunosuppression protocols as ABO-compatible transplantation (i.e., without desensitization), as long as anti-A titers are low [2]. Similarly, A_2B donor kidneys may be safely transplanted into blood type B recipients with low anti-A titers. The high degree of variability among labs and methods makes it difficult to compare titers between centers, but titer thresholds of 1:4 or 1:8 are usually considered acceptable.

In the United States, the allocation of deceased donor kidneys is based on ABO matching as opposed to ABO compatibility. In other words, while blood type O donors are universal donors and their kidneys may technically be transplanted into a recipient of any blood type, the current allocation system only allows allocation of these kidneys to blood type O candidates to prevent further lengthening of their waiting times. Similarly, while AB candidates can technically receive kidneys from any blood type, the allocation system only allows allocation of AB kidneys to AB recipients.

The waiting time for blood type B kidney transplant candidates is typically longer than for candidates with other blood types. In the United States, the blood type B kidney transplant candidate waitlist has the highest proportion of ethno-racial minority candidates, who are less likely to receive a living donor kidney transplant compared to white candidates, exacerbating longer waiting times for patients in these populations. With the goal of improving equity by improving access to transplantation for minority populations in the United States, the Kidney Allocation System (KAS) implemented by the Organ Procurement and Transplant Network (OPTN) in December 2014 now allows allocation of type A, non-A_1 and type AB, non-A_1B kidneys to blood type B candidates as long as anti-A titers are low, with the program's titer threshold defined in written policy [3]. However, the OPTN does not currently have a provision to direct kidneys from deceased type AB, non-A_1B donors to O candidates.

HLA Incompatibility

A recipient's immune system recognizes a kidney allograft as non-self predominantly through detecting mismatches in the major histocompatibility (MHC) molecules, also known as the human leucocyte antigens (HLA). Preformed antibodies in a potential recipient against a prospective donor's HLA define HLA incompatibility.

HLA genes are located on the short arm of chromosome 6 and are classified into class I and class II:

Major class I HLA genes include HLA-A, HLA-B, and HLA-C; these encode HLA A, B, and C molecules.

Class I HLA are comprised of a polymorphic alpha chain that is covalently associated with a non-polymorphic beta-2 microglobulin chain. These are expressed on all nucleated cells in the body.

Major class II HLA genes include HLA-DRA, HLA-DRB1, HLA-DRB3, HLA-DRB4, HLA-DRB5, HLA-DQA, HLA-DQB, HLA-DPA, and HLA-DPB. These genes encode HLA DR, DQ, and DP molecules. The DRB1 gene is present in all individuals. Allelic variants of DRB1 are linked with either none or one of DRB3, DRB4, and DRB5 genes. DRB3, DRB4, and DRB5 genes when present encode DR51, DR52, and DR53 molecules. As a result, in addition to the two DRs coded by the DRB1, an individual can express none, one, or two of the DR51, DR52, and DR53 antigens.

Class II HLA are heterodimers and consist of an alpha polypeptide chain and a beta-polypeptide chain. With the exception of the DR alpha, they are all highly polymorphic and can lead to formation of anti-HLA antibodies. Class II HLA are expressed primarily on antigen-presenting cells such as B cells and dendritic cells but are known to also be expressed under inflammatory conditions on other cell types including endothelial and epithelial cells.

Assessment of HLA Incompatibility and Crossmatch Techniques

The panel reactive antibody (PRA) provides an estimate of the percentage of potential donors against whom a transplant candidate has anti-HLA antibodies and ranges from 0% to 100%. Historically, PRA was assessed by testing recipient serum against a panel of lymphocyte cells whose HLA profile was felt to be representative of the donor population. Major limitations of this testing were variability in output depending on selection of cells used in the panel, poor sensitivity to detect antibodies to uncommon HLA, and ability to detect only relatively high-level antibodies. Since 2007, a calculated PRA (cPRA) has been used in the United States [4]. This combines the specificities of anti-HLA antibodies obtained from single-antigen bead (SAB) testing with the HLA frequencies in the United Network for Organ Sharing

(UNOS) database. For example, A_1 is present in 24% of the US donor population, and therefore having anti-A1 HLA antibodies alone gives a potential recipient a cPRA of 24%; i.e., this recipient will be immunologically incompatible with 24% of the donors. On the other hand, A24 is present in 2% of the US donor population, and having anti-A24 antibodies alone yields a cPRA of only 2%. Thus, someone who has many different antibodies to rare antigens may have a lower cPRA than someone who has a single antibody to a common antigen. The cPRA calculator is available on the OPTN website [5]. This provides a more uniform method of assessment of the degree of sensitization and predicts a positive crossmatch more accurately.

While the cPRA provides an assessment of the overall level of sensitization in a kidney transplant candidate, the following crossmatch techniques are available to determine whether donor-specific antibodies (DSA) are present against a specific donor:

Complement-dependent cytotoxic (CDC) crossmatch Recipient serum is added to donor lymphocytes, along with extrinsic complement. If a clinically significant DSA is present, cell lysis occurs, and the crossmatch is deemed positive. This is the least sensitive of all the crossmatch techniques but highly specific for predicting rejection posttransplant. T cells express class I HLA, and B cells express both class I and class II HLA. As a result, anti-class I HLA DSA should lead to both positive T-cell and B-cell crossmatches. A positive B-cell crossmatch with a negative T-cell crossmatch suggests presence of anti-class II DSA. It should be noted that B-cell crossmatch is more sensitive for detection of anti-class I DSA due to higher antigen expression on cell surface; as such, a low-level class I DSA can also result in an isolated positive B-cell crossmatch.

Anti-human globulin (AHG)-enhanced CDC crossmatch Addition of a complement-fixing AHG increases the sensitivity of this cell-based crossmatch assay in cases where the anti-HLA DSA are low titer. Additionally, since AHG also binds to non-complement-fixing DSA and subsequently activates complement, it allows detection of non-complement-binding DSA that would otherwise be missed by the unenhanced assay.

Flow cytometry crossmatch In this cell-based crossmatch technique, a secondary fluorochrome-conjugated anti-IgG antibody and subsequent flow cytometry is used to detect IgG DSA bound to donor lymphocytes. Since this test does not rely on cell lysis, this test is more sensitive but less specific than the enhanced CDC crossmatch. The methodology allows for detection of non-HLA DSA and non-complement-fixing DSA. Since the anti-human secondary antibody used detects only IgG DSA, IgM antibodies do not affect the flow crossmatch.

Virtual crossmatch This crossmatch is referred to as "virtual" as it does not involve an actual reaction between the serum of the potential recipient and donor lymphocytes. Rather, the spectrum of anti-HLA antibodies present in the potential recipient's serum, as determined by SAB assay, is compared with the donor HLA profile to determine whether DSA is present.

The SAB assay involves incubating the potential recipient's serum with microparticle beads with individual allele-specific HLA antigens presented on them. Since no cells are utilized, this is also referred to as a "solid phase assay." Subsequently, similar to cell-based flow cytometry, a secondary fluorochrome-conjugated anti-human IgG is added that helps detection of DSA bound to HLA targets on these beads when analyzed on a flow cytometer platform such as Luminex. This is a semi-quantitative test generating output in mean fluorescent intensity (MFI) units. This is the same technique that is used to calculate cPRA.

While extremely sensitive, major limitations of the SAB assays are [6]:

1. Difficulty in establishing a threshold above which the antibody level is clinically relevant
2. Semi-quantitative nature of the result obtained due to several factors such as variable antigen density on the bead surfaces and sharing of public epitopes between various beads
3. Conformational changes in the structure of proteins during the process of attachment to microparticle surfaces (false-positive output can result from expression of neo-antigens and false-negative output from masking of relevant epitopes)

SAB results combined with high-resolution typing allow for detection of allele-specific antibodies that will not react with an entire grouping based on low-resolution serologic typing. For example, a potential recipient may have antibodies to A_2:01 that do not cross-react with A_2:02. Exclusion of the entire A2 group would prevent this candidate from getting offers from A_2:02 donors. Widespread use of these techniques allows for a more detailed assessment of immunologic risk, which becomes especially relevant in the highly sensitized population where transplant options are very limited. One notable shortcoming is that the relative immunogenicity between antigens is not addressed [7]. For instance, a DQ2 → DQ5 transplant confers a 1 HLA mismatch as does a DQ6 → DQ5. At an epitope level, there are fewer structural differences between DQ5 and DQ6 than between DQ5 and DQ2. As a result, with a negative virtual crossmatch in both scenarios, a DQ6 → DQ5 transplant is associated with a lower immunologic risk than a DQ2 → DQ5 transplant.

CDC crossmatch, although not very sensitive for risk of rejection, is highly specific, and a positive CDC crossmatch generally precludes transplantation due to the high risk of hyperacute rejection (Fig. 10.1). Flow and virtual crossmatches, while more sensitive, are less specific. Positive results do not necessarily prevent proceeding with transplantation but do predict a higher risk of rejection-mediated graft injury and graft loss. Bentall et al. compared graft outcomes of 102 positive crossmatch (CDC or flow) living donor transplant recipients to 204 negative crossmatch recipients; 1-year graft survival was the lowest in the CDC crossmatch positive group at 82.4% [8]. In the positive crossmatch transplants with only class I DSA, 60% of graft losses occurred within the first year. In contrast, class II DSA was associated with a relatively low rate of early antibody-mediated rejection (ABMR) but a high rate of chronic injury, with 40% of grafts failing within 5-years of transplantation. Patients

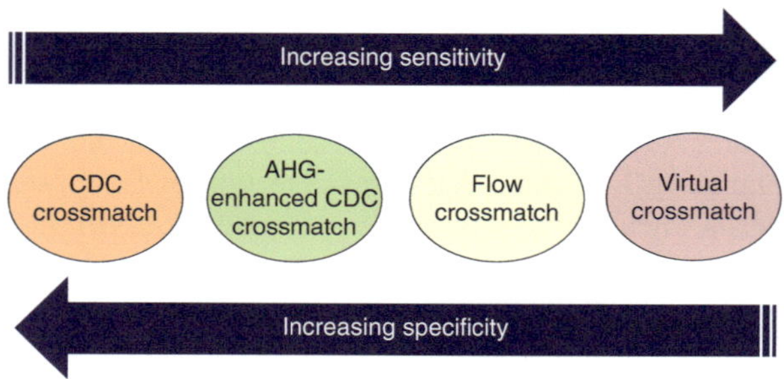

Fig. 10.1 Crossmatch techniques in sequence of increasing sensitivity and decreasing specificity for predicting rejection

with both class I and II DSA had outcomes similar to those with class II DSA only. Even in the absence of a positive crossmatch, DSA detected by SAB assays have been shown to significantly increase the risk of ABMR and graft loss [9].

Nearly 40% of wait-listed kidney transplant candidates in the United States are sensitized (i.e., having cPRA of greater than 1%), and 7% are highly sensitized (i.e., having cPRA of 98–100%.) [10]. In addition, based on ABO frequencies, it is estimated that about one-third of any two individuals will be ABO-incompatible [11]. Therefore, there are fewer opportunities for sensitized transplant candidates to find a blood type- and HLA-compatible donor. Although biologic incompatibility remains a significant barrier to transplantation, novel policies and programs have been developed to offer additional options for such patients. The OPTN KAS that went into effect in December 2014 now provides sensitized patients with a cPRA of 20 and above additional points toward organ allocation priority. Candidates with a cPRA of 100, 99, and 98 are provided 202.1, 50.09, and 24.4 additional points for allocation priority, with each point being equivalent to 1 year of wait-time [3]. In addition, candidates with cPRA of 100 receive priority for kidneys shared nationally, and those with cPRA of 99 receive priority regionally. These innovations have reduced waiting times for sensitized patients on the deceased donor waiting list [12]. However, living donor kidney transplantation remains the treatment of choice for transplant candidates as it typically provides more timely access to transplantation and superior long-term outcomes compared to deceased donor transplantation.

As outlined above, sensitized patients are less likely to identify a blood type- and HLA-compatible living kidney donor, which has significantly reduced access to living donor transplantation in this patient population. In the past, this may have been an insurmountable barrier to transplantation, but programs such as kidney paired donation (KPD) and desensitization now allow incompatible potential living donors to facilitate living donor transplantation for their intended recipient.

Kidney Paired Donation

KPD, or paired kidney exchange (PKE), is an approach to living donor kidney transplantation that was originally designed to overcome biologic incompatibility, wherein two or more incompatible donor-recipient pairs exchange kidneys and all recipients benefit by receiving compatible transplants. Since the first KPD

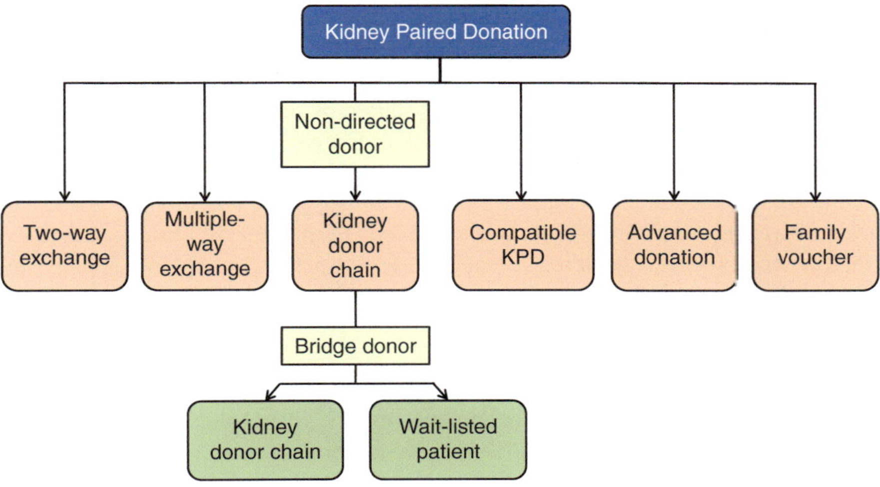

Fig. 10.2 Types of kidney paired donation

transplants performed in the United States in 2000, the scope of KPD has expanded significantly both within and outside the United States, especially with inclusion of non-directed living kidney donors [13]. The various types of transplants performed via KPD include (Fig. 10.2):

Two-way exchange This is the simplest form of KPD, where two pairs with incompatibilities exchange kidneys; the recipient in one incompatible pair receives a kidney from the donor in the second incompatible pair, and vice versa [14]. This requires pairs to have reciprocal or complementary incompatibilities.

Multiple-way exchange, which includes three or more pairs Entering more pairs into an exchange not only facilitates more transplants but also increases options for difficult-to-match patients, as complementary incompatibilities are not required.

Kidney donor chains These "chains" are typically initiated by non-directed donors (NDD), i.e., individuals who donate without an intended recipient. To maximize benefits to the transplant waitlist, a NDD is matched with a recipient with an incompatible living donor, who in turn donates his or her kidney to another incompatible pair. This generates a domino effect and keeps the chain going until the last donor donates to a recipient on the deceased donor waiting list or becomes a "bridge donor" who initiates another chain at a later time. Description of the first kidney donor chain in the United States of ten transplants initiated in July 2007 by a single NDD and coordinated over 8 months was published in the *New England Journal of Medicine* in 2009 [15]. Current practice recommends that all NDDs are routinely made aware of KPD as a donation option in order to maximize the utility of their gift, as opposed to directly donating to the deceased donor list [16, 17].

In simple two- or multiple-way exchanges, the donations are ideally performed simultaneously to avoid the possibility that a donor may fail to donate a kidney after one of the transplants has already occurred. Kidney donor chains initiated by NDDs and bridge donors add flexibility to the process in terms of scheduling transplants. Although reneging by a donor in the middle of the chain is still problematic, downstream affects are less dire as the chain was started by the "extra" NDD, and all the pending recipients still retain their respective donors [18]. An analysis of 1748 transplants facilitated by the National Kidney Registry (NKR) identified that broken chains are uncommon [19]. Medical issues in the approved donor while waiting to bridge was the most common reason identified. From over 400 bridge donors, 6 elected not to proceed, yielding a renege rate of 1.5%. All recipients affected by broken chains received a transplant, typically within 6 months from reactivation within the NKR.

Compatible KPD   A biologically compatible pair refers to a donor-recipient pair where there is no ABO or HLA incompatibility (i.e., direct donation is possible); however, they choose to pursue KPD, usually to obtain a more optimal kidney for the recipient and often also to facilitate additional transplants for other candidates with incompatible donors. For example, if a living donor is much older than the intended recipient and has extensive HLA mismatches, KPD may be used to obtain a kidney from a younger living donor with better kidney function and fewer HLA mismatches. Assessment of kidney quality and match with a particular donor is essential in these cases and is discussed below. Increasing the number of compatible pairs that enroll in KPD programs is believed to substantially increase the likelihood of incompatible pairs identifying a compatible donor through KPD.

Blood type O donors are rare within KPD programs, since only O donors who are HLA-incompatible with their intended recipient would need to enter KPD. This has created an imbalance where the number of blood type O transplant candidates in any KPD pool always exceeded the number of type O donors, leading to prolonged waiting times for these patients [20]. For this reason, a pair with a blood type O donor and non-blood type O recipient is considered a "favorable pair." Compatible pairs in KPD greatly help alleviate this imbalance, by making the KPD pool larger, and by infusing favorable pairs into the system. A recent analysis of 151 compatible pairs entered in NKR between 2/2008 and 11/2018, half of whom were favorable pairs, documented that each compatible pair facilitated two additional transplants, substantially benefiting the blood type O and the highly sensitized population [21].

Advanced donation   This type of KPD offers an option for "chronologically incompatible" pairs that enables living donation to occur when optimal for the donor and transplantation of the intended recipient to occur at a later time if and when needed. One intended recipient with documented kidney disease is identified in advanced donation. For example, a 50-year-old man with advanced kidney disease but not yet on dialysis is listed for transplantation. His wife is approved as a donor. However, due to their being the primary support person for each other, they prefer to separate their surgeries in time. Advanced donation allows the wife to donate to the KPD pool and the husband to receive a kidney several months later once the wife has recovered from her surgery. As in this case, the donor and recipient surgeries are usually separated by a few weeks to months; however, longer intervals are also possible. The latter scenario is illustrated by the case of a grandfather wanting to donate on behalf of his grandchild who has kidney disease but is not in imminent need of transplantation [22]. Here, the grandfather donates to the KPD pool, and in return, the grandchild may obtain a kidney from the KPD pool at a later time, if the need arises. This allows the grandfather to donate now, essentially as an NDD, without risking his candidacy as a donor being affected as he ages. If the intended recipient does not progress to end-stage kidney disease, or is deemed ineligible for transplantation for any reason, the "voucher" is not redeemed, and the donation remains as non-directed.

Family voucher   Another form of the voucher system recently introduced by the NKR is a "family voucher" that attempts to overcome a major barrier to non-directed donation, i.e., reluctance to donate for fear that one's currently healthy children or spouse or siblings will need a kidney in the future [23]. It allows naming up to five individuals to receive vouchers. If one or more of these individuals were to develop kidney failure in the future, the first one to need a kidney can redeem their voucher. While the details of voucher policies are still evolving, it is expected that this will further expand the KPD donor pool and facilitate more transplants.

Assessment of Quality of a Donor Kidney

Ensuring a "better" kidney for their intended recipient is an important driver for biologically compatible donors to consider donating through a KPD chain rather than donate directly to their intended recipient. While this may seem intuitive, one of the major challenges in increasing enrolment of compatible pairs in KPD chains is reliably quantifying the benefit of KPD for transplant candidates who have a compatible donor. The following key factors in donor assessment must be considered when weighing the potential benefits of compatible KPD for the recipient.

HLA mismatch   Even in the modern era of potent immunosuppression, there are clear benefits of HLA matching to graft survival. Several studies have documented the particularly important benefits of matching at HLA-DR and DQ loci in terms of long-term outcomes [24–27]. Donor-recipient pairs may be interested in KPD to obtain a better HLA match, especially at these class II loci (despite absence of pre-formed DSA).

Donor kidney function and comorbidities   It is not surprising that donor glomerular filtration rate (GFR) has an important impact on recipient outcomes [28]. Absolute (i.e., not adjusted for body surface area (BSA)) measured GFR of the donor candidate, when available, should be used to assess the kidney function that would be available to the recipient after transplantation. However, in the United States, creatinine clearance is used much more frequently [29]. A major limitation of creatinine clearance is the significant risk of under- or over-collections. Also, due to tubular secretion of creatinine, creatinine clearance overestimates true GFR by 10–20%.

The volume of the transplanted kidney also strongly correlates with recipient outcomes, even after adjustment for GFR [30]. However, there is significant inter-operator variability when assessing kidney volumes, and this measure is often not routinely available. Age and gender are frequently used surrogates for assessment of donor kidney function, but kidney volume and GFR have been shown to be better predictors of recipient outcomes than age and gender [30].

It should be emphasized that the absolute GFR should be used when considering impact on recipient outcomes, as is the case in compatible KPD. Also, when there is a significant difference in size between the two kidneys, assessment of single-kidney GFR using radionuclides or contrast agents that are excreted by glomerular filtration should be considered [17].

Additionally, risk factors for chronic kidney disease in the donor such as hypertension, race, and smoking also need to be considered. Currently, there is very limited data on how to weight these variables against each other when choosing between different donor candidates for a particular recipient.

Other variables Several other variables may be of relevance in specific cases, e.g., benefits of receiving a kidney from a cytomegalovirus (CMV) seronegative, rather than seropositive, donor in cases where the recipient is seronegative.

Cold ischemia time (CIT) There has been concern in the transplant community regarding shipping living donor kidneys over long distances through KPD programs, thereby adding significant CIT. An analysis by Treat et al. of 1267 shipped KPD, 205 non-shipped/internal KPD, and 4800 unrelated, non-shipped, non-KPD living donor kidney transplants showed that each hour of CIT was associated with a 5% increased odds of delayed graft function [31]. However, CIT was not significantly associated with graft or patient survival.

To better quantify and compare the risks and potential benefits associated with various living donor candidates for a potential recipient, Massie et al. created a living kidney donor profile index (LKDPI) on the same scale as the deceased donor kidney donor profile index or KDPI [28]. Notably, the c-statistic of this model is only 0.59. Subsequently, Ashby et al. published another model that provides estimates of graft survival at 5 and 10 years after transplantation while accounting for mismatches in age, gender, HLA, and body size [32]. While the c-statistic of their model was slightly better at 0.64, it did not use donor GFR but rather relied on surrogates such as age, gender, height, and weight. Another analysis documented that HLA matching had a larger impact on kidney life-years than donor age, sex, or biological sibling status [27]. Further research is needed to guide decision-making and patient counseling, especially in compatible KPD cases while paying heed to the logistics of each individual situation, especially the time it takes to get a "better kidney" and how that affects the total dialysis exposure in a particular recipient candidate.

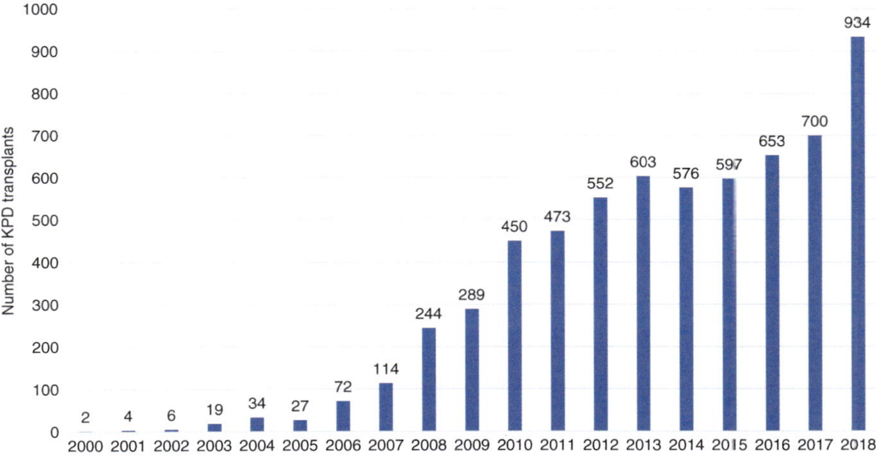

Fig. 10.3 LKDT performed via kidney paired donation in the United States, by year. (From Hart-Lentine et al. [33])

Scope of KPD

The practice of KPD in the United States has expanded exponentially, from two transplants in 2002 to 934 in 2018 (Fig. 10.3) [33]. A recent analysis of 9 years of transplants performed via NKR showed equal or better graft survival compared with several other living donor transplant subgroups, despite transplanting a higher proportion of highly sensitized patients [34]. Inclusion of compatible pairs in KPD has been a major advance as it adds to the pool of potential donors and facilitates transplants for blood type O and highly sensitized patients [21]. Several additional strategies are being considered to further expand the potential of KPD, for example, use of a deceased donor kidney to initiate a chain similar to kidney donor chains initiated by an NDD [35]. The first successful report of this approach was recently published from a transplant center in Italy [36]. Another innovative approach that was recently described is that of a pair in which a Filipino husband-wife pair underwent donation and transplantation in the United States via KPD that was financed by philanthropy [37]. In the process, a chain was initiated that facilitated a total of 11 transplants and ended in a bridge donor. This "global kidney exchange," although encompassing numerous logistical and ethical considerations, is an extraordinary example of the potential expansions of KPD.

Desensitization for Incompatible Living Donor Transplants

The availability of KPD has allowed circumventing the risk associated with ABO or HLA incompatibility and is usually the preferred option for transplant candidates with healthy, biologically incompatible potential donors. For incompatible pairs that are easy to match (e.g., where the donor blood type is O and recipient candidate

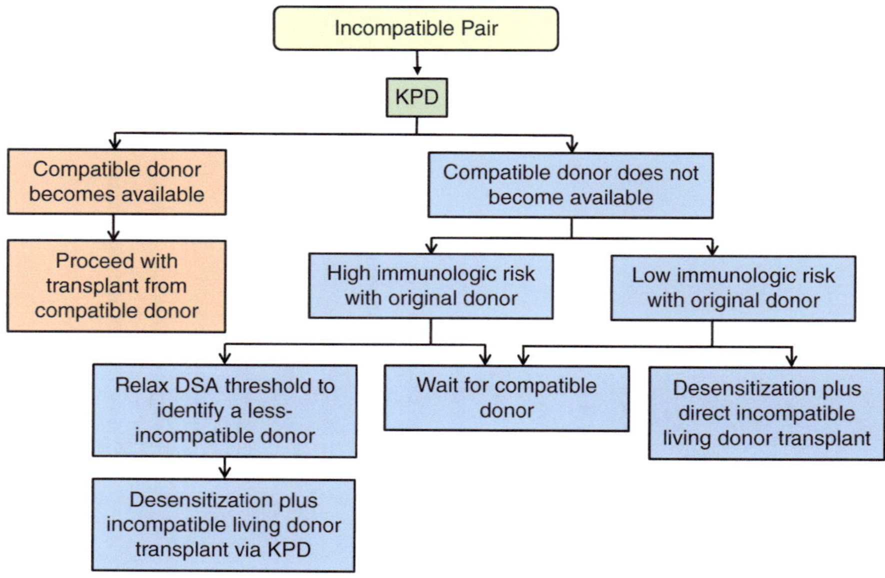

Fig. 10.4 Overall approach to KPD and desensitization

sensitization level is relatively low), a compatible donor would be expected to become available in a short time frame. For pairs that are difficult to match (e.g., a highly sensitized blood type O candidate with a non-blood type O donor), KPD may still find a compatible donor and is a desired option because transplant through KPD would avert the risk associated with incompatibility. However, if a compatible donor does not become available in a reasonable and predefined time frame, depending on assessment of risk associated with transplantation from the incompatible donor, options include (1) relaxing the DSA threshold in attempt to identify a donor in the KPD pool that is not fully compatible, but less incompatible than the original donor, (2) desensitization and proceeding with direct donation, or (3) continuing to wait for a compatible living or deceased donor. This framework is outlined in Fig. 10.4.

HLA desensitization refers to strategies aimed at reducing the amount of DSA present in the peritransplant period to reduce the risk of hyperacute or early ABMR. Various strategies have been used to achieve this goal:

Plasmapheresis followed by intravenous immunoglobulin (ivIg) with or without use of B-cell-depleting agents is the most commonly used strategy for desensitization.

In a study from Johns Hopkins, desensitization using a protocol of plasmapheresis and low-dose ivIg (100 mg/kg) followed by incompatible living donor transplantation was found to provide a substantial patient survival benefit compared with matched control groups of patients who continued to undergo dialysis and of patients who underwent dialysis or received HLA-compatible transplantation from a deceased donor [38]. Remarkably, 8-year patient survival in the desensitization plus incompatible living donor transplantation group was 80.6%, compared with 30.5% in the dialysis-only group and 49.1% in the dialysis or HLA-compatible transplantation group. These findings were subsequently validated from an analysis of over 1000 patients from 22 transplant centers [39]. It is important to highlight that the survival benefit compared with staying on dialysis while awaiting a compatible transplant was seen across all levels of DSA: positive virtual/negative flow, positive flow/negative CDC, and positive CDC crossmatch groups. Another analysis from the same cohort of patients showed that, when compared with compatible living donor transplantation, there was a 1.64- and 5.01-fold increase in risk of graft loss within the first year and 2.04- and 4.59-fold increase in the risk of death within the first year for positive flow/negative CDC and positive CDC crossmatch groups, respectively [40]. Interestingly, there was no difference in outcomes for the positive virtual/negative flow crossmatch group compared to compatible living donor transplants. To summarize, when compatible living donor transplant is not an option, desensitization and incompatible living donor transplant provide better outcomes than waiting on dialysis for a compatible deceased donor. When the DSA is low level, outcomes comparable to compatible living donor transplants can be achieved at the expense of desensitization and stronger induction immunosuppression therapies.

In another series of investigations from the Cedars Sinai Medical Center group, the combination of high-dose ivIg (2 g/kg) and the anti-CD20 antibody rituximab was reported to be safe and effective. In one study of 20 highly sensitized patients, receiving 2 doses of ivIg and 2 doses of rituximab over a 30-day period led to reduction of mean PRA from 77% to 44% and lowered mean time to living or deceased donor transplantation from 144 to 5 months [41, 42]. However, other groups have found limited benefits of this approach [43].

B-cell-depleting therapies   A study by Jackson et al. showed that rituximab alone reduced the incidence and magnitude of HLA antibody rebound, but there was no difference in ABMR or graft survival at 5 years [44]. On the contrary, another study randomizing patients to ivIg plus placebo vs. ivIg plus rituximab was terminated after enrolling only 15 patients due to three ABMRs and two graft losses among 7 patients in the former group [45]. An analysis of 54 transplant recipients by Loupy et al. comparing high-dose ivIg vs. ivIg, pheresis, and rituximab identified no difference in early outcomes; however, the latter group had fewer cases of subclinical ABMR and transplant glomerulopathy at 1 year [46]. These studies are limited by small sample sizes. Nonetheless, these data suggest a limited role of rituximab therapy alone in desensitization but potential benefit when used in conjunction with other therapies. A study evaluating obinutuzumab, another anti-CD20 antibody, for desensitization, is currently underway [47].

Several other drugs are being investigated for both desensitization and treatment of ABMR but are not part of standard of care regimens at most transplant centers. These include:

Proteasome inhibitors   Plasma cells make antibodies and are a logical target for suppression of antibody production. Bortezomib, a proteasome inhibitor, is a mainstay of treatment of multiple myeloma but has not been found to be effective for desensitization [48]. One possible hypothesis for this difference in response is that the plasma cells that produce anti-HLA antibodies are not as metabolically active as the malignant cells in multiple myeloma. Ixazomib is another proteasome inhibitor that is administered orally and is being evaluated as a desensitization agent in the Ixazomib for Desensitization (IXADES) study [49].

Complement inhibitors   Eculizumab is a humanized monoclonal antibody that binds to complement protein C5 and blocks generation of the terminal attack complex C5b-9. A trial of eculizumab compared to placebo as an add-on therapy to standard of care desensitization protocols in living donor transplantation did not identify any difference in the primary treatment failure endpoint, a composite of biopsy-proven Banff 2007 grade II or III ABMR, graft loss, patient death, or loss to follow-up [50]. When grade I ABMR was included, the treatment failure rate was significantly lower in the eculizumab arm compared to the standard of care arm (11.8% vs. 21.6%). C1 esterase inhibitor works more proximally in the complement cascade and is postulated to be more effective in controlling complement-mediated injury. In a trial of 20 sensitized patients desensitized with ivIg and rituximab, with or without plasmapheresis, C1 esterase inhibitor showed reduction in complement-fixing HLA antibodies [51]. Longer-term studies are needed to document benefit with patient and graft outcomes.

B-cell-activating factor (BAFF)/B-lymphocyte stimulator (BLyS) inhibitors   BAFF, also called BLyS, is a cytokine that promotes B-cell activation. Belimumab, an anti-BAFF antibody, is FDA-approved for treatment of systemic lupus erythematosus. While there is limited published literature with this agent in the kidney transplant population, there are a few ongoing trials investigating its role for desensitization [52, 53].

Interleukin (IL)-6 receptor inhibitor   IL-6 is a pleiotropic cytokine that has stimulates B cells and plasma cells and aids with antibody production. Tocilizumab is a monoclonal antibody directed against the IL-6 receptor that is being used for treatment of rheumatoid arthritis. In one pilot trial of ten transplant candidates who had failed desensitization with ivIg and rituximab and were subsequently treated with ivIg and tocilizumab, five were successfully transplanted [54]. Larger controlled studies are needed to prove its efficacy.

IgG-degrading enzyme derived from Streptococcus pyogenes (IdeS)   IdeS is an endopeptidase that cleaves all four subclasses of human IgG at the hinge region to Fab and Fc fragments, thereby preventing IgG-mediated complement-mediated cytotoxicity as well as antibody-dependent cellular cytotoxicity. It works extremely rapidly. In one study of 25 highly sensitized candidates, IdeS administered approximately 4–6 hours before transplantation essentially eliminated all anti-HLA antibodies until 7–14 days after transplantation, when new IgG synthesis was detected; 24 patients were successfully transplanted [55]. One major limitation of this therapy is that inactivating anti-IdeS antibodies appear very quickly, which severely limits the ability to re-dose. Future studies to evaluate using IdeS in combination with other therapies that prevent the rebound of antibodies after the initial week of quiescence are needed for success of this therapy [56].

Combining KPD and Desensitization

KPD and desensitization are not mutually exclusive strategies. Many highly sensitized individuals with biologically incompatible donors may not be able to find a completely compatible donor in a KPD pool [20]. However, KPD could still help such candidates by identifying a less incompatible donor and followed by desensitization and transplantation. For instance, a recipient candidate seeking retransplantation might have a high-level DSA against their original incompatible donor candidate, which is also a repeat mismatch with a previous transplant. The risk associated with this incompatible transplant would be high, and the pair would typically be entered into KPD. While a fully compatible donor might not be found, one to which the candidate has a low-level DSA and which is not a repeat mismatch might be available. The decision to pursue this "less incompatible" transplant would likely provide the patient with better survival than staying on dialysis and would also be preferable to proceeding with transplantation in the context of high-level DSA. These cases require frequent reevaluation by the transplant team and HLA personnel, especially if no offers become available after several months, and relaxing DSA acceptance thresholds needs to be considered.

Conclusion

KPD and desensitization are two available strategies for overcoming biological incompatibility in living donor kidney transplantation. Simple two-way and multiple-way exchanges allow overcoming incompatibilities for individual patients. Introducing non-directed donors and, more recently, compatible pairs enlarges the KPD pool consequently facilitating transplants for blood type O and the highly sensitized recipients. Several innovative approaches are being explored to expand the potential of KPD, such as advanced donation for the chronologically incompatible. More recently, a family voucher option has become available; this aims to overcome a major barrier to non-directed donation (i.e., concern that one's healthy loved ones will need a kidney in the future). In easy-to-match incompatible pairs, KPD to circumvent incompatibility is recommended. If a compatible donor does not become available for a difficult-to-match pair, options include reconsideration of acceptance criteria to identify a less incompatible donor followed by desensitization and transplantation, desensitization and direct donation from the original incompatible donor candidate, and continuing to wait for a compatible living or deceased donor. Most desensitization algorithms rely on plasmapheresis and ivIg, with or without B-cell-depleting therapies. Several new drugs borrowed from the oncology and rheumatology practice are being investigated for desensitization. In particular, IdeS has a promising mechanism of action. In combination with other agents, it may serve as an effective and reliable desensitization therapy option, thereby improving access to transplantation in the highly sensitized population.

References

1. Breimer ME, Samuelsson BE. The specific distribution of glycolipid-based blood group A antigens in human kidney related to A_1/A_2, Lewis, and secretor status of single individuals. A possible molecular explanation for the successful transplantation of A_2 kidneys into O recipients. Transplantation. 1986;42(1):88–91. https://pubmed.ncbi.nlm.nih.gov/3523889/.
2. Bryan CF, Cherikh WS, Sesok-Pizzini DA. A2 /A2 B to B renal transplantation: past, present, and future directions. Am J Transplant. 2016;16(1):11–20. https://doi.org/10.1111/ajt.13499.
3. Organ Procurement and Transplantation Network (OPTN) / United Network for Organ Sharing (UNOS). Policy 8: Allocation of Kidneys. Available at: https://optn.transplant.hrsa.gov/governance/policies/. Accessed: 7 Sept 2020.
4. Cecka JM. Calculated PRA (CPRA): the new measure of sensitization for transplant candidates. Am J Transplant. 2010;10(1):26–9. https://doi.org/10.1111/j.1600-6143.2009.02927.x.
5. Organ Procurement and Transplantation Network (OPTN) cPRA Calculator. Avaialable at: https://optn.transplant.hrsa.gov/resources/allocation-calculators/cpra-calculator/. Accessed: 7 Sept 2020.
6. Konvalinka A, Tinckam K. Utility of HLA antibody testing in kidney transplantation. J Am Soc Nephrol. 2015;26(7):1489–502. https://doi.org/10.1681/ASN.2014080837.
7. Sypek M, Kausman J, Holt S, Hughes P. HLA epitope matching in kidney transplantation: an overview for the general nephrologist. Am J Kidney Dis. 2018;71:720–31. https://doi.org/10.1053/j.ajkd.2017.09.021.
8. Bentall A, Cornell LD, Gloor JM, Park WD, Gandhi MJ, Winters JL, et al. Five-year outcomes in living donor kidney transplants with a positive crossmatch. Am J Transplant. 2013;13(1):76–85. https://doi.org/10.1111/j.1600-6143.2012.04291.x.
9. Mohan S, Palanisamy A, Tsapepas D, Tanriover B, Crew RJ, Dube G, et al. Donor-specific antibodies adversely affect kidney allograft outcomes. J Am Soc Nephrol. 2012;23(12):2061–71. https://doi.org/10.1681/ASN.2012070664.
10. Hart A, Smith JM, Skeans MA, Gustafson SK, Wilk AR, Castro S, et al. OPTN/SRTR 2017 annual data report: kidney. Am J Transplant. 2019;19 Suppl 2:19–123. https://doi.org/10.1111/ajt.15274.
11. Segev DL, Gentry SE, Warren DS, Reeb B, Montgomery RA. Kidney paired donation and optimizing the use of live donor organs. JAMA. 2005;293(15):1883–90. https://doi.org/10.1001/jama.293.15.1883.
12. Stewart DE, Kucheryavaya AY, Klassen DK, Turgeon NA, Formica RN, Aeder MI. Changes in deceased donor kidney transplantation one year after KAS implementation. Am J Transplant. 2016;16(6):1834–47. https://doi.org/10.1111/ajt.13770.
13. Faber DA, Joshi S, Ciancio G. Demographic characteristics of non-directed altruistic kidney donors in the United States. J Kidney. 2016;2(2):121. https://doi.org/10.4172/2472-1220.1000121.
14. Ellison B. A systematic review of kidney paired donation: Applying lessons from historic and contemporary case studies to improve the US model. 16 May 2014. Available at: http://repository.upenn.edu/wharton_research_scholars/107. Accessed: 7 Sept 2020.
15. Rees MA, Kopke JE, Pelletier RP, Segev DL, Rutter ME, Fabrega AJ, et al. A nonsimultaneous, extended, altruistic-donor chain. N Engl J Med. 2009;360(11):1096–101. https://doi.org/10.1056/NEJMoa0803645.

16. Melcher ML, Blosser CD, Baxter-Lowe LA, Delmonico FL, Gentry SE, Leishman R, et al. Dynamic challenges inhibiting optimal adoption of kidney paired donation: findings of a consensus conference. Am J Transplant. 2013;13(4):851–60. https://doi.org/10.1111/ajt.12140.

17. Lentine KL, Kasiske BL, Levey AS, Adams PL, Alberu J, Bakr MA, et al. KDIGO clinical practice guideline on the evaluation and care of living kidney donors. Transplantation. 2017;101(8S Suppl 1):S1–S109. https://doi.org/10.1097/TP.0000000000001769.

18. Roth AE, Sonmez T, Unver MU, Delmonico FL, Saidman SL. Utilizing list exchange and nondirected donation through 'chain' paired kidney donations. Am J Transplant. 2006;6(11):2694–705. https://doi.org/10.1111/j.1600-6143.2006.01515.x.

19. Cowan N, Gritsch HA, Nassiri N, Sinacore J, Veale J. Broken chains and reneging: a review of 1748 kidney paired donation transplants. Am J Transplant. 2017;17(9):2451–7. https://doi.org/10.1111/ajt.14343.

20. Gentry SE, Montgomery RA, Segev DL. Kidney paired donation: fundamentals, limitations, and expansions. Am J Kidney Dis. 2011;57(1):144–51. https://doi.org/10.1053/j.ajkd.2010.10.005.

21. Chipman VL, Lee B, Cooper M, Cuffy MC, Ronin M, Hil G, Flechner S, Thomas A, Mandelbrot DA, Waterman AD, Freise CE. Abstract: compatible pairs in paired kidney exchange - are there winners and loosers? Am J Transplant. 2019;19(Supplement 3):537. https://atcmeetingabstracts.com/abstract/compatible-pairs-in-paired-kidney-exchange-are-there-winners-and-loosers/.

22. Veale JL, Capron AM, Nassiri N, Danovitch G, Gritsch HA, Waterman A. et al. Vouchers for future kidney transplants to overcome "chronological incompatibility" between living donors and recipients. Transplantation. 2017;101(9):2115–9. https://doi.org/10.1097/TP.0000000000001744.

23. National Kidney Registry (NKR). Info about the voucher program. Available at: https://www.kidneyregistry.org/info/voucher-program. Accessed: 7 Sept 2020.

24. Coupel S, Giral-Classe M, Karam G, Morcet JF, Dantal J, Cantarovich D, et al. Ten-year survival of second kidney transplants: impact of immunologic factors and renal function at 12 months. Kidney Int. 2003;64(2):674–80. https://doi.org/10.1046/j.1523-1755.2003.00104.x.

25. Lee H, Min JW, Kim JI, Moon IS, Park KH, Yang CW, et al. Clinical significance of HLA-DQ antibodies in the development of chronic antibody-mediated rejection and allograft failure in kidney transplant recipients. Medicine (Baltimore). 2016;95(11):e3094. https://doi.org/10.1097/MD.0000000000003094.

26. Lim WH, Chapman JR, Coates PT, Lewis JR, Russ GR, Watson N, et al. HLA-DQ mismatches and rejection in kidney transplant recipients. Clin J Am Soc Nephrol. 2016;11(5):875–83. https://doi.org/10.2215/CJN.11641115.

27. Milner J, Melcher ML, Lee B, Veale J, Ronin M, D'Alessandro T, et al. HLA matching trumps donor age: donor-recipient pairing characteristics that impact long-term success in living donor kidney transplantation in the era of paired kidney exchange. Transplant Direct. 2016;2(7):e85. https://doi.org/10.1097/TXD.0000000000000597.

28. Massie AB, Leanza J, Fahmy LM, Chow EK, Desai NM, Luo X, et al. A risk index for living donor kidney transplantation. Am J Transplant. 2016;16(7):2077–84. https://doi.org/10.1111/ajt.13709.

29. Mandelbrot DA, Pavlakis M, Danovitch GM, Johnson SR, Karp SJ, Khwaja K, et al. The medical evaluation of living kidney donors: a survey of US transplant centers. Am J Transplant. 2007;7(10):2333–43. https://doi.org/10.1111/j.1600-6143.2007.01932.x.

30. Poggio ED, Hila S, Stephany B, Fatica R, Krishnamurthi V, del Bosque C, et al. Donor kidney volume and outcomes following live donor kidney transplantation. Am J Transplant. 2006;6(3):616–24. https://doi.org/10.1111/j.1600-6143.2005.01225.x.

31. Treat E, Chow EKH, Peipert JD, Waterman A, Kwan L, Massie AB, et al. Shipping living donor kidneys and transplant recipient outcomes. Am J Transplant. 2018;18(3):632–41. https://doi.org/10.1111/ajt.14597.

32. Ashby VB, Leichtman AB, Rees MA, Song PX, Bray M, Wang W, et al. A kidney graft survival calculator that accounts for mismatches in age, sex, HLA, and body size. Clin J Am Soc Nephrol. 2017;12(7):1148–60. https://doi.org/10.2215/CJN.09330916.

33. Hart A, Lentine KL, Smith JM, Miller JM, Skeans MA, Prentice M, et al. OPTN/SRTR 2019 Annual Data Report: Kidney. Am J Transplant. 2021;21(Suppl 2):21–137. https://doi.org/10.1111/ajt.16502.

34. Flechner SM, Thomas AG, Ronin M, Veale JL, Leeser DB, Kapur S, et al. The first 9 years of kidney paired donation through the National Kidney Registry: Characteristics of donors and recipients compared with National Live Donor Transplant Registries. Am J Transplant. 2018;18(11):2730–8. https://doi.org/10.1111/ajt.14744.

35. Brunner RF, Fumo D, Rees M. Novel approaches to expanding benefits from living kidney donor chains. Curr Transplant Rep. 2017;4(2):67–74.

36. Furian L, Cornelio C, Silvestre C, Neri F, Rossi F, Rigotti P, et al. Deceased-donor-initiated chains: First report of a successful deliberate case and its ethical implications. Transplantation. 2019;103:2196–200. https://doi.org/10.1097/TP.0000000000002645.

37. Rees MA, Dunn TB, Kuhr CS, Marsh CL, Rogers J, Rees SE, et al. Kidney exchange to overcome financial barriers to kidney transplantation. Am J Transplant. 2017;17(3):782–90. https://doi.org/10.1111/ajt.14106.

38. Montgomery RA, Lonze BE, King KE, Kraus ES, Kucirka LM, Locke JE, et al. Desensitization in HLA-incompatible kidney recipients and survival. N Engl J Med. 2011;365(4):318–26. https://doi.org/10.1056/NEJMoa1012376.

39. Orandi BJ, Luo X, Massie AB, Garonzik-Wang JM, Lonze BE, Ahmed R, et al. Survival benefit with kidney transplants from HLA-incompatible live donors. N Engl J Med. 2016;374(10):940–50. https://doi.org/10.1056/NEJMoa1508380.

40. Orandi BJ, Garonzik-Wang JM, Massie AB, Zachary AA, Montgomery JR, Van Arendonk KJ, et al. Quantifying the risk of incompatible kidney transplantation: a multicenter study. Am J Transplant. 2014;14(7):1573–80. https://doi.org/10.1111/ajt.12786.

41. Vo AA, Lukovsky M, Toyoda M, Wang J, Reinsmoen NL, Lai CH, et al. Rituximab and intravenous immune globulin for desensitization during renal transplantation. N Engl J Med. 2008;359(3):242–51. https://doi.org/10.1056/NEJMoa0707894.

42. Vo AA, Peng A, Toyoda M, Kahwaji J, Cao K, Lai CH, et al. Use of intravenous immune globulin and rituximab for desensitization of highly HLA-sensitized patients awaiting kidney transplantation. Transplantation. 2010;89(9):1095–102. https://doi.org/10.1097/TP.0b013e3181d21e7f.

43. Marfo K, Ling M, Bao Y, Calder B, Ye B, Hayde N, et al. Lack of effect in desensitization with intravenous immunoglobulin and rituximab in highly sensitized patients. Transplantation. 2012;94(4):345–51. https://doi.org/10.1097/TP.0b013e3182590d2e.

44. Jackson AM, Kraus ES, Orandi BJ, Segev DL, Montgomery RA, Zachary AA. A closer look at rituximab induction on HLA antibody rebound following HLA-incompatible kidney transplantation. Kidney Int. 2015;87(2):409–16. https://doi.org/10.1038/ki.2014.261.

45. Vo AA, Choi J, Cisneros K, Reinsmoen N, Haas M, Ge S, et al. Benefits of rituximab combined with intravenous immunoglobulin for desensitization in kidney transplant recipients. Transplantation. 2014;98(3):312–9. https://doi.org/10.1097/TP.0000000000000064.

46. Loupy A, Suberbielle-Boissel C, Zuber J, Anglicheau D, Timsit MO, Martinez F, et al. Combined posttransplant prophylactic IVIg/anti-CD 20/plasmapheresis in kidney recipients with preformed donor-specific antibodies: a pilot study. Transplantation. 2010;89(11):1403–10. https://doi.org/10.1097/TP.0b013e3181da1cc3.

47. A study of obinutuzumab to evaluate safety and tolerability in hypersensitized adult participants with end stage renal disease awaiting transplantation. Available at: s://clinicaltrials.gov/ct2/show/results/NCT02586051?term=obinutuzumab&cond=kidney+transplant&rank=1. Accessed: 7 Sept 2020.

48. Moreno Gonzales MA, Gandhi MJ, Schinstock CA, Moore NA, Smith BH, Braaten NY, et al. 32 doses of Bortezomib for desensitization is not well tolerated and is associated with only modest reductions in anti-HLA antibody. Transplantation. 2017;101(6):1222–7. https://doi.org/10.1097/TP.0000000000001330.

49. Ixazomib for Desensitization (IXADES). Available at: https://clinicaltrials.gov/ct2/show/NCT03213158. Accessed: 7 Sept 2020.

50. Marks WH, Mamode N, Montgomery RA, Stegall MD, Ratner LE, Cornell LD, et al. Safety and efficacy of eculizumab in the prevention of antibody-mediated rejection in living-donor kidney transplant recipients requiring desensitization therapy: a randomized trial. Am J Transplant. 2019;19:2876–88. https://doi.org/10.1111/ajt.15364.
51. Vo AA, Zeevi A, Choi J, Cisneros K, Toyoda M, Kahwaji J, et al. A phase I/II placebo-controlled trial of C1-inhibitor for prevention of antibody-mediated rejection in HLA sensitized patients. Transplantation. 2015;99(2):299–308. https://doi.org/10.1097/TP.0000000000000592.
52. Desensitization with belimumab in sensitized patients awaiting kidney transplant. Available at: https://clinicaltrials.gov/ct2/show/NCT01025193. Accessed: 7 Sept 2020.
53. A study of belimumab in the prevention of kidney transplant rejection. Available at: https://clinicaltrials.gov/ct2/show/NCT01536379. Accessed: 7 Sept 2020.
54. Vo AA, Choi J, Kim I, Louie S, Cisneros K, Kahwaji J, et al. A phase I/II trial of the interleukin-6 receptor-specific humanized monoclonal (tocilizumab) + intravenous immunoglobulin in difficult to desensitize patients. Transplantation. 2015;99(11):2356–63. https://doi.org/10.1097/TP.0000000000000741.
55. Jordan SC, Lorant T, Choi J, Kjellman C, Winstedt L, Bengtsson M, et al. IgG endopeptidase in highly sensitized patients undergoing transplantation. N Engl J Med. 2017;377(5):442–53. https://doi.org/10.1056/NEJMoa1612567.
56. Montgomery RA, Lonze BE, Tatapudi VS. IgG degrading enzyme of Streptococcus Pyogenes: an exciting new development in desensitization therapy. Transplantation. 2018;102(1):2–4. https://doi.org/10.1097/TP.0000000000002003.

Psychosocial Evaluation, Care and Quality of Life in Living Kidney Donation

11

Mary Amanda Dew, Andrea F. DiMartini, Jennifer L. Steel, and Sheila G. Jowsey-Gregoire

Introduction

One of the foremost goals in living donor transplantation is to protect donors from harm, and this goal encompasses not only medical but psychosocial outcomes. The imperative to protect living donors has led to guidelines, policy, and regulations to promote donor safety [1–15], as well as to a growing evidence base on postdonation adverse events and their risk factors [16–18]. The evaluation of prospective donors is the cornerstone for helping to ensure donor safety, and the psychosocial component of the evaluation provides transplantation programs with a key opportunity to identify risk factors for poor donor psychosocial outcomes. Moreover, in concert with the medical work-up of prospective donors, the psychosocial evaluation provides critical information necessary to achieve the objectives for donor selection stated almost 20 years ago:

> *The person who gives consent to be a live organ donor should be competent, willing to donate, free from coercion, medically and psychosocially suitable, fully informed of the risks and benefits as a donor, and fully informed of the risks, benefits, and alternative treatment available to the recipient* [1].

M. A. Dew (✉)
Departments of Psychiatry, Psychology, Epidemiology, Biostatistics and the Clinical and Translational Science Institute, University of Pittsburgh, Pittsburgh, PA, USA
e-mail: dewma@upmc.edu

A. F. DiMartini
Departments of Psychiatry and Surgery and the Clinical and Translational Science Institute, University of Pittsburgh, Pittsburgh, PA, USA

J. L. Steel
Departments of Surgery, Psychiatry and Psychology, University of Pittsburgh, Pittsburgh, PA, USA

S. G. Jowsey-Gregoire
Department of Psychiatry, Mayo Clinic, Rochester, MN, USA

© Springer Nature Switzerland AG 2021
K. L. Lentine et al. (eds.), *Living Kidney Donation*,
https://doi.org/10.1007/978-3-030-53618-3_11

The predonation evaluation and transplant team decisions about donor selection are not the endpoints in the process of protecting donors from harm. Follow-up care after donation and routine monitoring of health-related quality of life (HRQOL) outcomes are also essential for promoting donor safety and maximizing donor well-being. Such activities allow early signs of problems to be addressed in a timely manner. Moreover, evidence collected through follow-up care and monitoring may help to augment existing descriptive, longitudinal research findings, thereby leading to better understanding of risk factors and further refinements of the predonation evaluation.

In this chapter, we summarize the domains that should be addressed in the psychosocial evaluation of living kidney donor candidates, as well as process issues relevant to conducting, reporting, and acting on psychosocial evaluation findings. We consider how the evaluation can inform the care of donors as well as individuals who do not go on to donate. Although we necessarily focus on kidney donors, the issues we consider concerning evaluation content and process are relevant to all types of living donors. In addition, we consider living donors' postdonation psychosocial care needs, and review evidence from large and growing qualitative and quantitative research literatures on kidney donors' HRQOL outcomes. We consider the implications of those data for clinical care and for intervention development.

The Content of the Psychosocial Evaluation

The content of the psychosocial evaluation is dictated by its several major goals [7, 16, 19–25]. First, as noted above, it provides critical information relevant for the selection of donors, with a focus on identification and appraisal of risks for poor psychosocial outcomes, and assessment of donor candidates' capacity to understand information and make decisions without undue pressure from others. Second, it enables the identification of factors requiring intervention before donation can occur. Third, it facilitates postdonation care to support optimal psychosocial and medical outcomes. Fourth, should donor candidates be found ineligible to donate for either medical or psychosocial reasons, the information collected in the psychosocial evaluation may be relevant for identifying other resources and care that these individuals may need.

Table 11.1 lists nine domains to be addressed in the psychosocial evaluation and describes the components of each. The domains reflect the areas noted to be critical in a variety of consensus statements, expert commentaries, and reviews reported over the past 20 years [4, 7, 8, 10, 16, 19–32], and are consistent with the elements currently required by Organ Procurement and Transplantation Network (OPTN) policy in the United States [13], as well as those recommended by the European Platform on the Ethical, Legal and Psychosocial Aspects of Organ Transplant (ELPAT) of the European Society for Organ Transplantation [30] and Kidney Disease: Improving Global Outcomes (KDIGO) Living Kidney Donor Work Group [10]. The specific components of each domain, as detailed in Table 11.1, suggest the areas of questioning that should be undertaken to ensure that the domains are

Table 11.1 Domains to be assessed in the psychosocial evaluation of living donor candidates

Evaluation domain	Components comprising the domain
Donation and decision-making about donation	
Motivation for donation	• Rationale and reasons for donation, how the decision to come forward for donation was made • Evidence of undue pressure, inducement (financial or otherwise), or exploitation by others • Expectations about donation • Ambivalence about donation
Relationship with the transplant candidate	• Type of relationship (e.g., family member, spouse, friend, no previous relationship) • If a relationship exists, degree of emotional closeness and relationship quality • Evidence that donation or inability to donate would adversely affect relationship, or that donation would impose expectations or obligations on the part of the donor or recipient
Knowledge and understanding of donation surgery and recovery	• Knowledge and understanding of alternative treatments (included deceased donor transplantation) available to transplant candidate, potential for short- and long-term benefits to recipient, risks for surgical complications and adverse health outcomes for recipient • Knowledge and understanding of short- and long-term risks for donor surgical complications, potential for negative impact on health outcomes, employability, lifestyle, and ability to obtain or maintain health, disability or life insurance • Understanding of postdonation recovery time; willingness to participate in postdonation clinical follow-up care • For anonymous donation, acceptance of program protocols for if and when donors and recipients can communicate with each other
Cognitive status and capacity	• Evidence of impairment that could limit capacity to comprehend information and engage in decision-making about donation • Capacity to make decisions voluntarily and without exploitation by or undue pressure from others
Risk factors for adverse donor outcomes after donation	
Mental health history	• Past and current psychiatric disorders, including mood, anxiety, or other disorders including personality disorders • Current psychiatric symptom severity and chronicity • Past and current mental health treatment including hospitalizations; adherence to and response to treatment; willingness to seek treatment • Current or past suicidal ideation or self-injurious behaviors • Current life stressors; history and responses to loss/bereavement; exposures to trauma including physical or psychological abuse • Evidence of ability to cope with health-related and other stressors
Substance use history	• Tobacco, alcohol, other substance frequency, amount, duration of use and any periods of abstinence • Diagnosable disorder, degree of impairment, and any legal issues • Past and current substance use treatment; insight into any substance use problems, willingness to seek treatment; skills and supports for undertaking treatment and for abstinence

(continued)

Table 11.1 (continued)

Evaluation domain	Components comprising the domain
Donor social, environmental, and personal circumstances and resources	
Social support and attitudes of others	• Availability of emotional and practical assistance from spouse/partner, family, friends, employer on a routine basis and during recovery from donation; willingness of employer or school to accommodate leave from responsibilities • Support, opposition, and other positive or negative reactions from spouse/partner, children, other family, friends
Financial status and preparation	• Financial resources and ability to cover financial obligations for expected/unexpected donation-related expenses • Arrangements made to address role responsibilities (e.g., at work, school, or home) during donation surgery and recovery period; financial impact of time away from role responsibilities • Health, disability, and life insurance coverage
Demographic and social history	• Demographic characteristics including education, literacy and health literacy, occupation, employment history, citizenship, cultural background including religious/faith practices • Marital/partnership status, living arrangements and number of dependents • Community and volunteer activities and service • History of legal issues • History of behaviors that increase the risk of disease transmission to the transplant recipient

thoroughly covered. We have grouped the domains and their components into three critical areas: (a) donation-related factors, encompassing how and why prospective donors came forward and elements relevant for their decision-making about donation; (b) factors that could increase risk for adverse medical and psychosocial outcomes after donation; and (c) factors related to donor candidates' personal, social, and environmental circumstances and resources (which could buffer against other risk factors' effects, although some may serve as risk factors in their own right).

The type of relationship between the prospective donor and the transplant candidate must be considered when determining the specific nature and depth of questioning required in order to fully examine each domain during the evaluation. Although biologically and/or emotionally related donors have long been the most common types of living donors, it is increasingly common for donors to be unrelated, that is, to have limited or even no preexisting relationship with their intended recipient. Examples of types of unrelated donors that have raised concerns among living donor transplant professionals in recent years include individuals who (a) come forward due to social media appeals, (b) are in either a subordinate or superior position relative to the intended recipient (e.g., employees/employers), (c) are foreign nationals, (d) have very low socioeconomic status for whom financial gains may be of concern, (e) share membership in organizations/faith communities with the intended recipient, and (f) seek to make an anonymous donation (directed or nondirected, including starting chains in exchange donation) [7, 19]. For such individuals, key domains of concern pertain to motivation and evidence of any undue pressure, their anticipations about their future relationship (if any) with the recipient, knowledge about the donation process, social supports including attitudes of others about the donation, and their understanding of potential financial implications of donation [19].

Of course, these domains must also be evaluated in biologically and emotionally related donors—the issue is that attention to certain features of these domains is heightened during the evaluation of unrelated donors. For example, individuals coming forward as unrelated donors sometimes have less knowledge about the transplantation process than prospective donors who have seen their loved one live with life-threatening chronic illness. Unrelated prospective donors may have also been swayed by the emotional appeal of a case in the media or an acquaintance who has become ill, without knowing that treatment alternatives might exist or that organ donation carries its own risks, including both health-related risks and unanticipated financial issues for the donor [19, 22]. They may minimize those risks and feel frustrated at facing opposition from family and colleagues regarding their decision to come forward as a donor [33]. Some unrelated donors may believe or hope that their donation will prompt recipients to want a close—or closer—relationship with the donor, or unrelated donors may harbor wishes for the kind of public recognition that they have seen in other cases in the media.

Case vignette

A man in his mid-forties presented for an evaluation to be a kidney donor. He had heard at his church about a child who was a member of his congregation who needed a kidney transplant. He contacted the girl's mother who was eager that he be evaluated as soon as possible. He learned that no one else had come forward and he felt he was called to do so. During the evaluation he revealed that he hoped that donating would help him to make amends, in an indirect way, for an alcohol-related driving under the influence charge a few years back, in which he had injured a young child crossing a road. He felt that he had been given the opportunity to donate so he could make up for his past. He no longer consumed any alcohol and he had become very involved in his church. When asked how he would feel if he could not donate, he said he would feel personally defeated. He also acknowledged that if the young girl's body rejected his kidney, he would be devastated and would take it as an indication that he had not yet been successful in atoning for his past. Due to donor program concerns about the combination of his motives for donation plus possible reactions to unfavorable outcomes in the transplant recipient, a decision was made by the living donor program that he would not be a suitable donor at the present time.

In contrast, some lines of questioning must necessarily be pursued in greater depth for related donors than for unrelated donors. For example, related donors may be subject to greater—or, at least, different—feelings of psychological pressure to donate relative to psychological pressures experienced by unrelated donors. They may view donation as helping them to improve their relationship with the transplant candidate or with other family members, or make up for past problems [16, 31, 34]. Family members may have expectations for which member should initially come forward for evaluation, and that individual may feel unable to decline this type of request or expectation, either to their family or in discussion with the living donor transplantation team [35]. Expectations of other friends and associates may be powerful as well. For example, parents of a child in need of a transplant may feel that everyone they know assumes that they, the parents, should be eager to be evaluated as donors [36]. Similarly, transplant candidates may expect that their own spouse/partner would naturally want to donate, even while the spouse/partner donor feels very uncertain about such a prospect but is fearful of damaging their relationship if they do not proceed with the evaluation [33].

Case vignette

A woman in her early 30s presented for an evaluation to serve as a kidney donor for her father. She stated that she had three other siblings but that she was fully committed to donating. On additional questioning, she indicated that her family got together and mutually agreed that she was at the best stage in her life, compared to her brothers and sister, to donate: she was single and still in school (as a graduate student), while they needed to either focus on career advancement or taking care of their own young families. She admitted she worried about how she would finish school according to her original ambitious timeline and how this might affect her level of personal debt and student loan situation. She also acknowledged that, while she loved her father, he always seemed to look more favorably on her siblings, given their career successes and the fact that they now had their own families. She thought that perhaps the current situation would give her a chance to show him that she could do something worthwhile as well. Nevertheless, she did feel ambivalent about donating. During the medical evaluation, it was determined that she needed some additional testing and that there were some medical comorbidities that would make her a less than ideal candidate. The donor program decided that she should not go forward with donation at the present time secondary to potential medical contraindications and concerns about her psychosocial circumstances. The plan would be to identify another family member who could be brought in for evaluation. The donor program informed the woman that they would inform the transplant candidate that she could not serve as a donor due to medical contraindications and that all specific information that she revealed in the psychosocial and medical evaluations would be kept confidential.

Exploration of motivations, psychosocial history, and reactions to family members' and others' attitudes about potential donation can thus be critical for establishing related donor candidates' capacity to voluntarily decide whether to donate. Overall, then, while all domains listed in Table 11.1 should be considered with all donor candidates, regardless of their connection to the transplant candidate, the nature of questioning must remain flexible to accommodate the very different and unique situations and circumstances that have led prospective donors—both related and unrelated—to seek evaluation.

The Psychosocial Evaluation Process and Predonation Care

The psychosocial evaluation is best considered as a process rather than a one-time event. Although the extensive interview that addresses the domains in Table 11.1 may indeed take place during a single session, there are additional parts of the psychosocial evaluation process that also are important and can affect donor selection decisions by the living donor transplantation program. The optimal scenario is for each program to develop its own protocol and set of procedures to undertake to ensure that a consistent approach is taken to complete the psychosocial evaluation process. The process usually begins with screening of potential donors, continues through the evaluation interview, and may lead to referrals for additional assessments and interventions. Ultimately, a summary of the psychosocial evaluation is provided to the living donor transplantation team, and this information, along with any new results of assessments and interventions, is used by the team in making decisions about donor candidacy. Table 11.2 summarizes important process and care issues to be considered.

The Screening of Prospective Donors

Many, if not most, living donor programs complete a telephone screening before potential donors are asked to schedule any other evaluations or tests. The screening includes medical and psychosocial questions and is most commonly conducted by a living donor transplantation program nurse coordinator [2, 19, 25, 26, 37]. With respect to psychosocial issues, screening questions typically ascertain the prospective donor's relationship (if any) to the transplant candidate and how they learned of the need for an organ donor. Although screening can often lead to automatic exclusions of individuals due to medical factors, from a psychosocial standpoint, the goal is usually less about ruling out prospective donors and more about obtaining information that may help to identify issues that may require more extensive consideration in the full-scale psychosocial evaluation. We have discussed some of those issues for both related and unrelated donors earlier in this chapter. The screening also provides the program's first opportunity to educate prospective donors about donation. If it is not immediately clear that a prospective donor is unsuitable for or uninterested in living donation, then the individual is typically asked to come in for a comprehensive medical and psychosocial evaluation.

The Psychosocial Evaluation Interview

Role and Qualifications of the Evaluator

Living donor transplantation programs should carefully consider which professional will conduct the evaluation. Although the evaluator is typically a member of the program's team, the evaluator is sometimes an external consultant. In some

Table 11.2 Considerations related to the process of the psychosocial evaluation and predonation care

Process factor	Strategies for addressing process factor
Donor candidate screening	Aside from medical factors to be assessed, the donor candidate's relationship to transplant candidate should be documented. Psychosocial issues that require special consideration in psychosocial evaluation should be noted. The donor education process should begin during the screening.
Performance of the psychosocial evaluation interview	**Role and qualification of evaluator** • Either a member of the living donor transplantation program team or an external consultant should be designated to conduct the evaluation. • The evaluator must not only conduct the evaluation but report on its findings, provide recommendations for any assessments or interventions needed by the donor candidate, and determine that the recommendations have been successfully carried out. • The evaluator should have training in behavioral health assessments, particularly those relevant to the content of the psychosocial evaluation for donation, and, in some countries, must be trained in a specific discipline (e.g., social work, psychology, psychiatry in the United States). • The evaluator should have opportunities for continued education and training in psychosocial issues related to living organ donation. • When possible, the evaluator should not also conduct the transplant candidate's psychosocial evaluator in order to avoid actual or perceived bias and potential conflicts of interest. **Interview logistics** • Unless precluded by the urgency of the transplant candidate's medical condition, the timing of the interview should be such that the donor candidate does not feel rushed and all evaluation components can be adequately addressed. • The donor candidate must be informed of the purpose of the psychosocial evaluation interview and that its results will be reviewed by the living donor transplantation team. • The interview should be conducted in private without the transplant candidate, family members, or other friends/associates present. Collateral information should be sought from these individuals or from other sources (e.g., other healthcare providers) as needed. • The interview should be conducted a language that allows the donor candidate to fully participate. If an interpreter is required, this person should have no personal connection to the donor candidate. • Interview questions should be asked in a nonconfrontational manner without leading the donor candidate toward desired answers, and efforts should be undertaken to build rapport with the donor candidate so that he/she will be willing to engage in open and honest discussion. • The interview may need to be repeated if donation is delayed due to transplant candidate medical factors or if the evaluator judges that the donor candidate requires additional assessments and interventions. **Use of checklists as adjuncts for conducting or summarizing interview findings** • The evaluator should consider employing checklists or templates that have been developed to assist the evaluator to ensure that all psychosocial domains in the interview are thoroughly covered.

Table 11.2 (continued)

Process factor	Strategies for addressing process factor
Communication with living donor transplantation team about evaluating findings	• A written report summarizing evaluation findings should be prepared and entered into the donor candidate's medical record. • The report should include recommendations for any additional psychosocial assessments and interventions that should be completed by the donor candidate. • The evaluator should attend team meetings in which discussion and selection of donor candidates occurs.
Referral for psychosocial assessments or interventions	• The evaluator, alone or in consultation with the ILDA and living donor transplantation team, is responsible for making these referrals. • The evaluator should review the results of any assessments and interventions before making further recommendations to the team about living donor candidate selection. • If the donor candidate is required to complete any psychosocial interventions, the evaluator should specify what constitutes intervention success.
Communication with the donor candidate after team decisions are mad about donor candidacy	• The evaluator should provide further recommendations for care or education of individuals that the team selects as donor candidates. • If a donor candidate is not approved to donate, the evaluator, alone or in consultation with the ILDA, should offer recommendations for any care the donor candidate may need and provide referrals as needed for local counseling or support resources. • Unless the situation is urgent, the evaluator, in consultation with the ILDA, should advocate for a "cooling off period" for donor candidates to allow them to reflect on their decision before donation occurs.

Abbreviation: ILDA independent living donor advocate

programs, the evaluator may also serve as the program's independent living donor advocate (ILDA). It has been strongly recommended, and is a requirement in the United States, for example, that programs have an ILDA, whose obligation is to protect the interests of living donors, including living donor candidates [1, 2, 5, 7, 10, 13, 19]. Even if the ILDA does not conduct the evaluation, the psychosocial evaluator should bear in mind that the ILDA will review its results and will also meet with the donor candidate to help ensure that the individual understands the donation process and to facilitate the individual's informed decision-making about donation. As we discuss further below, the evaluator is charged not only with conducting the psychosocial evaluation interview but with reporting on its findings to the living donor transplantation team, and with making and monitoring the implementation of recommendations for additional psychosocial assessments, treatments, or interventions required by the donor candidate.

Internationally, programs vary in terms of the psychosocial evaluator's discipline or original field of training, although some countries such as the United States have specific requirements for discipline of training. In general, the evaluator should have training and expertise in psychosocial and behavioral health assessments, and is typically (or, in the United States, must be) a social worker, psychologist, or psychiatrist [13]. Even more important, the evaluator must be knowledgeable and have experience in assessing the domains listed in Table 11.1. Moreover, evaluators should be encouraged to take advantage of opportunities for education and training in living donor evaluation to build skills and learn from other clinicians experienced in the psychosocial evaluation process. When possible, the individual who evaluates the prospective donor should be different from the transplant candidate's psychosocial evaluator in order to avoid bias and potential conflicts of interest.

Interview Logistics

The psychosocial evaluation interview must be conducted in keeping with the following central tenets, as delineated in expert reviews, commentaries, and consensus statements [2, 4, 7, 16, 19, 22–24, 27, 31]. First, the interview may be conducted in one single session or across several sessions, depending not only on complexity but on timing of the medical components of the donor evaluation. It is important that the face-to-face interview is not rushed and provides sufficient time to build trust so that the donor candidate feels able to answer the evaluator's questions openly. Although timeline to complete the evaluation can sometimes be short, especially for donors who are related (either biologically or emotionally) to their recipient related donors, due to the urgency of the transplant candidate's medical condition, time pressures may be less severe or are minimal with many types of unrelated donors, particularly anonymous nondirected donors.

Second, the evaluator must inform donor candidates about the purpose of the evaluation and that it is one of the components considered in the selection of living donors. Although selection may be a primary goal, the prospective donor should also be told that the evaluation may help to identify areas for which intervention may address and remove potential barriers to donation. For example, if a prospective donor has significant psychiatric symptomatology, treatment of the symptoms may lead to their resolution and the individual could then be reconsidered as a donor candidate. Thus, it is important for the evaluator to bear in mind—and explain to the donor candidate—that the evaluation is not only a "veto" tool but an assessment that could lead to treatment recommendations to improve the likelihood that the individual will be found to be a suitable donor.

Third, it is optimal to conduct the evaluation interview in private. Neither the transplant candidate nor other family members or friends and associate of the prospective donor should be present. Although it can sometimes be helpful to corroborate some information with other family members, friends, etc. [23, 27, 29, 31], the interview must provide an opportunity for the prospective donor to speak freely without concern about others' reactions. In addition, the evaluator must ensure that the donor candidate is able to fully participate in the interview, without language barriers. If an interpreter is needed, the interpreter should have no personal connection to the prospective donor in order to avoid potential influence or bias (conscious or otherwise) during the interpretation process.

Despite efforts to facilitate trust and rapport, the evaluator must keep in mind that donor candidates may not answer all questions truthfully or may withhold relevant information. Often, it is not their intent to mislead. Most people want to "put their best foot forward." This effort at self-presentation occurs in most first-time social interactions. In addition, prospective donors may attempt to state what they think the evaluator wants to hear or what they hope will enable them to be approved as donors [16, 19, 22, 24]. Efforts at self-presentation may be heightened if donor candidates feel pressured to consider donation by other people or by circumstances (including but not limited to the transplant candidate's medical urgency). Hence, questioning about motives for wanting to donate—asked in a nonconfrontational manner that does not imply that certain answers are best—becomes critical for helping to ascertain that prospective donors have freely chosen to consider donation.

Finally, if the psychosocial evaluation is completed but the donation surgery is unable to be scheduled (because, for example, the transplant candidate develops other medical problems precluding immediate transplantation), the evaluator may need to repeat the psychosocial evaluation interview closer to the time at which donation may be likely to occur. A repeat evaluation may also be required should the evaluator recommend that the donor candidate complete any needed interventions, as we discuss further below.

Use of Checklists as Adjuncts when Conducting or Summarizing the Evaluation

There are no regulations or policy in the United States or elsewhere regarding the specific structure or ordering of questioning within the psychosocial evaluation interview. This is appropriate given the evaluator's need to adjust the depth of focus depending on issues that may need greater or lesser attention [2, 4, 29, 32]. However, it can be of great benefit for evaluators to employ one of several tools available to help ensure that they (a) cover all of the domains in Table 11.1), (b) record notes systematically, and (c) prepare a summary of the evaluation to provide to the living donor transplantation team. Three such checklists or templates to be used by evaluators are the Live Donor Assessment Tool (LDAT) [28], a tool developed by Leo et al. [29], and a checklist of questions proposed by Fisher [27]. The LDAT and the Leo et al. measures focus on evaluator ratings of donors' strengths and liabilities across areas of the evaluation. Of the three tools, the LDAT has received more extensive testing and it has been found to be reliable across evaluators [37, 38].

It is noteworthy that the LDAT and the Leo et al. and Fisher strategies are designed to assist the evaluator—they are not completed by patients. The evaluator might also consider administering self-report questionnaires to donor candidates to assess areas such as motivation to donate, social supports, coping styles, and psychological symptomatology. For example, Rodrigue et al. [39] and Wirken et al. [40] provide examples of two brief self-report measures that could be used immediately before the evaluation interview to assess prospective donors' expectations, motives for donating, and perceptions of donation. In addition, Massey et al. propose use of the ELPAT Psychosocial Assessment Tool (EPAT) [30], a very lengthy package of many self-report measures that they suggest should be included as part of the interview. However, given that survey tools and their psychometrics are under continuous development, plus time constraints that may preclude the use of the EPAT battery, we believe the choice of whether and which such questionnaires should be administered should be left to the evaluator.

Communication with the Living Donor Transplantation Team About Psychosocial Evaluation Findings

The evaluator should prepare a written report to be entered into the donor candidate's medical record, as well as attend meetings in which donor selection decisions are made [23]. The impact of a clearly written summary cannot be overestimated. It is the starting point for discussions regarding whether, from a psychosocial perspective, the prospective donor should proceed with donation. It also provides a key opportunity to delineate any recommendations concerning additional psychosocial assessments or interventions that a donor candidate is deemed to need before a decision is made regarding the possibility of donating. Attendance at donor selection meetings provides opportunities for the evaluator not only to present his/her perspective but to address any concerns that team members may raise and reach consensus on whether additional psychosocial assessments or interventions are warranted.

Referral for Additional Assessments or for Psychosocial Treatments or Interventions

Should the evaluator have concerns about donor candidates' capacity to engage in informed decision-making and consent, or if areas are identified that either require more in-depth evaluation (e.g., determination of the presence of psychiatric disorders including substance use disorders) or require treatment before donation can safely proceed (e.g., mental health treatment), the evaluator should refer these individuals for additional care. In some cases, prospective donors may already be receiving care for such issues. No matter whether new assessments and care are required, or ongoing care is already in place, it is important that the evaluator review any additional assessments and information on the outcomes of treatment before making recommendations to the living donor transplantation program about the prospective donor. If the prospective donor required new or additional treatment, the evaluator should specify what criteria must be met for treatment to be considered successful and sufficient. The evaluator may also wish to reevaluate the donor candidate after any assessments or treatments have been completed.

Communication with the Prospective Donor After Team Decisions Are Made About Donor Candidacy

Although the psychosocial evaluator is not generally the living donor program member who communicates candidacy decisions to the donor candidate, the evaluator may be called upon to make recommendations for further care or education. This may be particularly likely should a prospective donor be informed that they cannot be accepted as a donor by the program. Individuals declined for donation may experience disappointment, elevated psychological distress and a feeling of a loss of purpose in life in the wake of being turned down [41], and they may experience anticipatory grief should the transplant candidate be unlikely to survive until another living donor or a deceased donor is identified. The ILDA and the living donor coordinator are also likely to be in contact with prospective donors who are turned down. Alone or in consultation with these team members, the psychosocial evaluator should provide the individual with recommendations for local care providers or for other support resources to cope with issues surrounding their reaction to being turned down [10, 42].

The psychosocial evaluator may also be called upon to provide options for counseling or other resources to individuals approved as donors but whose transplant candidate does not survive to transplantation or who succumbs after transplantation. Although the living donor transplantation program may offer some resources such as support groups for such individuals, it is likely that these donors would also benefit from recommendations for local care providers and resources.

Finally, for individuals whom the team approves as donors, the evaluator should support and advocate for a "cooling off" period, in which these individuals are given some time to reconsider the decision to donate [16, 19, 22, 25]. This period is particularly critical for donor candidates who may have lingering concerns or hesitation about proceeding with donation, despite informing the team that they are willing to donate. There is some evidence that the use of motivational interviewing with donor candidates before donation can lessen such ambivalence and thereby improve postdonation psychosocial outcomes [43]. Whether or not such an intervention is offered, the evaluator and the ILDA should be available to donor candidates after they are approved to donate, so that any remaining questions relevant to psychosocial aspects of the donation process can be addressed.

Postdonation Psychosocial Care and HRQOL Outcomes

Psychosocial Care

There is consensus in the transplantation community that donors require lifelong follow-up care in order to maximize their health and well-being and to provide timely identification of any adverse effects of donation [1–4, 6, 8–12]. Face-to-face follow-up care is often provided by the living donor transplantation program during the first year after donation. Donors may be contacted by the donor program by telephone rather than through face-to-face visits and/or may be referred back to their primary care physician for follow-up care. Postdonation follow-up includes a medical evaluation, and donors are also typically questioned about psychosocial well-being, including, for example, resumption of social roles (e.g., return to work).

Although recommendations for the content of the medical component of follow-up evaluations are available [10], there has been limited consideration of the psychosocial areas that should be addressed [10, 15]. It is important to assess or at least screen for clinically significant psychiatric distress [32, 44], and brief screeners for both depression and anxiety are readily available [45, 46]. Among donors who have had contact with their recipients or recipients' families, this type of screening takes on added importance if the recipients have had medical complications, graft failure, or have not survived. However, even donors not faced with poor recipient outcomes may experience emotional distress postdonation, as we discuss later in this chapter, and thus should receive ongoing screening as well. Whether such distress was definitively caused by donation or by recipient outcomes is often unclear. However, this does not preclude the need to offer appropriate care to donors. This is especially important for donors who had received mental health interventions before donation and had been well-stabilized: it is important that they continue such care (e.g., pharmacotherapy, psychotherapy, or a combination of both) after donation [47].

Beyond psychiatric distress, it has been suggested that brief measures that consider multiple domains of HRQOL (e.g., physical functioning, pain, emotional functioning, social relationships, global perceptions of well-being) should also be administered as a routine part of follow-up care [10, 15, 48]. Such measures should be used both for monitoring and for the identification of donors who may be at risk for future psychosocial difficulties [48]. Impaired HRQOL observed during routine postdonation psychosocial screening should, as for psychiatric distress, lead to appropriate referrals for interventions or resources to assist donors. The individual who conducted the psychosocial evaluation before donation should be consulted regarding referral options for both HRQOL issues and psychosocial concerns more generally (including psychiatric distress); this evaluator may also be asked to see the donor at a follow-up visit to further evaluate postdonation psychosocial needs [23].

Follow-up care of living donors is entwined with the systematic collection and reporting of follow-up data. Follow-up data collection is essential because it can lead to (a) better understanding the risks of donation and (b) improved education and informed consent for future living donors [11, 12, 47, 49, 50]. To work toward these goals, living kidney (and liver) donor transplantation programs in the United States are required to submit to the OPTN follow-up information about living donor medical and psychosocial status at regular intervals through 2 years postdonation [51]. Notably, donor programs' data submissions must be complete and without missing data fields for a majority of their donors (i.e., donors must be assessed and cannot simply be noted as not located or contacted). The data elements that must be submitted include some psychosocial information (physical functional status, work status, perceived pain, loss of insurance due to donation), but do not address important areas such as depression and anxiety symptoms or impaired global HRQOL.

In addition to the collection of data from living donors, Kasiske et al. [50] emphasize that there is good reason to institute the reporting of follow-up information on individuals who do not donate, either because they were judged not to be medically and psychosocially suitable to donate, or because they decided not to donate, the transplant candidate did not survive, or the candidate received a deceased donor organ or an organ from another living donor. Among these nondonors, individuals who were judged suitable to donate but did not do so for other reasons constitute a particularly important potential comparison group for research attempting to determine which medical and psychosocial donor outcomes are attributable to donation. In the United States, the Scientific Registry of Transplant Recipients (SRTR) has established the Living Donor Collective, an effort to create a national registry that includes both donors and donor candidates who did not donate, and to collect not only annual medical but psychosocial information prospectively for the lifetimes of these individuals [50]. Notably, the project intends to assess HRQOL domains including physical functional status, mental health, role impairments, and global well-being.

Psychosocial and HRQOL Outcomes

The careful and extensive evaluation process for the selection of living donors helps to ensure that donors do not have physical, psychological, or social liabilities that would cause them to be at heightened risk for adverse medical or psychosocial outcomes after donation. Given this, plus donors' generally high levels of motivation and desire to donate, it is not surprising that the vast majority of kidney donors (exceeding 90–95% in most studies) do not regret having donated, would donate again if that were possible, and experience deep gratification at having donated [16, 52, 53]. A qualitative literature dating back five decades has provided powerful evidence of the many layers of personal meaning and significance that living donors assign to the donation experience [54–56]. In addition, quantitative studies show that both pre- and postdonation (after the initial perioperative period), kidney donors' HRQOL is, on average, very high and generally exceeds that of the general population across all assessed domains [16, 17, 49, 52, 57–59]. In fact, this would be expected, given the careful selection of living donor candidates.

However, beyond average levels of HRQOL, it is also noteworthy that some donors report specific difficulties and impaired HRQOL. It is important to understand how common such negative outcomes are and whether donors at risk for such outcomes could be proactively identified in order to offer protective interventions. In the sections below, we summarize the two relevant literatures on these concerns: qualitative studies that ask donors in an open-ended manner about the consequences of donation, and quantitative reports using structured assessments to determine rates and risk factors for psychosocial difficulties experienced by donors.

Qualitative Research

A large and still growing qualitative literature describes both short- and longer-term psychosocial consequences of kidney donation for the donor, including impact on their HRQOL. This literature is valuable for at least two reasons. First, it documents donors' experiences in their own words, embodying the perspective that donors—rather than the researchers—are the experts on their psychosocial outcomes [60]. Second, qualitative research can suggest possible risk factors for adverse donation experiences that may have previously been overlooked.

Three systematic reviews—two focused on kidney donors and one considering multiple types of living donors—have summarized much of the published evidence [35, 56, 61]. (A fourth review concerned donors for pediatric transplantation but focused on liver donors and did not report the qualitative data in detail [62].) The three reviews converge in numerous respects, and some dominant themes that emerged have been consistently noted in the living donor literature for the past 50 years and continue to appear in qualitative research published even after these reviews. One of these themes pertains to the donation as a life-changing event, giving donors a new appreciation of life and leading to personal growth and an enhanced sense of self-worth. Kidney donor statements illustrative of this theme include:

- *"It was the best thing I have done in my life. I feel proud of myself."* [63]

- *"In every way I am better. For realizing how far I could go for others. I am up a notch in life...I value things more, big and small things."* [54]

- *"For me, being a donor means personal growth. Being a donor makes me so proud. Maybe one becomes less selfish and focuses bit more on others. I hope so!"* [64].

Another theme is a heightened sense of connection with the recipient (whether or not the donor had met this person), as well as with other people.

- *"In a way, we are closer now."* [64]

- *"It's just like a brotherhood."* [65]

- *"I suppose we've got closer in a sense, where we communicate much more than we would've in the past. It has been generalised to other things [than the transplant]."* [66]

- *"In all...the relationships I have, have been made better by this experience. I think...it [the reason] was me because people talk to me differently, people spoke to me more emotionally and more honestly because of the experience...it was like it was inviting them in and I think once you've done that it's continuous, the benefit just continues to grow."* [65].

Unfortunately, an equally recurrent theme over many decades pertains to donors' feelings of abandonment by the living donor transplant program after donation—what has been called "medical dismissiveness" [67].

- *"I felt neglected after the operation was over. My brother got all the publicity and I was left on my own."* [68]

- *"I felt very much like a spare part... and not like a real patient."* [69]

- *"I have to remind the hospital to call me up for my medical follow-up...They confirmed that I could have my medical follow-up at the transplant centre, but after discharge they never contacted me."* [70]

Also consistent across the reviews are themes related to physical, psychological, and social HRQOL-related costs of donation. For example, donors may experience the physical impact of the surgery to be considerably greater than what they expected, with consequent unanticipated limitations to their ability to resume daily activities.

- *"The transplant coordinators beforehand are busy telling you how many people are walking around after a few days and bounce back. And you kind of have this impression that, not that it's easy, but that most people recover quickly. I don't know that that's true for everyone. [71]*

- *"I don't regret it. But I'm not fine. I'm not 100%. It's a frustrating position to be in because I don't fit what the ranges are…I definitely felt there was an expectation that I wouldn't have any needs past 6 weeks. It was a magical number." [72]*

Emotional costs of donation typically described include, for example, worries about future health, feelings of sadness or depression, and—if the recipient was doing poorly—guilt.

- *"Well, one of my concerns was…the risk of losing my kidney and going on dialysis myself." [73]*

- *"Afterward…about five months…I just felt different…I just didn't feel right. Like I'd be…wanting to cry all the time when I don't cry and…stuff like that, and then I thought, 'Oh maybe the whole experience…I've come down off this big high, and now it's just hitting me…booff!' You know, "This is what you've done'…I don't know if it's a psychological thing after an operation that you go through." [74]*

- *"The fact that [the recipient's] kidney disease recurred after the transplantation is quite tough for me. Life is tough, you know! I returned to work too early…It was quite a busy period at work, and in the middle of the summer I felt entirely empty. I was depressed, had no energy and felt wholly out of it." [70].*

Social costs include impacts on role responsibilities and relationships, employability, and concerns over financial issues.

- *"It's hard being a donor and a carer and a mother." [74]*

- *"I was actually fired for the amount of time that I was about to take off…apart from the actual firing itself, I found it very hard after the recovery of about 2 months to get another job. People just didn't want to look at me." [72]*

- *"…There needs to be more, post-op, operation medical coverage, you know, whatever, for the person going through, who's donated. Because, you know, I had to pay $100 to see the emergency doctor, because I didn't have my own doctor at the time, which is a bit stupid, but…that certainly took a toll." [75]*

Donors may also experience what Tong et al. [35] have referred to as "proprietorial concern" regarding the donation, that is, worries regarding the status of the transplanted kidney, whether recipients were taking care of it, and general worries about the recipient's health.

- *"I knew [the rejection episode] was not my fault but I still felt emotionally anxious and semi-responsible."* [76]

- *"When you see the recipient not doing...the right thing, it's hard being a donor...it's real hard when you see the recipient abusing [the kidney]."* [74]

Interestingly, Kisch et al. [56], who included not only kidney donors but donors of other organs and hematopoietic stem cells, found that these types of themes transcended the specific type of donation. They did identify some differences in themes between donors who had some relationship to their recipient (even if they were only casually acquainted) versus those who donated anonymously. However, these differences largely pertained to predonation factors (e.g., motives for donation) rather than postdonation outcomes. Postdonation costs and benefits were described similarly, even concerning areas such as perceived closeness with the recipient. For example, both related and anonymous, nondirected donors described unique and strengthened ties to their recipients, even though, for nondirected donors, the feelings of connection were not necessarily manifested in a tangible relationship.

One suggestion made based on the qualitative literature is that kidney donor reactions and outcomes after donation might be improved by increasing efforts to help ensure that donor candidates have realistic expectations about potential effects on their physical, psychological, and social functioning [35]. However, modification of expectations, by itself, is not likely to be sufficient: strategies are also needed to lower the risk of negative donor psychosocial outcomes themselves. For example, the negative potential financial impact of donation is a well-recognized problem across multiple countries and healthcare systems [17, 53, 77–80] and it cannot, and should not, be addressed only by changing donor expectations. The qualitative body of research also supports the need for postdonation care strategies, including the use of screening tools—as we have discussed above—to identify donors who are experiencing difficulties so that timely referrals and interventions can be offered. In addition, donors themselves, who are obviously key stakeholders in the donation process, should be consulted regarding what outcomes are most important and relevant to them [81]. In fact, Hanson et al. [72] have initiated such work with donors from Australia and Canada. They found that donors perceived the most important outcome domain to be donors' own kidney health, followed by recovery time and surgical complications; relationships with family and with the recipient; life satisfaction; and lifestyle restrictions.

Quantitative Research

Descriptive Findings A recent systematic review and meta-analysis examined a portion of the very large quantitative literature on kidney donor psychosocial outcomes, with a focus on studies examining the course of physical functioning, psychological status, and social activity limitations from before to after donation (generally through the first year after the surgery) [58]. Results indicated that, by 3 months postdonation, HRQOL in all three domains had returned to baseline (predonation) levels, except for some evidence of slight elevations in fatigue. However, the authors could document no differences between donors and general population norms for fatigue, suggesting that, after the initial recovery from surgery, donors should expect no marked negative impact on their well-being.

There has been increasing interest in longer-term (i.e., beyond the first 1–3 years) postdonation outcomes [17, 57]. Thus, a growing number of reports have conducted follow-up assessments of kidney donors' HRQOL [59, 82–90]. Donors in these studies range from an average of 5–17 years postdonation, with some donors having donated as many as 48 years earlier. For example, the multicenter Renal and Lung Living Donors Evaluation (RELIVE) Study in the United States reported that kidney donors' average level of satisfaction with life was similar to or better than that of other community-based samples [91], and their average level of depressive symptoms was very low [92]. Results from RELIVE [59] as well as six other such studies published in the last 10 years [82–84, 86, 88, 90] are shown in Fig. 11.1, which depicts each study's findings on donors' average physical composite summary score and mental composite summary score from the SF-36, a widely used generic (non-donation-specific) HRQOL measure. The figure shows that in virtually all studies,

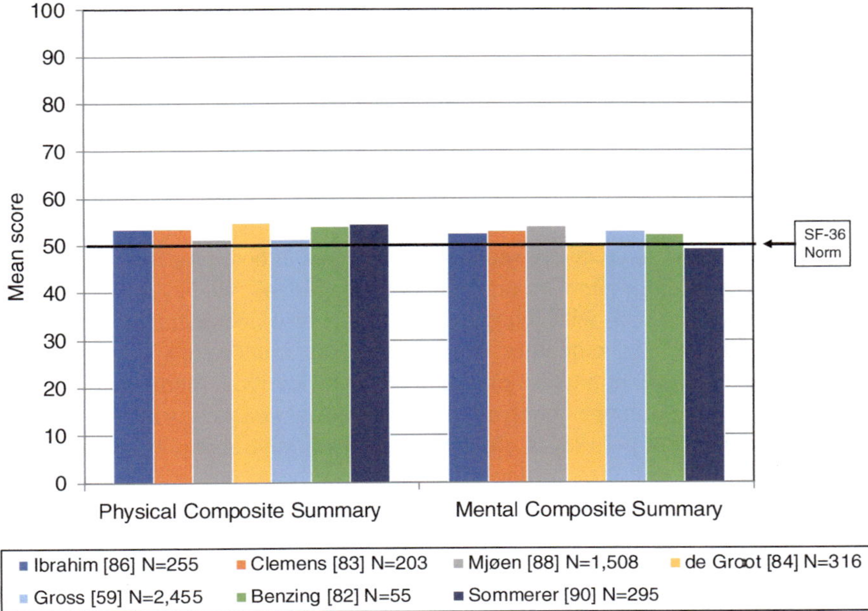

Fig. 11.1 Mean SF-36 composite summary scores across seven studies examining long-term health-related quality of life in kidney donors. Studies shown in temporal order of publication, from 2009 to 2015. Numbers in brackets in figure legend refer to reference numbers

donors' average HRQOL scores were at or above the community-based normative level (a score of 50). One report [83] additionally compared donors to a healthy nondonor cohort and found no differences in HRQOL levels. The SF-36 also yields eight subscales (which are combined to yield the composite scores in Fig. 11.1). Similar to the data in Fig. 11.1, the studies reporting on the subscales show that donors are similar to or exceed normative levels on physical functioning, pain, vitality, general health perceptions, mental health, role functioning in relation to physical functioning, role functioning in relation to emotional status, and social functioning [59, 82–85, 87–90]. In a few studies examining levels of fatigue in the long term after donation, average fatigue levels are generally similar to normative data [84, 90], and some longitudinal evidence suggests that any elevations compared to predonation levels slowly resolve over time after donation [87].

The evidence discussed above focuses average values computed across all donors in a given study. Such a focus may obscure equally important evidence that at least some donors experience physical functional difficulties and emotional distress [18, 47, 49, 52]. For example, up to one-third of donors describe their health to be fair to poor or substantially worse than predonation; they show clinically significant impairments in physical functional HRQOL and—despite improvements over time for most donors—fatigue appears to be an enduring problem for some individuals [47, 49, 52, 93]. In the RELIVE Study, for example, from 14% to 20% of donors showed impairments on the physical functional-related subscales of the SF-36 [59]. In addition, across studies, one-quarter or more of donors have been found to have clinically significant psychological distress [47, 49, 52]. The frequency of depression has been variably reported as approximately 10–16% within the first 2–5 years postdonation [44, 94], with point prevalence estimates of 4–20% [92, 95, 96]. Point prevalence for anxiety has ranged from 5% to 67% [95–97]. It is often difficult to conclude that such HRQOL indicators are necessarily related to donation, given the cross-sectional nature of much of the research in this area and the absence of comparison groups. However, findings that these types of outcomes are experienced by sizable proportions of donors are at least suggestive of important areas that should be considered in both preparing individuals to donate and providing follow-up care after donation [18, 47, 49, 52, 98].

Survey-based research with living kidney donors also documents donor reports of adverse psychosocial outcomes that appear more immediately attributable to donation. For example, donors endorse enduring worries about their health because of the donation, body image concerns, and donation-related strains in relationships with family members [47, 93]. Consistent with qualitative research, the RELIVE Study documented that 20% of donors felt that healthcare professionals were not supportive after the donation surgery and 9% felt that they were ignored after surgery [53]. The negative financial repercussions experienced by at least one-quarter to one-third of donors (including unreimbursed costs, loss of income due to time off from work, and problems obtaining or keeping health, life, or disability insurance) have received increasing attention and are among the major psychosocial risks linked to kidney donation [53, 77–80, 99]. One daunting finding was that kidney donors' out-of-pocket expenses were estimated to be greater than 1 month's income for 76% of donors [100]. It is encouraging that, in the United States, the Department of Health and Human Services has launched a new initiative that seeks to address financial burdens on living donors [101].

Prediction of Poor Donor Psychosocial and HRQOL Outcomes It has been surprisingly difficult to identify reliable risk factors for poor psychosocial and HRQOL outcomes after kidney donation. There are marked inconsistencies in findings across studies [16, 43, 49, 52, 58], perhaps because many studies utilize cross-sectional/retrospective designs (so that the direction of prediction is unclear), and do not include healthy nondonor comparison groups. In their systematic review, Wirken et al. [58] examined nine studies on putative risk factor-psychosocial outcome linkages among living donors. Overall, they found little to no evidence that factors related to donors' predonation physical health status (e.g., body mass index, renal function, other comorbidities, tobacco use), demographics (e.g., age, sex), or factors related to the recipient (e.g., type of donor relationship to the recipient, recipient complications) predicted either physical functional or emotional HRQOL outcomes. Wirken et al. stated that poor psychological functioning before donation was "the most consistent predictor" but the studies were almost evenly split in terms of whether this factor did or did not predict outcomes (three studies found such effects while two did not; the remaining four studies did not examine this factor). However, it is noteworthy that Rodrigue et al. [93] also found that mental health before donation predicted postdonation mental health in a recent multisite study, and it is well-known that mental health history is always a strong predictor of future mental health in epidemiologic studies of community samples. Moreover, although Wirken et al. found that only three of the nine studies examined recipient complications as a potential risk factor, two of the three found that such complications increased risk for psychological (but not physical) limitations in donor HRQOL.

This last finding is noteworthy because it speaks to a clinical concern that living donors may not only be devastated in the aftermath of poor recipient outcomes but may never recover. However, while living donors are indeed deeply affected by poor recipient outcomes, including recipient death [16, 35, 36, 70, 102], they also consistently note that they take comfort in having done all they could for the recipient. Moreover, the experience of grief in the aftermath of a recipient's death does not necessarily imply that a donor will meet criteria for psychiatric disorder. In short, it is natural to experience grief—even very profound grief—after loss of the recipient. Yet most individuals, including living donors, appear to recover and do not appear to show HRQOL decrements when assessed years afterwards [16, 102, 103]. In fact, recipient graft loss without death may have more enduring impact than recipient death, possibly because donors experience an ongoing grieving process with uncertainty about the ultimate endpoint [103]. Overall, no matter what the nature of recipient adverse outcomes, and whether or not most donors' HRQOL would be expected to eventually return to normal levels, living donor transplantation programs should reach out to donors in the wake of such events in order to provide any resources or referrals that these individuals might need in order to facilitate their adaptation and the recovery process.

Another factor that has raised clinical concerns in terms of its potential for impact on donor psychosocial outcomes is whether and how closely donors are related to their recipients [19]. For example, donors with close relationships with their recipients would be able to observe the benefits of the transplantation, in comparison to donors who have little connection or no connection to the recipient (nondirected donors). At the same time, related donors may be more adversely affected by poor recipient outcomes. Alternatively, because unrelated donors may have little to no opportunity to observe how their recipients have benefitted from transplantation, unrelated donors may feel even more devastated at learning, for example, of the recipient's death because this might be the only information they have about post-transplant outcomes. The empirical literature, however, generally provides little indication that donor outcomes vary by type of relationship to the recipient [49]. For example, Rodrigue et al. compared related kidney donors to anonymous donors (including nondirected and directed donors) [104] and found no differences in donor perceptions of general HRQOL; psychological benefits and satisfaction with having donated; and health or financial consequences of donation. Other reports have obtained similar findings [105, 106]. However, anonymous donors may be more likely than other donors to experience and be distressed by others' negative reactions concerning their decision to donate, and they may not have the financial supports that related donors have [104–107]. Additionally, small reports of kidney exchange donor participants found no evidence that their psychosocial outcomes differed from that of other types of donors or that such donors needed additional psychosocial services or practical or emotional support after donation [108, 109]. One study did find differences across related versus unrelated donors: Lentine et al. [108] observed that recipient death and death-censored graft failure were associated with over twice the relative risk of a subsequent depressive disorder diagnosis in unrelated donors, while there was no evidence of such associations in biologically or emotionally related donors [44].

Lastly, the empirical literature suggests that if living donor candidates have unresolved ambivalence about donation, they are at increased risk for poor psychosocial outcomes [16, 43, 52]. This type of ambivalence refers to lingering feelings of hesitation and uncertainty that remain even shortly before donation, and is distinct from feelings of indecision so great that an individual would be excluded as a donor [43]. Lingering ambivalence is relatively common in donor candidates [16, 43]. A small study suggested that a predonation intervention to reduce ambivalence in kidney donor and liver donor candidates resulted in fewer physical symptoms, lower rates of fatigue and pain, shorter recovery time, fewer unexpected medical problems, less anxiety and fewer family-related problems in the first 3 months postdonation [43]. There was no impact on depression levels, feelings about donation or family relationship quality. These results suggest that other predonation preventive interventions targeting risk factors for poor psychosocial outcomes should be developed and tested. For example, given that predonation mental health appears to be a potent risk factor for postdonation psychosocial outcomes, predonation interventions to optimize emotional well-being—tailored to the specific context of living donation—could be empirically evaluated for efficacy and potential for use in routine clinical care.

Conclusion

The psychosocial evaluation process for prospective living donors is the starting point for living donor transplantation programs to ensure that donor psychosocial and HRQOL outcomes postdonation are as favorable as possible. The content of the evaluation is necessarily comprehensive and, as such, provides information critical not only for selection of donors but for the identification of risk factors requiring intervention before donation and for addressing donors' needs postdonation. Although extensive research shows that donors, on average, have very favorable outcomes in terms of physical functional, emotional, and social functioning aspects of HRQOL, some donors experience HRQOL difficulties as well as other psychosocial problems, including significant financial burdens related to donation. The nature of these problems reinforces the importance of key components of the evaluation, including the assessment of expectations, understanding, and decision-making about donation; emotional preparation for donation and risk factors related to mental health history; and donor candidates' practical preparations in terms of such factors as available social supports during their postsurgical recovery and planning for possible short- and long-term financial burdens.

Research documenting the prevalence of adverse HRQOL and psychosocial outcomes is important for reasons beyond informing the content of the psychosocial evaluation. Empirical evidence on outcomes can help to refine the education provided to potential donors, anticipate their postdonation care needs, and facilitate the timely provision of interventions to avert or remediate postdonation psychosocial problems. However, we have noted that research on donor outcomes to date has been limited due to lack of appropriate nondonor comparison groups and the cross-sectional (as opposed to prospective) design of much of the work in this area. In this regard, the registry under development by the SRTR Living Donor Collective has considerable potential to provide a more accurate and complete understanding of whether and how the donation experience affects donor well-being. But beyond collecting quantitative evidence, we also must listen to what donors themselves have to say: qualitative research that allows donor voices to be heard and that identifies outcomes that matter most to donors is equally important in advancing our understanding. Such work is essential for further refining the evaluation process, the care that is provided to prospective and actual donors, and the research questions that are addressed in the future.

References

1. Abecassis M, Adams M, Adams P, Arnold RM, Atkins CR, Barr ML, et al. Consensus statement on the live organ donor. JAMA. 2000;284(22):2919–26. https://doi.org/10.1001/jama.284.22.2919.
2. Adams PL, Cohen D, Danovitch G, Edington RM, Gaston RS, Jacobs CL, et al. The nondirected live-kidney donor: ethical considerations and practice guidelines: a national conference report. Transplantation. 2002;74:582–9. https://doi.org/10.1097/00007890-200208270-00030.

3. Barr ML, Belghiti J, Villamil FG, Pomfret EA, Sutherland DS, Gruessner RW, et al. A report of the Vancouver Forum on the care of the live organ donor: lung, liver, pancreas, and intestine data and medical guidelines. Transplantation. 2006;81(10):1373–85. https://doi.org/10.1097/01.tp.0000216825.56841.cd.

4. Canadian Council for Donation and Transplantation. Enhancing living donation: a Canadian forum. Edmonton, AB: The Council; 2006.

5. Department of Health and Human Services (HHS), Centers for Medicare & Medicaid Services (CMS). 42 CFR Parts 405, 482, 488, and 498 Medicare Program; Hospital Conditions of Participation: Requirements for Approval and Re-Approval of Transplant Centers to Perform Organ Transplants; Final Rule. Available at: https://www.cms.gov/Medicare/Provider-Enrollment-and-Certification/GuidanceforLawsAndRegulations/Downloads/TransplantFinalLawandReg.pdf. Accessed: 7 Sept 2020.

6. Delmonico F, Council of the Transplantation Society. A report of the Amsterdam Forum on the care of the live kidney donor: data and medical guidelines. Transplantation. 2005;79(6 Suppl):S53–66. https://pubmed.ncbi.nlm.nih.gov/15785361/.

7. Dew MA, Jacobs CL, Jowsey SG, Hanto R, Miller C, Delmonico FL, et al. Guidelines for the psychosocial evaluation of living unrelated kidney donors in the United States. Am J Transplant. 2007;7(5):1047–54. https://doi.org/10.1111/j.1600-6143.2007.01751.x.

8. Ethics Committee of the Transplantation Society. The consensus statement of the Amsterdam Forum on the care of the live kidney donor. Transplantation. 2004;78(4):491–2. https://doi.org/10.1097/01.tp.0000136654.85459.1e.

9. Kanellis J, CARI (Caring for Australasians with Renal Impairment) Group. The CARI guidelines: justification of living donor kidney transplantation. Nephrology. 2010;15(Suppl 1):S72–9. https://doi.org/10.1111/j.1440-1797.2009.01212.x.

10. Kidney Disease: Improving Global Outcomes (KDIGO) Living Kidney Donor Work Group. KDIGO clinical practice guideline on the evaluation and care of living kidney donors. Transplantation. 2017;101(Suppl 8S):S1–109. https://kdigo.org/wp-content/uploads/2017/07/2017-KDIGO-LD-GL.pdf.

11. LaPointe Rudow D, Hays R, Baliga P, Cohen DJ, Cooper M, Danovitch GM, et al. Consensus conference on best practices in live kidney donation: recommendations to optimize education, access, and care. Am J Transplant. 2015;15(4):914–22. https://doi.org/10.1111/ajt.13173.

12. Living Kidney Donor Follow-Up Conference Writing Group, Leichtman A, Abecassis M, Barr M, Charlton M, Cohen D, et al. Living kidney donor follow-up: state-of-the-art and future directions, conference summary and recommendations. Am J Transplant. 2011;11(12):2561–8. https://doi.org/10.1111/j.1600-6143.2011.03816.x.

13. Organ Procurement and Transplantation Network (OPTN) / United Network for Organ Sharing (UNOS). Policy 14: Living Donation. Available at: https://optn.transplant.hrsa.gov/governance/policies/. Accessed: 7 Sept 2020.

14. Lentine KL, Segev DL. Understanding and communicating medical risks for living kidney donors: a matter of perspective. J Am Soc Nephrol. 2017;28(1):12–24. https://doi.org/10.1681/ASN.2016050571.

15. Tong A, Chapman JR, Wong G, de Bruijn J, Craig JC. Screening and follow-up of living kidney donors: a systematic review of clinical practice guidelines. Transplantation. 2011;92:962–72. https://doi.org/10.1097/TP.0b013e3182328276.

16. Dew MA, Switzer GE, DiMartini AF, Myaskovsky L, Crowley-Matoka M. Psychosocial aspects of living organ donation. In: Tan HP, Marcos A, Shapiro R, editors. Living donor organ transplantation. New York: Taylor and Francis; 2007. p. 7–26.

17. Matas AJ, Hays RE, Ibrahim HN. Long-term non-end-stage renal disease risks after living kidney donation. Am J Transplant. 2017;17(4):893–900. https://doi.org/10.1111/ajt.14011.

18. Lentine KL, Lam NN, Segev DL. Risks of living kidney donation: current state of knowledge on outcomes important to donors. Clin J Am Soc Nephrol. 2019;14(4):597–608. https://doi.org/10.2215/CJN.11220918.

19. Dew MA, Boneysteele G, DiMartini AF. Unrelated donors. In: Steel JL, editor. Living donor advocacy: an evolving role within transplantation. New York: Springer; 2014. p. 149–67.

20. DiMartini AF, Shenoy A, Dew MA. Organ transplantation. In: Levenson JL, editor. The American Psychiatric Publishing Textbook of psychosomatic medicine and consultation-liaison psychiatry. 3rd ed. Washington, DC: American Psychiatric Publishing, Inc; 2019. p. 859–906.
21. DiMartini AF, Dew MA, Crone C. Organ transplantation. In: Sadock BJ, Sadock VA, Ruiz P, editors. Kaplan and Sadock's Comprehensive textbook of psychiatry. 10th ed. Philadelphia: Wolters Kluwer; 2017. p. 2357–73.
22. Jowsey SG, Schneekloth TD. Psychosocial factors in living organ donation: clinical and ethical challenges. Transplant Rev. 2008;22(3):192–5.
23. LaPointe Rudow D, Swartz K, Phillips C, Hollenberger J, Smith T, Steel JL. The psychosocial and independent living donor advocate evaluation and post-surgery care of living donors. J Clin Psychol Med Settings. 2015;22(2–3):136–49.
24. Olbrisch ME, Benedict SM, Haller DL, Levenson JL. Psychosocial assessment of living organ donors: clinical and ethical considerations. Prog Transplant. 2001;11(1):40–9. https://doi.org/10.1016/j.trre.2008.04.008.
25. Shenoy A. The psychosocial evaluation of live donors. In: Sher Y, Maldonado J, editors. The psychosocial care of end-stage disease and transplant patients. New York: Springer; 2019. p. 49–59.
26. Duerinckx N, Timmerman L, Van Gogh J, van Busschbach J, Ismail SY, Massey EK, et al. Predonation psychosocial evaluation of living kidney and liver donor candidates: a systematic literature review. Transpl Int. 2014;27(1):2–18. https://doi.org/10.1111/tri.12154.
27. Fisher MS Sr. Psychosocial evaluation interview protocol for living related and living unrelated kidney donors. Soc Work Health Care. 2003;38(1):39–61. https://doi.org/10.1300/j010v38n01_03.
28. Iacoviello BM, Shenoy A, Braoude J, Jennings T, Vaidya S, Brouwer J, et al. The Live Donor Assessment Tool: a psychosocial assessment tool for live organ donors. Psychosomatics. 2015;56(3):254–61. https://doi.org/10.1016/j.psym.2015.02.001.
29. Leo RL, Smith BA, Mori DL. Guidelines for conducting a psychiatric evaluation of the unrelated kidney donor. Psychosomatics. 2003;44(6):452–60. https://doi.org/10.1176/appi.psy.44.6.452.
30. Massey EK, Timmerman L, Ismail SY, Duerinckx N, Lopes A, Maple H, et al. The ELPAT living organ donor Psychosocial Assessment Tool (EPAT): from 'what' to 'how' of psychosocial screening-a pilot study. Transpl Int. 2018;31(1):56–70. https://doi.org/10.1111/tri.13041.
31. Schroder NM, McDonald LA, Etringer G, Snyders M. Consideration of psychosocial factors in the evaluation of living donors. Prog Transplant. 2008;18:41–9. https://pubmed.ncbi.nlm.nih.gov/18429581/.
32. van Hardeveld E, Tong A, CARI Group. The CARI guidelines: psychosocial care of living kidney donors. Nephrology. 2010;15(suppl 1):S80–7. https://doi.org/10.1111/j.1440-1797.2009.01213.x.
33. Hanson CS, Ralph AF, Manera KE, Gill JS, Kanellis J, Wong G, et al. The lived experience of "being evaluated" for organ donation: focus groups with living kidney donors. Clin J Am Soc Nephrol. 2017;12(11):1852–61. https://doi.org/10.2215/CJN.03550417.
34. Ralph AF, Butow P, Hanson CS, Chadban SJ, Chapman JR, Craig JC, et al. Donor and recipient views on their relationship in living kidney donation: thematic synthesis of qualitative studies. Am J Kidney Dis. 2017;69(5):602–16. https://doi.org/10.1053/j.ajkd.2016.09.017.
35. Tong A, Chapman JR, Wong G, Kanellis J, McCarthy G, Craig JC. The motivations and experiences of living kidney donors: a thematic synthesis. Am J Kidney Dis. 2012;60:15–26. https://doi.org/10.1053/j.ajkd.2011.11.043.
36. Crowley-Matoka M, Siegler M, Cronin DC 2nd. Long-term quality of life issues among adult-to-pediatric living liver donors: a qualitative exploration. Am J Transplant. 2004;4(5):744–50. https://doi.org/10.1111/j.1600-6143.2004.00377.x.
37. Iacoviello BM, Shenoy A, Hunt J, Filipovic-Jewell Z, Haydel B, LaPointe Rudow D. A prospective study of the reliability and validity of the Live Donor Assessment Tool. Psychosomatics. 2017;58(5):519–26. https://doi.org/10.1016/j.psym.2017.03.012.

38. Kook YWA, Shenoy A, Hunt J, Desrosiers F, Gordon-Elliott JS, Jowsey-Gregoire S, et al. Multicenter investigation of the reliability and validity of the Live Donor Assessment Tool as an enhancement to the psychosocial evaluation of living donors. Am J Transplant. 2019;19(4):1119–28. https://doi.org/10.1111/ajt.15170.

39. Rodrigue JR, Guenther R, Kaplan B, Mandelbrot DA, Pavlakis M, Howard RJ. Measuring the expectations of kidney donors: initial psychometric properties of the Living Donation Expectancies Questionnaire. Transplantation. 2008;85(9):1230–4. https://doi.org/10.1097/TP.0b013e31816c5ab0.

40. Wirken L, van Middendorp H, Hooghof CW, Sanders JSF, Dam RE, van der Pant KAMI, et al. Pre-donation cognitions of potential living organ donors: the development of the Donation Cognition Instrument in potential kidney donors. Nephrol Dial Transplant. 2017;32:573–80. https://doi.org/10.1093/ndt/gfw421.

41. Reese PP, Allen MB, Carney C, Leidy D, Levsky S, Pendse R, et al. Outcomes for individuals turned down for living kidney donation. Clin Transpl. 2018;32:e13408. https://doi.org/10.1111/ctr.13408.

42. Allen MB, Abt PL, Reese PP. What are the harms of refusing to allow living kidney donation? An expanded view of risks and benefits. Am J Transplant. 2014;14(3):531–7. https://doi.org/10.1111/ajt.12599.

43. Dew MA, DiMartini AF, DeVito Dabbs AJ, Zuckoff A, Tan HP, McNulty ML, et al. Preventive intervention for living donor psychosocial outcomes: feasibility and efficacy in a randomized controlled trial. Am J Transplant. 2013;13(10):2672–84. https://doi.org/10.1111/ajt.12393.

44. Lentine KL, Schnitzler MA, Xiao H, Axelrod D, Davis CL, McCabe M, et al. Depression diagnoses after living kidney donation: linking U.S. Registry data and administrative claims. Transplantation. 2012;94:77–83. https://doi.org/10.1097/TP.0b013e318253f1bc.

45. National Council for Behavioral Health. Center for Integrated Health Solutions. Screening tools. https://www.integration.samhsa.gov/clinical-practice/screening-tools#anxiety. Accessed: 7 Sept 2020.

46. Rush AJ Jr, First MB, Blacker D, editors. Handbook of psychiatric measures. 2nd ed. Washington, DC: American Psychiatric Association Press; 2008.

47. Tan JC, Gordon EJ, Dew MA, LaPointe Rudow D, Steiner RW, Woodle ES, et al. Living donor kidney transplantation: facilitating education about live kidney donation-recommendations from a consensus conference. Clin J Am Soc Nephrol. 2015;10(9):1670–7. https://doi.org/10.2215/CJN.01030115.

48. Organ Procurement and Transplantation Network (OPTN). Procedures to collect post-donation follow-up data from living donors. Available at: https://optn.transplant.hrsa.gov/resources/guidance/procedures-to-collect-post-donation-follow-up-data-from-living-donors/. Accessed: 7 Sept 2020.

49. Dew MA, Jacobs CL. Psychosocial and socioeconomic issues facing the living kidney donor. Adv Chronic Kidney Dis. 2012;19(4):237–43. https://dx.doi.org/10.1053%2Fj.ackd.2012.04.006.

50. Kasiske BL, Asrani SK, Dew MA, Henderson ML, Henrich C, Humar A, et al. The Living Donor Collective: a scientific registry for living donors. Am J Transplant. 2017;17(12):3040–8. https://doi.org/10.1111/ajt.14365.

51. Organ Procurement and Transplantation Network (OPTN) / United Network for Organ Sharing (UNOS). Policy 18: Data Submission Requirements. Available at: https://optn.transplant.hrsa.gov/governance/policies/. Accessed: 7 Sept 2020.

52. Dew MA, Zuckoff A, DiMartini AF, DeVito Dabbs AJ, McNulty ML, Fox KR, et al. Prevention of poor psychosocial outcomes in living organ donors: from description to theory-driven intervention development and initial feasibility testing. Prog Transplant. 2012;22(3):280–93. https://doi.org/10.1053/j.ackd.2012.04.006.

53. Jacobs CL, Gross CR, Messersmith EE, Hong BA, Gillespie BW, Hill-Callahan P, et al. Emotional and financial experiences of kidney donors over the past 50 years: the RELIVE Study. Clin J Am Soc Nephrol. 2015;10(12):2221–31. https://doi.org/10.2215/CJN.07120714.

54. Fellner CH, Marshall JR. Twelve kidney donors. JAMA. 1968;206(12):2703–7. https://pubmed.ncbi.nlm.nih.gov/4880430/.

55. Simmons RG, Klein SD, Simmons RL. Gift of life: the social and psychological impact of organ transplantation. Brunswick, NJ: Transaction Books; 1987. http://hdl.handle.net/10822/1034762.

56. Kisch AM, Forsberg A, Fridh I, Almgren M, Lundmark M, Lovén C, et al. The meaning of being a living kidney, liver or stem cell donor-a meta-ethnography. Transplantation. 2018;102:744–56. https://doi.org/10.1097/TP.0000000000002073.

57. Slinin Y, Brasure M, Eidman K, Bydash J, Maripuri S, Carlyle M, et al. Long-term outcomes of living kidney donation. Transplantation. 2016;100(6):1371–86. https://doi.org/10.1097/TP.0000000000001252.

58. Wirken L, van Middendorp H, Hooghof CW, Rovers MM, Hoitsma AJ, Hilbrands LB, et al. The course and predictors of health-related quality of life in living kidney donors: a systematic review and meta-analysis. Am J Transplant. 2015;15:3041–54. https://doi.org/10.1111/ajt.13453.

59. Gross CR, Messersmith EE, Hong BA, Jowsey SG, Jacobs C, Gillespie BW, et al. Health-related quality of life in kidney donors from the last five decades: results from the RELIVE study. Am J Transplant. 2013;13:2924–34. https://doi.org/10.1111/ajt.12434.

60. Dew MA, Switzer GE. Listening to living donors. Transplantation. 2018;102(5):718–9. https://doi.org/10.1097/TP.0000000000002074.

61. Ralph AF, Butow P, Hanson CS, Chadban SJ, Chapman JR, Craig JC, et al. Donor and recipient views on their relationship in living kidney donation: thematic synthesis of qualitative studies. Am J Kidney Dis. 2017;69:602–16. https://doi.org/10.1053/j.ajkd.2016.09.017.

62. Thys K, Schwering KL, Siebelink M, Dobbels F, Borry P, Schotsmans P, et al. Psychosocial impact of pediatric living-donor kidney and liver transplantation on recipients, donors, and the family: a systematic review. Transpl Int. 2015;28:270–80. https://doi.org/10.1111/tri.12481.

63. Franklin PM, Crombie AK. Live related renal transplantation: psychological, social, and cultural issues. Transplantation. 2003;76(8):1247–52. https://doi.org/10.1097/01.TP.0000087833.48999.3D.

64. Andersen MH, Mathisen L, Øyen O, Wahl AK, Hanestad BR, Fosse E. Living donors' experiences 1 wk after donating a kidney. Clin Transpl. 2005;19(1):90–6. https://doi.org/10.1111/j.1399-0012.2004.00304.x.

65. Clarke A, Mitchell A, Abraham C. Understanding donation experiences of unspecified (altruistic) kidney donors. Br J Health Psychol. 2014;19(2):393–408. https://doi.org/10.1111/bjhp.12048.

66. Ralph AF, Butow P, Craig JC, Wong G, Chadban SJ, Luxton G, et al. Living kidney donor and recipient perspectives on their relationship: longitudinal semi-structured interviews. BMJ Open. 2019;9(4):e026629. https://doi.org/10.1136/bmjopen-2018-026629.

67. Garcia MC, Chapman JR, Shaw PJ, Gottlieb DJ, Ralph A, Craig JC, et al. Motivations, experiences, and perspectives of bone marrow and peripheral blood stem cell donors: thematic synthesis of qualitative studies. Biol Blood Marrow Transplant. 2013;19(7):1046–58. https://doi.org/10.1016/j.bbmt.2013.04.012.

68. Sharma VK, Enoch MD. Psychological sequelae of kidney donation: a 5-10 year follow up study. Acta Psychiatr Scand. 1987;75(3):264–7. https://doi.org/10.1111/j.1600-0447.1987.tb02787.x.

69. Duffy MA. Intrafamilial kidney transplants: the impact on the sibling relationship among donors, recipients and volunteers. 2009. Available from ProQuest Dissertations & Theses Global-305174960. http://pitt.idm.oclc.org/login?url=https://search-proquest-com.pitt.idm.oclc.org/docview/305174960?accountid=14709. Accessed: 7 Sept 2020.

70. Andersen MH, Bruserud F, Mathisen L, Wahl AK, Hanestad BR, Fosse E. Follow-up interviews of 12 living kidney donors one yr after open donor nephrectomy. Clin Transpl. 2007;21(6):702–9. https://doi.org/10.1111/j.1399-0012.2007.00726.x.

71. Shaw RM. Rethinking elements of informed consent for living kidney donation: findings from a New Zealand study. Health Sociol Rev. 2015;24(1):109–22.
72. Hanson CS, Chapman JR, Gill JS, Kanellis J, Wong G, Craig JC, et al. Identifying outcomes that are important to living kidney donors: a nominal group technique study. Clin J Am Soc Nephol. 2018;13(6):916–26. https://doi.org/10.2215/CJN.13441217.
73. Lunsford SL, Shilling LM, Chavin KD, Martin MS, Miles LG, Norman ML, et al. Racial differences in the living kidney donation experience and implications for education. Prog Transplant. 2007;17(3):234–40.
74. Williams AM, Colefax L, O'Driscoll CT, Dawson S. An exploration of experiences of living renal donors following donation. Nephrol Nurs J. 2009;36(4):423–7. https://pubmed.ncbi.nlm.nih.gov/19715110/.
75. Shaw RM, Bell LJM. 'Because you can't live on love': living kidney donors' perspectives on compensation and payment for organ donation. Health Expect. 2015;18(6):3201–12. https://doi.org/10.1111/hex.12310.
76. Hildebrand L, Melchert TP, Anderson RC. Impression management during evaluation and psychological reactions post-donation of living kidney donors. Clin Transpl. 2014;28(8):855–61. https://doi.org/10.1111/ctr.12390.
77. Tushla L, LaPointe RD, Milton J, Rodrigue JR, Schold JD, Hays RE, et al. Reducing financial barriers to live kidney donation: resources available and policy changes needed to improve access. Clin J Am Soc Nephrol. 2015;10(9):1696–702. https://doi.org/10.2215/CJN.01000115.
78. Barnieh L, Kanellis J, McDonald S, Arnold J, Sontrop JM, Cuerden M, et al. Direct and indirect costs incurred by Australian living kidney donors. Nephrology. 2018;23(12):1145–51. https://doi.org/10.1111/nep.13205.
79. Przech S, Garg AX, Arnold JB, Barnieh L, Cuerden MS, Dipchand C, et al. Financial costs incurred by living kidney donors: a prospective cohort study. J Am Soc Nephrol. 2018;29(12):2847–57. https://doi.org/10.1681/ASN.2018040398.
80. Rodrigue JR, Schold JD, Morrissey P, Whiting J, Vella J, Kayler LK, et al. Direct and indirect costs following living kidney donation: findings from the KDOC study. Am J Transplant. 2016;16(3):869–76. https://doi.org/10.1111/ajt.13591.
81. Hanson CS, Tong A. Outcomes of interest to living kidney donors. Curr Transplant Rep. 2019;6:177–83.
82. Benzing C, Hau HM, Kurtz G, Schmelzle M, Tautenhahn HM, Morgül MH, et al. Long-term health-related quality of life of living kidney donors: a single-center experience. Qual Life Res. 2015;24(12):2833–42. https://doi.org/10.1007/s11136-015-1027-2.
83. Clemens K, Boudville N, Dew MA, Geddes C, Gill JS, Jassal V, et al. The long-term quality of life of living kidney donors: a multicenter cohort study. Am J Transplant. 2011;11(3):463–9. https://doi.org/10.1111/j.1600-6143.2010.03424.x.
84. de Groot IB, Stiggelbout AM, van der Boog PJM, Baranski AG, Marang-van de Mheen PJ, PARTNER-study group. Reduced quality of life in living kidney donors: association with fatigue, societal participation and pre-donation variables. Transpl Int. 2012;25(9):967–75. https://doi.org/10.1111/j.1432-2277.2012.01524.x.
85. Dols LFC, IJzermans JNM, Wentink N, Tran TCK, Zuidema WC, Dooper IM, et al. Long-term follow-up of a randomized trial comparing laparoscopic and mini-incision open live donor nephrectomy. Am J Transplant. 2010;10:2481–7. https://doi.org/10.1111/j.1600-6143.2010.03281.x.
86. Ibrahim HN, Foley R, Tan L, Rogers T, Bailey RF, Guo H, et al. Long-term consequences of kidney donation. N Engl J Med. 2009;360:459–69. https://doi.org/10.1056/NEJMoa0804883.
87. Janki S, Klop KWJ, Dooper IMM, Weimar W, Ijzermans JNM, Kok NFM. More than a decade after live donor nephrectomy: a prospective cohort study. Transpl Int. 2015;28(11):1268–75. https://doi.org/10.1111/tri.12589.
88. Mjøen G, Stavem K, Westlie L, Midtvedt K, Fauchald P, Norby G, et al. Quality of life in kidney donors. Am J Transplant. 2011;11(6):1315–9. https://doi.org/10.1111/j.1600-6143.2011.03517.x.

89. Meyer K, Wahl AK, Bjørk IT, Wisløff T, Hartmann A, Andersen MH. Long-term, self-reported health outcomes in kidney donors. BMC Nephrol. 2016;17:8. https://doi.org/10.1186/s12882-016-0221-y.

90. Sommerer C, Feuerstein D, Dikow R, Rauch G, Hartmann M, Schaier M, et al. Psychosocial and physical outcome following kidney donation-a retrospective analysis. Transpl Int. 2015;28(4):416–28. https://doi.org/10.1111/tri.12509.

91. Messersmith EE, Gross CR, Beil CA, Gillespie BW, Jacobs C, Taler SJ, et al. Satisfaction with life among living kidney donors: a RELIVE Study of long-term donor outcomes. Transplantation. 2014;98(12):1294–300. https://doi.org/10.1097/TP.0000000000000360.

92. Jowsey SG, Jacobs C, Gross CR, Hong BA, Messersmith EE, Gillespie BW, et al. Emotional well-being of living kidney donors: findings from the RELIVE Study. Am J Transplant. 2014;14(11):2535–44. https://doi.org/10.1111/ajt.12906.

93. Rodrigue JR, Schold JD, Morrissey P, Whiting J, Vella J, Kayler LK, et al. Mood, body image, fear of kidney failure, life satisfaction, and decisional stability following living kidney donation: findings from the KDOC study. Am J Transplant. 2018;18(6):1397–407. https://doi.org/10.1111/ajt.14618.

94. Rodrigue JR, Fleishman A, Schold JD, Morrissey P, Whiting J, Vella J, et al. Patterns and predictors of fatigue following living donor nephrectomy: findings from the KDOC Study. Am J Transplant. 2020;20(1):181–9. https://doi.org/10.1111/ajt.15519.

95. Holscher CM, Leanza J, Thomas AG, Waldram MM, Haugen CE, Jackson KR, et al. Anxiety, depression, and regret of donation in living kidney donors. BMC Nephrol. 2018;19(1):218. https://doi.org/10.1186/s12882-018-1024-0.

96. Weidebusch S, Reiermann C, Steinke FA, Muthny HJ, Pavenstaedt B, Schoene-Seifert N, et al. Quality of life, coping, and mental health status after living kidney donation. Transplant Proc. 2009;41(5):1483–8. https://doi.org/10.1016/j.transproceed.2009.02.102.

97. Lopes A, Frade IC, Teixeira L, Oliveira C, Almeida M, Dias L, et al. Depression and anxiety in living kidney donation: evaluation of donors and recipients. Transplant Proc. 2011;43(1):131–6. https://doi.org/10.1016/j.transproceed.2010.12.028.

98. Kroencke S. The relevance of donor satisfaction after living kidney donation-a plea for a routine psychosocial follow-up. Transpl Int. 2018;31(12):1330–1. https://doi.org/10.1111/tri.13355.

99. Menjivar A, Torres X, Paredes D, Avinyo N, Peri JM, De Sousa-Amorim E, et al. Assessment of donor satisfaction as an essential part of living donor kidney transplantation: an eleven-year retrospective study. Transpl Int. 2018;31(12):1332–44. https://doi.org/10.1111/tri.13334.

100. Gill JS, Gill J, Barnieh L, Dong J, Rose C, Johnston O, et al. Income of living kidney donors and the income difference between living kidney donors and their recipients in the United States. Am J Transplant. 2012;12(11):3111–8. https://doi.org/10.1111/j.1600-6143.2012.04211.x.

101. Lentine KL, Mannon RB. The Advancing American Kidney Health (AAKH) Executive Order: Promise and Caveats for Expanding Access to Kidney Transplantation. Kidney360. 2020;1(6):557–560. https://doi.org/10.34067/KID.0001172020.

102. Dew MA, Butt Z, Liu Q, Simpson MA, Zee J, Ladner DP, et al. Prevalence and predictors of patient-reported long-term mental and physical health after donation in the Adult-to-Adult Living-Donor Liver Transplantation Cohort Study. Transplantation. 2018;102(1):105–18. https://doi.org/10.1097/TP.0000000000001942.

103. Watson JM, Behnke MK, Fabrizio MD, McCune TR. Recipient graft failure or death impact on living kidney donor quality of life based on the living organ donor network database. J Endourol. 2013;27(12):1525–9. https://doi.org/10.1089/end.2013.0189.

104. Rodrigue JR, Schutzer ME, Paek M, Morrissey P. Altruistic kidney donation to a stranger: psychosocial and functional outcomes at two US transplant centers. Transplantation. 2011;91(7):772–8. https://doi.org/10.1097/TP.0b013e31820dd2bd.

105. Maple H, Chilcot J, Burnapp L, Gibbs P, Santhouse A, Norton S, et al. Motivations, outcomes, and characteristics of unspecified (nondirected altruistic) kidney donors in the United Kingdom. Transplantation. 2014;98(11):1182–9. https://doi.org/10.1097/TP.0000000000000340.

106. Massey EK, Kranenburg LW, Zuidema WC, Hak G, Erdman RAM, Hilhorst M, et al. Encouraging psychological outcomes after altruistic donation to a stranger. Am J Transplant. 2010;10:1445–52. https://doi.org/10.1111/j.1600-6143.2010.03115.x.
107. Jacobs C, Berglund DM, Wiseman JF, Garvey C, Larson DB, Voges M, et al. Long-term psychosocial outcomes after nondirected donation: a single-center experience. Am J Transplant. 2019;19(5):1498–506. https://doi.org/10.1111/ajt.15179.
108. Kranenburg L, Zuidema W, Vanderkroft P, Duivenvoorden H, Weimar W, Passchier J, et al. The implementation of a kidney exchange program does not induce a need for additional psychosocial support. Transpl Int. 2007;20(5):432–9. https://doi.org/10.1111/j.1432-2277.2007.00461.x.
109. Serur D, Charlton M, Lawton M, Sinacore J, Gordon-Elliot J. Donors in chains: psychosocial outcomes of kidney donors in paired exchange. Prog Transplant. 2014;24(4):371–4. https://doi.org/10.7182/pit2014222.

Risk Assessment Tools and Innovations in Living Kidney Donation

12

Abimereki D. Muzaale, Allan B. Massie, and Dorry L. Segev

Introduction

One of the cornerstones of donor evaluation is the exclusion of candidates who are projected to have a high risk of kidney failure in their lifetime. The 2017 Kidney Disease: Improving Global Outcomes (KDIGO) Clinical Practice Guideline on the Evaluation and Care of Living Kidney Donors featured an accessible online risk calculator that providers and prospective donors may use to facilitate projection of the 15-year and lifetime risk of end-stage kidney disease (ESKD) based on ten baseline demographic and health factors [1]. To generate projections, all the user has to do is populate the drop-down menus in the tool for age (18–80 years), sex, race (white or black), estimated glomerular filtration rate (eGFR), systolic blood pressure, hypertension medication (if any), body mass index (BMI), non-insulin dependent diabetes (yes/no), urine albumin-to-creatinine ratio, and smoking history (yes/ no) to get the projected 15-year and lifetime incidence of kidney failure [2]. Of note, this tool estimated "predonation risk," meaning risk for the individual based on these characteristics, without the additional risk related to kidney donation.

A threshold of *predonation* risk may inform the decision on whether or not to proceed with donation. Among those who proceed with donation, it must be understood that additional risks attributable to nephrectomy are superimposed on the risks one has before they donate to yield a postdonation risk [3]. This is because donation leads to a 50% loss of renal mass, a 25–40% decrease in renal function, and, as such, a step closer to kidney failure (de novo kidney disease may sooner reach kidney failure in donors than in their healthy nondonor peers, due to lower renal reserve) [4]. Depending on race and sex, the impact of donation is equivalent to a three- to fivefold higher risk when compared with predonation risk. Beyond considerations of race and sex, donation has been associated with substantive risks

A. D. Muzaale (✉) · A. B. Massie · D. L. Segev
Johns Hopkins University, Baltimore, MD, USA
e-mail: amuzaal1@jhmi.edu; amassie1@jhmi.edu; dorry@jhmi.edu

© Springer Nature Switzerland AG 2021
K. L. Lentine et al. (eds.), *Living Kidney Donation*,
https://doi.org/10.1007/978-3-030-53618-3_12

in donors who are obese and biologically related to their recipient [5, 6]; the magnitude of the risk observed among obese donors compared with non-obese donors has not been seen in healthy obese nondonors compared with healthy non-obese donors, suggesting that nephrectomy might modify this risk.

Risk calculators that inform an individual about their risk in the absence of donation and postdonation are freely available online to guide discussions with prospective donors [1, 7]. Importantly, at the present time, these calculators do not consider identical risk factors. While the healthy donor candidate calculator considered ten risk factors (see above), the postdonation risk calculator includes only age (18–80 years), sex, race (white/black), BMI (18–30 kg/m^2), and relationship to the recipient (yes/no for first-degree biological relative). Various potentially important risk factors including renal risk alleles, adverse perinatal conditions, granular assessment of family history, and single-nephron GFR are not considered by the current calculators. It is thus acknowledged that precision medicine has not arrived for risk prediction in kidney donors and iterative improvements of these calculators will be necessary as insights from new research are incorporated [8]. This chapter provides an overview of current understanding of the risks faced by the living kidney donor. Please see Chap. 2 for a discussion of Informed Consent and Chap. 15 for ethical considerations in donor evaluation.

Perioperative Risks

Perioperative mortality is extremely rare following living kidney donor nephrectomy (3 per 10,000 at 90 days). Surgical mortality is higher in men vs. women (5.1 vs. 1.7 per 10,000; risk ratio [RR], 3.0; 95% confidence interval [CI], 1.3–6.9; $P = 0.007$), black vs. white and Hispanic (7.6 vs. 2.6 and 2.0 per 10,000 donors; RR, 3.1; 95% CI, 1.3–7.1; $P = 0.01$), and in donors with hypertension vs. without hypertension (36.7 vs. 1.3 per 10,000 donors; RR, 27.4; 95% CI, 5.0–149.5; $P = 0.001$) [9]. Transplant professionals might be less concerned about perioperative risks because adverse events are extremely rare. But it is worth noting that donor surveys have identified time to recovery, surgical complications, and effect on family as their foremost concerns [10].

Long-Term Risks

A US national study that quantified the risk of ESKD among 96,217 donors compared with 20,024 healthy nondonors over median of 7 years found an eightfold higher risk among donors compared with healthy nondonors (risk of ESKD 15 years after donation was 30.8 per 10,000 vs. 3.9 per 10,000 in nondonors; $P < 0.001$) [4]. This difference was observed across race (74.7 per 10,000 black donors vs. 23.9 per 10,000 black nondonors; 32.6 per 10,000 Hispanic donors vs. 6.7 per 10,000; and 22.7 per 10,000 white donors vs. 0.0 per 10,000 white nondonors). Estimated lifetime risk of ESKD was 90 per 10,000 donors, 326 per 10,000 unscreened nondonors (general population), and 14 per 10,000 healthy nondonors). A Norwegian national study with a comparable study design reached similar inferences in finding an 11-fold higher risk in donors compared with healthy nondonors [11].

From a multinational meta-analysis including over 4 million individual records from Canada, the United States, and Israel, long-term ESKD risk estimates based on simultaneous consideration of each candidate's profile have been incorporated into an online risk calculator [2]. Importantly, the initial tools provide a proof of concept and starting point that need to be advanced and refined in ongoing research. Available calculators consider risk factors such as race/ethnicity as binary (white/black), and yet recent evidence points to high risks among individuals with Han-Chinese ancestry who have a family history of kidney failure [12]. Furthermore, within each race/ethnicity, the specific nature of the donor-recipient relationship is important in refining long-term risk estimates [6].

Thus for Asian donors, risks compared with unrelated donors were:

- 259.4-fold greater for identical twins (95% CI, 19.5–3445.6)
- 4.7-fold greater for full siblings (95% CI, 0.5–41.0)
- 3.5-fold greater for offspring (95% CI, 0.6–39.5)
- 1.0 for parents, and 1.0 for half-sibling or other biological relatives.

For black donors, risks were:

- 22.5-fold greater for identical twin donors (95% CI, 4.7–107.0)
- 4.1-fold for full siblings (95% CI, 2.1–7.8)
- 2.7-fold for offspring (95% CI, 1.4–5.4)
- 3.1-fold for parents (95% CI, 1.4–6.8), and
- 1.3-fold for half-sibling or other biological relatives (95% CI, 0.5–3.3).

For white donors, risks were:

- 3.5-fold greater for identical twin donors (95% CI, 0.5–25.3), 2.0-fold for full siblings (95% CI, 1.4–2.8)
- 1.4-fold for offspring (95% CI, 0.9–2.3)
- 2.9-fold for parents (95% CI, 2.0–4.1), and
- 0.8- fold for half-sibling or other biological relatives (95% CI, 0.3–1.6).

Relatives of African Americans with nondiabetic ESKD have high odds of carrying apolipoprotein L1 (*APOL1*) renal risk variants [13]. Likewise, related donors with ancestries other than African might be enriched for some other increased risk variants. Because none of the online calculators account for the variation in risk across race/ethnicity and donor-recipient relationship, clinical judgment during risk assessment will remain crucial for the foreseeable future.

Various other risk factors for ESKD and other health outcomes after donation have been reported in the living donor literature and are summarized in Table 12.1.

Unknown Risks

Genetic factors may predispose otherwise healthy, screened donors to postdonation kidney disease. But the pathways from gene expression through to kidney disease remain unknown. The notion of a "second hit" has been proposed, but "second hits" have not been empirically identified in the donor population [14]. As such, the

Table 12.1 Summary of recent studies identifying risk factors for health out

Timeline	Risk factor or "hit" (outcome of interest)	Population referenced in literature	
		Healthy nondonor	Kidney donor
Genetic	ADPKD (ESKD)	–	Zand 2001 [22]
	APOL1 renal risk variants (ESKD)	–	Mena-Gutierrez 2020 [23]
	MCKD (ESKD)	–	Muzaale 2020 [6]
Perinatal	Underweight at birth/preterm as marker of reduced nephron endowment [15] (ESKD)	NA	NA
Life course	Older age (ESKD)	Grams 2016 [2]	Massie 2017 [3]
	Sex (ESKD)	Grams 2016 [2]	Massie 2017 [3]
	Race/ethnicity (ESKD)	Grams 2016 [2]	Massie 2017 [3]
	Familial risk (ESKD)	NA	Muzaale 2020 [6]
	Hyperglycemia (ESKD)	Grams 2016 [2]	NA
	Hypertension (ESKD)	Grams 2016 [2]	Al Ammary 2019 [24]
	Urinary albumin: creatinine (ESKD)	Grams 2016 [2]	NA
	Kidney function, GFR (ESKD)	Grams 2016 [2]	Massie 2017 [3, 18]
	Functional reserve, snGFR (NA)	NA	Steiner 2018 [17]
	Blood pressure (ESKD)	Grams 2016 [2]	Al Ammary 2019 [24]
	Body mass index (ESKD)	Grams 2016 [2]	Locke 2017 [5]
	Smoking (ESKD)	Grams 2016 [2]	NA
	HIV infection (ESKD)	Muzaale 2017 [25]	Martin 2019 [26]
	Histological renal abnormalities (GFR)	–	Fahmy 2016 [27]
	Donor ESKD (recipient graft failure)	–	Muzaale 2016 [19]
	Declined as kidney donor (psychosocial harm)	–	Allen 2014 [20]
Postdonation nephrectomy	Donation-attributable (perioperative and long-term mortality)	–	Segev 2010 [9]
	Donation-attributable (ESKD)	–	Muzaale 2014/2017 [4, 28]
	Donation-attributable (psychosocial benefit)	–	Rasmussen 2017 [21]
	Donation-attributable (postdonation SBP elevation)		Boudville 2006 [29]
	Post donation HTN (recipient graft failure)	–	Holscher 2019 [30]
	Post donation GFR (ESKD)	–	Massie 2020 [18]
	Donation-attributable (gestational HTN/preeclampsia)	–	Garg 2015 [31]
	Missed opportunity for early detection (ESKD due to *de novo* GN, HTN or DM)	–	Anjum 2016 [32]
	Missed opportunity for early detection (long-term ESKD/ mortality)	–	Mjøen 2014 [11]

Abbreviations: *ADPKD* autosomal dominant polycystic kidney disease, *APOL1* apolipoprotein L1 gene, *DM* diabetes mellitus, *ESKD* end-stage kidney disease, *GFR* glomerular filtration rate, *GN* glomerulonephritis, *HTN* hypertension, *MCKD* medullary cystic kidney disease, *NA* not available, *snGFR* single-nephron glomerular filtration rate finding of high-risk genetic profiles, such as the presence of two *APOL1* renal risk variants, during donor evaluation, may not offer all the necessary information about an individuals' nephrectomy-attributable risk. This is an area of risk assessment and communication that has room for improvement.

Perinatal factors such as preeclampsia or maternal smoking are strongly associated with low birth weight, which in turn is associated with a substantially lower nephron endowment in each kidney [15]. While this has been established quite thoroughly in the nondonor literature, the implications for the kidney donor remain unknown. Because of a lifetime of adaptive hyperfiltration in such a population, a single-nephron glomerular filtration rate (snGFR) assessment might be more useful for this subgroup of prospective donors [16, 17]. And since the information regarding birth weight may not be available at donor evaluation, this might mean that every donor should ideally be assessed for snGFR. The emergent phenotype association with higher snGFR might be that of a lower adaptive response following nephrectomy [18].

Life-course events like kidney trauma, acute kidney injury, or various other subclinical phenomena have the potential to damage nephrons and reduce the nephron endowment in a manner similar to perinatal events. The kidneys might "keep track" of these life-course subclinical events, which might escape detection during donor evaluation, but subsequently manifest not only in donor kidney failure but also in adverse recipient outcomes [19]. Such upstream factors that are clinically latent are more likely to become clinically salient in donors than in their healthy nondonor counterparts.

Known Benefits

Very often a kidney donated is directed to a spouse/partner, sibling, offspring, or parent. Since such donors are likely to share a household with the recipient, their well-being is closely tied to the recipient, and these have been termed "interdependent donors." A risk-benefit approach that combines risk assessment with benefits to interdependent donors will contribute to donor evaluation and selection in a manner that accurately reflects what is at stake for donors. This in turn may allow some donors to accept greater risk in donation decisions [20, 21].

Summary

The goal of providing donor candidates with individually tailored risk assessment is an important goal. Recent research has provided a step in the right direction, by enabling descriptions of average risks for various subgroups of donors and explanations of the considerable variations in risk observed from one group to the next. Innovative tools provide a framework for supplying point-of-care risk projection based on limited sets of known demographic and health factors that can be validated and refined as more data become available. Fortunately, the absolute risks faced by the majority of donors are low, a tribute to the rigor in the current practice standards. Future work should continue to advance the science of risk prediction to move the field closer toward tailored risk prediction to inform donor candidate evaluation, selection, and counseling.

References

1. ESRD Risk Tool for Kidney Donor Candidates. http://www.transplantmodels.com/esrdrisk/. Accessed: 7 Sept 2020.
2. Grams ME, Sang Y, Levey AS, Matsushita K, Ballew S, Chang AR, et al. Kidney-failure risk projection for the living kidney-donor candidate. N Engl J Med. 2016;374(5):411–21. https://doi.org/10.1056/NEJMoa1510491.
3. Massie AB, Muzaale AD, Luo X, Chow EKH, Locke JE, Nguyen AQ, et al. Quantifying postdonation risk of ESRD in living kidney donors. J Am Soc Nephrol. 2017;28(9):2749–55. https://doi.org/10.1681/ASN.2016101084.
4. Muzaale AD, Massie AB, Wang MC, Montgomery RA, McBride MA, Wainright JL, et al. Risk of end-stage renal disease following live kidney donation. JAMA. 2014;311(16):579–86. https://doi.org/10.1001/jama.2013.285141.
5. Locke JE, Reed RD, Massie A, MacLennan PA, Sawinski D, Kumar V, et al. Obesity increases the risk of end-stage renal disease among living kidney donors. Kidney Int. 2017;91(3):699–703. https://doi.org/10.1016/j.kint.2016.10.014.
6. Muzaale AD, Massie AB, Al Ammary F, et al. Donor-recipient relationship and risk of ESKD in live kidney donors of varied racial groups. Am J Kidney Dis. 2020;75:333–41. https://doi.org/10.1053/j.ajkd.2019.08.020.
7. Postdonation Risk of ESRD in Living Kidney. http://www.transplantmodels.com/donesrd/. Accessed: 7 Sept 2020.
8. Poggio ED, Reese PP. The quest to define individual risk after living kidney donation. Ann Intern Med. 2018;168(4):296–7. https://doi.org/10.7326/M17-3249.
9. Segev DL, Muzaale AD, Caffo BS, Mehta SH, Singer AL, Taranto SE, et al. Perioperative mortality and long-term survival following live kidney donation. JAMA. 2010;303(10):959–66. https://doi.org/10.1001/jama.2010.237.
10. Lentine KL, Lam NN, Segev DL. Risks of living kidney donation: current state of knowledge on outcomes important to donors. Clin J Am Soc Nephrol. 2019;14(4):597–608. https://doi.org/10.2215/CJN.11220918.
11. Mjoen G, Hallan S, Hartmann A, Foss A, Midtvedt K, Oyen O, et al. Long-term risks for kidney donors. Kidney Int. 2014;86(1):162–7. https://doi.org/10.1038/ki.2013.460.
12. Wu HH, Kuo CF, Li IJ, Weng CH, Lee CC, Tu KH, et al. Family aggregation and heritability of ESRD in Taiwan: a population-based study. Am J Kidney Dis. 2017;70(5):619–26. https://doi.org/10.1053/j.ajkd.2017.05.007.
13. Freedman BI, Langefeld CD, Turner J, Nunez M, High KP, Spainhour M, et al. Association of APOL1 variants with mild kidney disease in the first-degree relatives of African American patients with non-diabetic end-stage renal disease. Kidney Int. 2012;82(7):805–11. https://doi.org/10.1038/ki.2012.217.
14. Chang JH, Husain SA, Santoriello D, Stokes MB, Miles CD, Foster KW, et al. Donor's APOL1 risk genotype and "second hits" associated with de novo collapsing glomerulopathy in deceased donor kidney transplant recipients: a report of 5 cases. Am J Kidney Dis. 2019;73(1):134–9. https://doi.org/10.1053/j.ajkd.2018.05.008.
15. Vikse BE, Irgens LM, Leivestad T, Hallan S, Iversen BM. Low birth weight increases risk for end-stage renal disease. J Am Soc Nephrol. 2008;19(1):151–7. https://doi.org/10.1681/ASN.2007020252.

16. Denic A, Mathew J, Lerman LO, Lieske JC, Larson JJ, Alexander MP, et al. Single-nephron glomerular filtration rate in healthy adults. N Engl J Med. 2017;376(24):2349–57. https://doi.org/10.1056/NEJMoa1614329.

17. Steiner RW. Increased single-nephron GFR in normal adults: too much of a good thing … or maybe not? Am J Kidney Dis. 2018;71(3):312–4. https://doi.org/10.1053/j.ajkd.2017.11.005.

18. Massie AB, Holscher CM, Henderson ML, Fahmy LM, Thomas AG, Al Ammary F, et al. Association of early postdonation renal function with subsequent risk of end-stage renal disease in living kidney donors. JAMA Surg. 2020;155(3):e195472. https://doi.org/10.1001/jamasurg.2019.5472.

19. Muzaale AD, Massie AB, Anjum S, Liao C, Garg AX, Lentine KL, et al. Recipient outcomes following transplantation of allografts from live kidney donors who subsequently developed end-stage renal disease. Am J Transplant. 2016;16(12):3532–9. https://doi.org/10.1111/ajt.13869.

20. Allen MB, Abt PL, Reese PP. What are the harms of refusing to allow living kidney donation? An expanded view of risks and benefits. Am J Transplant. 2014;14(3):531–7. https://doi.org/10.1111/ajt.12599.

21. Van Pilsum Rasmussen SE, Henderson ML, Kahn J, Segev D. Considering tangible benefit for interdependent donors: extending a risk-benefit framework in donor selection. Am J Transplant. 2017;17(10):2567–71. https://doi.org/10.1111/ajt.14319.

22. Zand MS, Strang J, Dumlao M, Rubens D, Erturk E, Bronsther O. Screening a living kidney donor for polycystic kidney disease using heavily T2-weighted MRI. Am J Kidney Dis. 2001;37(3):612–9. https://pubmed.ncbi.nlm.nih.gov/11228187/.

23. Lentine KL, Mannon RB. Apolipoprotein L1: role in the evaluation of kidney transplant donors. Curr Opin Nephrol Hypertens. 2020;29(6):645–55. https://doi.org/10.1097/MNH.0000000000000653.

24. Al Ammary F, Luo X, Muzaale AD, Massie AB, Crews DC, Waldram MM, et al. Risk of ESKD in older live kidney donors with hypertension. Clin J Am Soc Nephrol. 2019;14(7):1048–55. https://doi.org/10.2215/CJN.14031118.

25. Muzaale AD, Althoff KN, Sperati CJ, Abraham AG, Kucirka LM, Massie AB, et al. Risk of end-stage renal disease in HIV-positive potential live kidney donors. Am J Transplant. 2017;17(7):1823–32. https://doi.org/10.1111/ajt.14235.

26. 1st Living HIV-Positive Organ Donor Wants To Lift 'The Shroud Of HIV Related Stigma'. https://www.npr.org/2019/04/06/710247561/1st-living-hiv-positive-organ-donor-wants-to-lift-the-shroud-of-hiv-related-stig. Accessed: 7 Sept 2020.

27. Fahmy LM, Massie AB, Muzaale AD, Bagnasco SM, Orandi BJ, Alejo JL, et al. Long-term renal function in living kidney donors who had histological abnormalities at donation. Transplantation. 2016;100(6):1294–8. https://doi.org/10.1097/TP.0000000000001236.

28. Muzaale AD, Massie AB, Segev DL. Concerns about the long-term safety of live kidney donors are justified. Eur J Epidemiol. 2017;32(2):91–3. https://doi.org/10.1007/s10654-017-0241-3.

29. Boudville N, Prasad GV, Knoll G, Muirhead N, Thiessen-Philbrook H, Yang RC, et al. Meta-analysis: risk for hypertension in living kidney donors. Ann Intern Med. 2006;145(3):185–96. https://doi.org/10.7326/0003-4819-145-3-200608010-00006.

30. Holscher CM, Ishaque T, Haugen CE, Jackson KR, Garonzik Wang JM, Yu Y, et al. Association between living kidney donor post-donation hypertension and recipient graft failure. Transplantation. 2020;104(3):583–90. https://doi.org/10.1097/TP.0000000000002832.

31. Garg AX, Nevis IF, McArthur E, Sontrop JM, Koval JJ, Lam NN, et al. Gestational hypertension and preeclampsia in living kidney donors. N Engl J Med. 2015;372(2):124–33. https://doi.org/10.1056/NEJMoa1408932.

32. Anjum S, Muzaale AD, Massie AB, Sontrop JM, Koval JJ, Lam NN, et al. Patterns of end-stage renal disease caused by diabetes, hypertension, and glomerulonephritis in live kidney donors. Am J Transplant. 2016;16(12):3540–7. https://doi.org/10.1111/ajt.13917.

Living Donor Nephrectomy: Approaches, Innovations, and Outcomes

Jonathan Merola, Matthew Cooper, and Sanjay Kulkarni

Surgical Considerations

Living Donor Eligibility

Evaluation of individuals for living donation involves ensuring a candidate is donating voluntarily, assessing all the medical, surgical, and socioeconomic risks of donation, providing donor education and counseling, and devising a plan for follow-up care. Evidence-based clinical practice guidelines for each of these aspects of evaluation have been put forth in the 2017 Kidney Disease: Improving Global Outcomes (KDIGO) 'Guideline for the Evaluation and Care of Living Donors' [1]. Utilization of a multidisciplinary team helps ensure a comprehensive evaluation, an iterative informed consent process, and extensive patient education on all aspects of the living donation process.

As described in accompanying chapters, all donor candidates undergo a thorough medical evaluation including assessment of blood pressure, kidney function, and metabolic health. Over the past several decades, however, criteria for donor eligibility have evolved. Older persons and those with medically managed hypertension, prediabetes, known nephrolithiasis, and obesity who were once considered ineligible as living donor candidates are increasingly accepted for donation [2]. The 2017 KDIGO guideline advances a framework for replacing decisions based on assessments of single risk factors in isolation with a comprehensive approach to risk assessment based on simultaneous consideration of each candidate's demographic profile and health characteristics [1]. Accurate assessment of kidney function is

J. Merola · S. Kulkarni (✉)
Department of Surgery, Yale School of Medicine, New Haven, CT, USA
e-mail: Jonathan.Merola@yale.edu; Sanjay.Kulkarni@yale.edu

M. Cooper
Medstar Georgetown Transplant Institute, Washington, DC, USA
e-mail: Matthew.Cooper@gunet.georgetown.edu

© Springer Nature Switzerland AG 2021
K. L. Lentine et al. (eds.), *Living Kidney Donation*,
https://doi.org/10.1007/978-3-030-53618-3_13

necessary to ensure adequate renal reserve after donation and assess expected function in relation to recipient needs. Despite evolving trends in donor acceptance, however, the absolute risk of end-stage renal disease after donation is overall less than 1% at 15 years [3].

Technical Factors

All living donor candidates should have renal imaging in the form of computed tomography (CT) or magnetic resonance (MR) angiography to assess their renal vasculature as well as screen for nephrolithiasis or occult mass lesions preoperatively. Both modalities have been shown to reveal relevant anatomy with a high degree of accuracy [4]. While MR avoids contrast enhancement and spares potential donors' radiation exposure, newer low-dose radiation CT protocols have successfully been employed for evaluating potential living donors [5]. Vascular multiplicity can be anticipated in 30–50% of cases, while duplicated collecting systems are identified in approximately 1% of the population [6]. While any accessory veins and arteries supplying a minor portion of the upper pole can often be safely sacrificed, arteries supplying the lower pole and proximal ureter require reconstruction following nephrectomy. Accessory arteries are not considered prohibitive for donation, though some reports show an association with increased operative time and urologic complications [7–9]. These findings have recently been challenged by newer reports that fail to show an association with increased donor complications in experienced living donor programs [10, 11].

While preoperative imaging is an important part of living donor evaluation, it should be noted that up to 25% of potential donors have incidental radiographic abnormalities, including kidney stones, scarring, fibromuscular dysplasia, and atherosclerosis [12]. These findings rarely disqualify a potential living donor but can affect both transplant outcomes and dictate the choice of laterality in living donor nephrectomy. Generally, it is preferable to procure the smaller kidney for donation to minimize adaptive hyperfiltration in the donor postoperatively. While adaptive hyperfiltration may potentially lead to glomerular hypertension as seen in animal studies, recent studies evaluating donors several years post-nephrectomy have not found evidence that this occurs in humans [13]. Volumetric analyses obtained from imaging are often utilized for accurate renal size assessment and prediction of split renal function, shown to highly correlate with post-nephrectomy kidney function [14]. For the majority of kidney donors, small differences in renal size have not resulted in appreciable changes in post-donation renal function. However, volumetric analyses are likely to be of greater importance in patients with suboptimal levels of kidney function and older donors, as size differences of 10% in higher risk populations may lead to differences in post-nephrectomy kidney function [1].

Data from several recent meta-analyses have shown that, with adequate experience, laterality has no significant effect on donor complications or graft survival [15, 16]. However, in the absence of compelling indications for right-sided nephrectomy (e.g., significant split function difference, multiple cysts, solid lesions), left nephrectomy is often preferred. Technical advantages to left-sided nephrectomy include a longer venous pedicle, a lower rate of thrombotic complications, and the ability to avoid injury to the liver [15]. The 2017 KDIGO guideline recommends that when asymmetry in renal function, parenchymal abnormalities, vascular abnormalities, or urological abnormalities are present but do not preclude donation, the more severely affected kidney should be used for donation [1].

Approaches

Open Retroperitoneal Donor Nephrectomy

The open approach has long been considered the gold standard for donor nephrectomy to which newer techniques are compared. Open donor nephrectomy dates back to the first kidney transplant performed by Joseph Murray between two identical twins in 1954 [17]. This procedure poses risks of significant morbidity associated with a large flank incision. At times, a 12th rib resection is required, and donors often reported significant pain, requiring prolonged hospital convalescence, and may experience complications including pneumothorax or incisional hernia. However, there are circumstances in which the open technique may still be preferred, particularly in patients with extensive intraperitoneal adhesions due to prior surgery and in the setting of short renal vessels, when obtaining adequate length for successful transplantation is critical (e.g., right renal vein <1.5 cm). The surgeon should have adequate training and experience for the decided surgical approach for the donor nephrectomy, and the risks and benefits of the recommended approach should be carefully discussed with the donor candidate as part of informed consent.

In the open approach, the patient is placed in the lateral decubitus position with the operating table flexed and in slight Trendelenburg position such that the flank is parallel to the floor. An axillary roll is placed to avoid pressure on the brachial plexus, and the patient's legs are padded. An incision of 15–18 cm is made between the 11th and 12th rib. The retroperitoneum is entered, dissecting the diaphragm and pleura free from the lateral aspect of the 11th rib. The retroperitoneal space is developed, and the ureter is identified with care to preserve the surrounding areolar tissue as it is dissected down to the level of the iliac vessels. Gerota's fascia is entered, and the kidney is mobilized and dissected free from the adrenal gland. Dissection of the renal hilum is then carried out. In the case of right nephrectomy, the renal artery is identified in a retrocaval position. On the left side, the renal artery is identified following ligation of the left adrenal vein coursing more superficially along the upper pole of the kidney. The ureter is then divided with care to preserve the ureteral blood supply located within the triangle of tissue bordered by the lower pole of the kidney, the inferior vena cava, and the renal hilum. The renal artery is doubly ligated and divided, and subsequently the renal vein is then clamped and its remaining stump oversewn with non-absorbable suture. The flank incision is then closed in multiple layers.

Laparoscopic Transperitoneal Donor Nephrectomy

The introduction of laparoscopy led to significant advances in living donor nephrectomy. This less invasive technique offers less pain, faster recovery, and more cosmetically favorable results compared to the open technique [18]. Initially described by Clayman et al. in 1990 for treatment of renal cancer in an elderly patient, the first laparoscopic donor nephrectomy was performed by Kavoussi and implanted by Ratner at Johns Hopkins Bayview Medical Center in 1995 [19].

The traditional technique for laparoscopic left donor nephrectomy involves placement of the patient in a right lateral decubitus position with the hips slightly rotated posteriorly [19]. The operating surgeon faces the abdomen while the assistant stands to the right and caudad to the surgeon. Two 12-mm ports are placed in the periumbilical position and laterally along the semilunar line (Fig. 13.1). A third 5-mm port is placed in the midline 3 cm below the xiphoid process. An overall schematic of the dissection is shown in Fig. 13.2a. Dissection is begun by dividing the peritoneal reflection along the white line of Toldt from the splenic flexure to the pelvic inlet. The spleen is mobilized lateral to medial, creating a plane between the spleen and upper renal pole. Mobilization of the colon is continued medially along the plane between Gerota's fascia and the mesentery of the descending colon until the left gonadal vein is encountered (Fig. 13.2b). The left gonadal vein is dissected along its lateral aspect cranially to its insertion into the left renal vein with care to identify the left ureter and preserve tributaries coursing on the medial aspect of the left gonadal vein. The gonadal vein, ureter, and lower pole of the kidney are then elevated anterolaterally off the psoas muscle to expose the renal vein and artery (Fig. 13.2c). Lumbar veins coursing posteriorly to the left renal vein are ligated and divided. Branches of the adrenal vein are identified and divided (Fig. 13.2d). The left renal artery is then dissected circumferentially from investing lymphatics and neural tissue from the renal hilum proximally to the aorta. One important principle

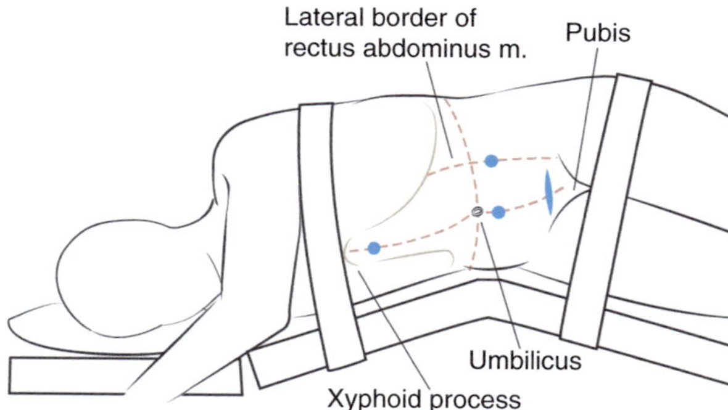

Fig. 13.1 Patient positioning and laparoscopic port placement for transperitoneal laparoscopic donor nephrectomy. Two 12 mm ports are placed in the periumbilical and along the lateral border of the rectus abdominis muscle 2 cm below the level of the umbilicus. One 5 mm port is placed in the upper midline 3 cm below the xiphoid. A 6 cm Pfannenstiel incision is used for extraction

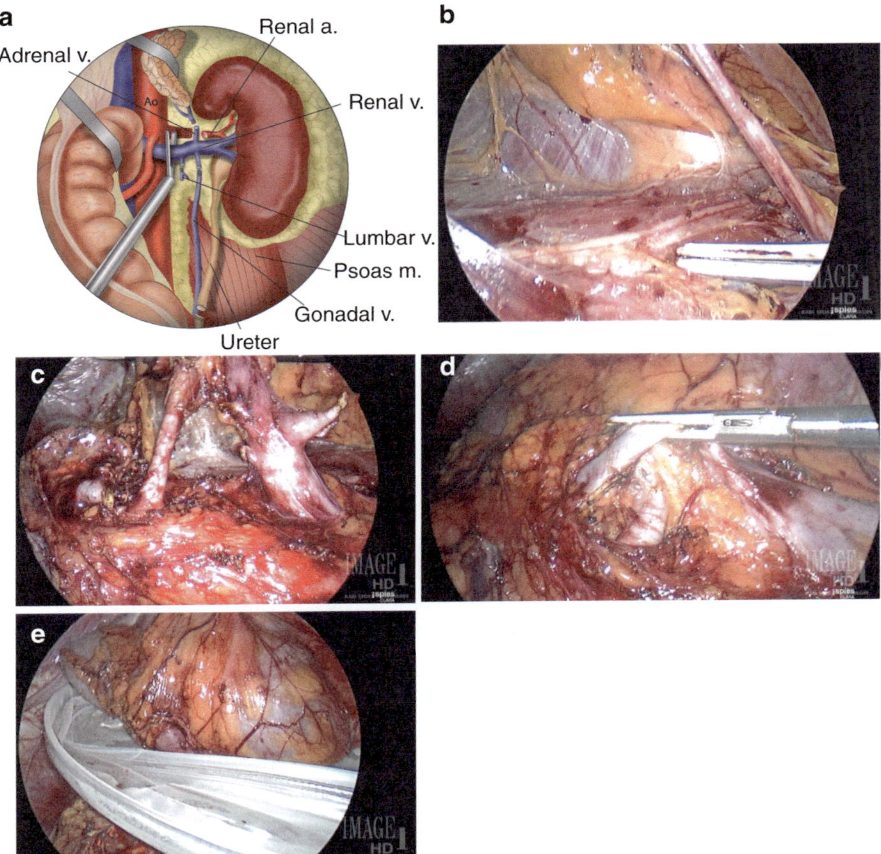

Fig. 13.2 Operative dissection for left laparoscopic donor nephrectomy. (**a**) Overall schematic of laparoscopic left kidney dissection. (**b**) The gonadal vein is dissected with care to preserve ureteral blood supply medially. (**c**) Lower pole of kidney is elevated off the psoas muscle to expose the left renal artery and vein. (**d**) The lumbar and adrenal venous branches are divided from the left renal vein. (**e**) The kidney is extracted through a Pfannenstiel incision. *Abbreviations: a* artery; *m* muscle; *v* vein

in division of renal vein tributaries is the avoidance of clips, which can result in subsequent stapler malfunction if incorporated into the staple line. The kidney is then mobilized off the retroperitoneum and extracted using a 10 mm Endo Catch bag through a 6 cm transverse Pfannenstiel incision approximately 2 cm above the pubis (Fig. 13.2e). The abdominal wall fascia and skin are then reapproximated with sutures.

Importantly, ligation of the renal vessels should be performed with tissue transfixion by suture ligation or vascular staples. Use of non-transfixing vascular clips (such as Weck Hem-O-Lock) have been associated with hemorrhagic deaths due to clip dislodgement, particularly when placed on the renal artery

[20]. A black box warning has been issued for use of such clips for the ligation of renal arteries during laparoscopic donor nephrectomy [21]. The 2017 KDIGO guidelines emphasize the critical importance of renal artery transfixation by suture ligature or anchored staples within the vessel wall. Non-transfixing clips to ligate the renal artery in living donor nephrectomy should be avoided [1].

Modifications of Laparoscopic Nephrectomy

Hand-Assisted Laparoscopy

One of the major shortcomings of laparoscopic surgery that has hindered its widespread use was the learning curve required among surgeons without advanced laparoscopic experience that led to long operative times and greater blood loss. Recent studies have demonstrated that reduced intraoperative complications and adequate proficiency are gained following performance of a minimum case volume of 25–35 among advanced trainees [22]. As a modification of the pure laparoscopic approach, a "mini-open" or hand-assisted approach using a hand port was introduced, championed as reducing operative time and complications while facilitating wider adoption of the laparoscopic technique [23]. Initially described by Wolf et al., a 9–10 cm occlusive sleeve was used to maintain pneumoperitoneum while taking advantages of manual assistance. The sleeve may be placed in the lower or upper midline or through a lower transverse incision [23].

Advocates of the hand-assisted approach note that tissue planes may be more easily retracted, particularly facilitating colonic flexion in exposure of the left kidney. Additionally, the hand port facilitates tactile feedback, absent in pure laparoscopy, and also allows for manual compression of readily controllable bleeding. Several initial studies comparing the hand-assisted and pure laparoscopic approaches have noted lower warm ischemia time and transfusion rates with addition of the hand port [24, 25]. However, as laparoscopy has become more widely adopted, recent studies have noted no significant differences in outcomes in operative time, warm ischemia time, transfusion rate, analgesic requirement, or hospital length of stay. Both approaches remain widely accepted and utilized [26, 27].

Robotic-Assisted Laparoscopy

The use of robotic-assisted laparoscopy was first reported in 2002 by Benedetti and colleagues [28]. Early adopters of this approach note decreased analgesic requirements, shorter hospital length of stay, and the ability to preserve longer arterial length on the right side [29]. However, the expense of the robot systems such as DaVinci, coupled with longer retrieval and warm ischemia time, has hindered widespread use of this technology. Moreover, the additional training required for use of the robotic system without established advantages in outcomes has led to its limited expansion.

Retroperitoneoscopic Donor Nephrectomy

In patients with prior transabdominal surgery or increased body mass index, a retroperitoneoscopic approach may offer a more successful approach than open nephrectomy, while minimizing risks of enterotomy with intra-abdominal laparoscopy. This approach is particularly advantageous with right nephrectomy, where transabdominal exposure is limited by the liver. In this approach, the patient is placed in the lateral decubitus position with the operating table flat [30]. Two 12-mm ports are inserted, the first along the mid-axillary line between the iliac crest and the 12th rib and the second at the angle of the 12th rib and the lateral margin of the rectus abdominis muscle. A third port is inserted 3 cm above the anterior superior iliac spine. A balloon dilator is inserted to create a retroperitoneal working space deep to the thoracolumbar fascia and insufflated to a pressure of 5–10 mmHg. The psoas muscle is identified and the fascia is opened. The renal artery and vein are identified and freed from surrounding lymphatic tissues with an ultrasonic knife or LigaSure device. The renal vein is then identified and dissected. A GIA vascular stapler is used to divide gonadal or lumbar veins >7 mm in diameter. The ureter is dissected with care to avoid damage to feeding arteries and veins and transected at level of the common iliac artery. A 5 cm flank incision below the 11th rib is then created for kidney removal (Fig. 13.3).

Single-Port Surgery and Transvaginal Extraction

New modifications have been introduced to further improve cosmesis as well as limit postoperative pain and hasten recovery heralded by traditional laparoscopic approaches. Laparoendoscopic single-site surgery has been described to accomplish these aims by utilizing a GelPort device placed within a 5 cm vertical periumbilical incision. Three or four trocars can be placed within this device to perform an identical surgical dissection that is described in the total laparoscopic technique. Decreased morbidity with this technique is therefore achieved in eliminating extra-umbilical trocar sites. Advocates for this technique note greater patient satisfaction with cosmesis while achieving similar operative times and postoperative recipient renal function [31, 32]. However, opposition to the use of this technique exists among some who feel that compromised visibility and intra-abdominal access are not justified in the absence of objective improvement in outcome measures. As retrieval of the kidney may be more arduous and a learning curve for utilization of specialized articulating instruments required, further objective assessments of single-port surgery are needed to justify greater adoption [33].

Mitigation of postoperative pain associated with laparoscopic donor nephrectomy has also been recently accomplished by use of natural orifice transluminal surgery (NOTES), employed by performing surgery through natural orifices including the vagina, mouth, and rectum. Donor nephrectomy with transvaginal extraction was described in 2010 using a robotic-assisted laparoscopic technique, allowing for ergonomic dissection of the renal vascular pedicle, while affording superior cosmetic and analgesic outcomes [34]. Greater adoption of these approaches requires validation of postoperative complication rates among experienced surgeons in the setting of controlled clinical trials.

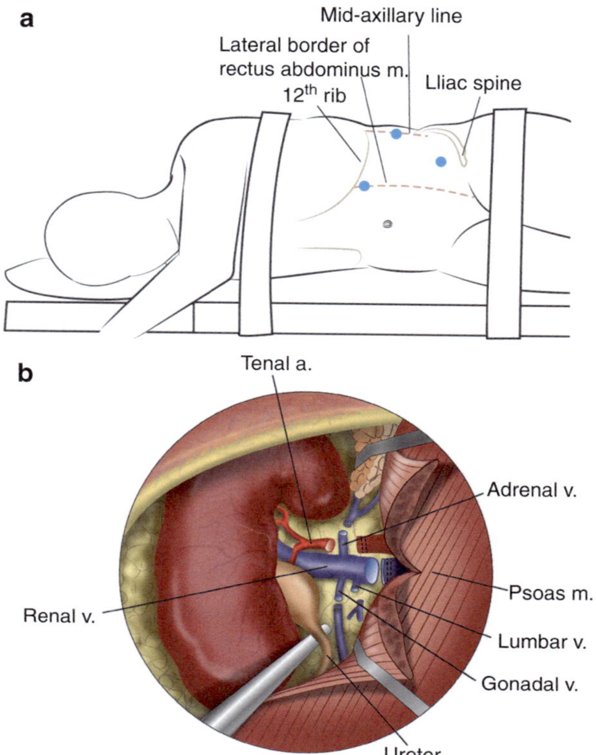

Fig. 13.3 Retroperitoneoscopic donor nephrectomy. (**a**) Port placement and (**b**) schematic of dissection achieved for retroperitoneoscopic donor nephrectomy. *Abbreviations: a* artery; *m* muscle; *v* vein

Donor Outcomes

Living donor nephrectomy is a safe operation with an overall 0.03% 90-day mortality [35]. Advantages and disadvantages to the described approaches are summarized in Table 13.1. Morbidity associated with donor nephrectomy is overall lower with laparoscopic compared to open approaches. The most common complications of donor nephrectomy include bleeding (2.6% laparoscopic vs. 1.4% open), wound infection (1.9% laparoscopic vs. 3.2% open), hernia (1.1% laparoscopic vs. 3.1% open), chronic pain (1.1% laparoscopic vs. 6.4% open), and post-operative pneumonia (2.7% laparoscopic vs. 3.4% open). Overall, patients undergoing laparoscopic nephrectomy benefit from a shorter length of stay, decreased analgesic requirement, and faster return to work and normal activities. Recipients demonstrate similar graft functional outcomes [36, 37]. Given a lower morbidity profile, higher degree of patient satisfaction, and equivalent outcomes, the laparoscopic approach has become the standard method for living donor nephrectomy [38].

Table 13.1 Comparison of surgical approaches for donor nephrectomy

	Advantages	Disadvantages
Open	• Best vascular control • Lower intraoperative blood loss	• Higher rates of wound complications (infection, hernia, pain) • Higher postoperative pneumonia • Longer length of hospital stay • Longer time to recovery
Laparoscopic	• Excellent visualization • Reduced wound complications • Short length of stay • Lower analgesic requirement • Faster return to work	• Lack of tactile feedback • Longer warm ischemic time
Retroperitoneoscopic	• Lower risk of enterotomy and intra-abdominal organ injury	• Higher intraoperative blood loss • Technically challenging, smaller working area
Robotic-assisted	• Lower intraoperative blood loss • Ergonomically favorable	• Higher cost • Lack of tactile feedback

Several small studies comparing retroperitoneoscopic donor nephrectomy with standard laparoscopic approaches have found similar rates of complications, length of hospital stay, and quality of life [39, 40]. While such reports have been published by experienced centers, higher rates of intraoperative blood loss have been noted with the retroperitoneoscopic approach [40]. Robotic-assisted laparoscopic nephrectomies have similarly been shown to have similar length of stay, postoperative graft outcomes, and in some reports lower blood loss and warm ischemic time compared to pure laparoscopic donor nephrectomy [41]. At present, however, retroperitoneoscopic and robotic-assisted nephrectomy require further clinical studies for validation.

Pending more evidence, the 2017 KDIGO guideline recommends that, at this time, robotic, single-port, and natural orifice transluminal nephrectomy should generally not be used for living donor nephrectomy [1] in the routine clinical setting.

Conclusions

Advancements in surgical techniques and laparoscopy have made laparoscopic living donor nephrectomy a safe and more feasible operation over the last two decades. Minimizing analgesic requirements and time to recovery have removed significant disadvantages for donors. While novel approaches such as robotic-assisted, total robotic, and single-port nephrectomies are not currently standard of care, approaches to donor nephrectomy will likely continue to evolve with innovations in the available range of techniques and surgical instruments. The overall goal remains to reduce risks and morbidity for the altruistic persons who undergo kidney donation to provide the life-saving benefit of transplantation to patients with renal failure.

Acknowledgments   Illustrations were created and reproduced with permission by Wendolyn Hill.

References

1. Lentine KL, Kasiske BL, Levey AS, Adams PL, Alberu J, Bakr MA, et al. KDIGO clinical practice guideline on the evaluation and care of living kidney donors. Transplantation. 2017;101(8S Suppl 1):S1–S109. https://doi.org/10.1097/TP.0000000000001769.
2. Reese PP, Boudville N, Garg AX. Living kidney donation: outcomes, ethics, and uncertainty. Lancet. 2015;385(9981):2003–13. https://doi.org/10.1016/S0140-6736(14)62484-3.
3. Muzaale AD, Massie AB, Wang MC, Montgomery RA, McBride MA, Wainright JL, et al. Risk of end-stage renal disease following live kidney donation. JAMA. 2014;311(6):579–86. https://doi.org/10.1001/jama.2013.285141.
4. Blankholm AD, Pedersen BG, Ostrat EO, Andersen G, Stausbol-Gron B, Laustsen S, et al. Noncontrast-enhanced magnetic resonance versus computed tomography angiography in preoperative evaluation of potential living renal donors. Acad Radiol. 2015;22(11):1368–75. https://doi.org/10.1016/j.acra.2015.06.015.
5. Davarpanah AH, Pahade JK, Cornfeld D, Ghita M, Kulkarni S, Israel GM. CT angiography in potential living kidney donors: 80 kVp versus 120 kVp. AJR Am J Roentgenol. 2013;201(5):W753–60. https://doi.org/10.2214/AJR.12.10439.
6. Gay SB, Armistead JP, Weber ME, Williamson BR. Left infrarenal region: anatomic variants, pathologic conditions, and diagnostic pitfalls. Radiographics. 1991;11(4):549–70. https://doi.org/10.1148/radiographics.11.4.1887111.
7. Ahmadi AR, Lafranca JA, Claessens LA, Imamdi RM, JN IJ, Betjes MG, et al. Shifting paradigms in eligibility criteria for live kidney donation: a systematic review. Kidney Int. 2015;87(1):31–45. https://doi.org/10.1038/ki.2014.118.
8. Rahnemai-Azar AA, Gilchrist BF, Kayler LK. Independent risk factors for early urologic complications after kidney transplantation. Clin Transpl. 2015;29(5):403–8. https://doi.org/10.1111/ctr.12530.
9. Kok NF, Dols LF, Hunink MG, Alwayn IP, Tran KT, Weimar W, et al. Complex vascular anatomy in live kidney donation: imaging and consequences for clinical outcome. Transplantation. 2008;85(12):1760–5. https://doi.org/10.1097/TP.0b013e318172802d.
10. Fehrman-Ekholm I. Living donor kidney transplantation. Transplant Proc. 2006;38(8):2637–41. https://doi.org/10.1016/j.transproceed.2006.07.027.
11. Benedetti E, Troppmann C, Gillingham K, Sutherland DE, Payne WD, Dunn DL, et al. Short- and long-term outcomes of kidney transplants with multiple renal arteries. Ann Surg. 1995;221(4):406–14. https://doi.org/10.1097/00000658-199504000-00012.
12. Lorenz EC, Vrtiska TJ, Lieske JC, Dillon JJ, Stegall MD, Li X, et al. Prevalence of renal artery and kidney abnormalities by computed tomography among healthy adults. Clin J Am Soc Nephrol. 2010;5(3):431–8. https://doi.org/10.2215/CJN.07641009.
13. Lenihan CR, Busque S, Derby G, Blouch K, Myers BD, Tan JC. Longitudinal study of living kidney donor glomerular dynamics after nephrectomy. J Clin Invest. 2015;125(3):1311–8. https://doi.org/10.1172/JCI7888578885[pii].
14. Wahba R, Franke M, Hellmich M, Kleinert R, Cingoz T, Schmidt MC, et al. Computed tomography volumetry in preoperative living kidney donor assessment for prediction of Split renal function. Transplantation. 2016;100(6):1270–7. https://doi.org/10.1097/TP.0000000000000889.
15. Khalil A, Mujtaba MA, Taber TE, Yaqub MS, Goggins W, Powelson J, et al. Trends and outcomes in right vs. left living donor nephrectomy: an analysis of the OPTN/UNOS database of donor and recipient outcomes–should we be doing more right-sided nephrectomies? Clin Transpl. 2016;30(2):145–53. https://doi.org/10.1111/ctr.12668.
16. Liu N, Wazir R, Wang J, Wang KJ. Maximizing the donor pool: left versus right laparoscopic live donor nephrectomy–systematic review and meta-analysis. Int Urol Nephrol. 2014;46(8):1511–9. https://doi.org/10.1007/s11255-014-0671-8.
17. Merrill JP, Murray JE, Harrison JH, Guild WR. Successful homotransplantation of the human kidney between identical twins. J Am Med Assoc. 1956;160(4):277–82. https://doi.org/10.1001/jama.1956.02960390027008.

18. Fonouni H, Mehrabi A, Golriz M, Zeier M, Muller-Stich BP, Schemmer P, et al. Comparison of the laparoscopic versus open live donor nephrectomy: an overview of surgical complications and outcome. Langenbeck's Arch Surg/Deutsche Gesellschaft fur Chirurgie. 2014;399(5):543–51. https://doi.org/10.1007/s00423-014-1196-4.

19. Ratner LE, Ciseck LJ, Moore RG, Cigarroa FG, Kaufman HS, Kavoussi LR. Laparoscopic live donor nephrectomy. Transplantation. 1995;60(9):1047–9. https://pubmed.ncbi.nlm.nih.gov/7491680/.

20. Friedman AL, Peters TG, Ratner LE. Regulatory failure contributing to deaths of live kidney donors. Am J Transplant. 2012;12(4):829–34. https://doi.org/10.1111/j.1600-6143.2011.03918.x.

21. Friedman AL, Peters TG, Jones KW, Boulware LE, Ratner LE. Fatal and nonfatal hemorrhagic complications of living kidney donation. Ann Surg. 2006;243(1):126–30. https://doi.org/10.1097/01.sla.0000193841.43474.ec.

22. Serrano OK, Bangdiwala AS, Vock DM, Berglund D, Dunn TB, Finger EB, et al. Defining the tipping point in surgical performance for laparoscopic donor nephrectomy among transplant surgery fellows: a risk-adjusted cumulative summation learning curve analysis. Am J Transplant. 2017;17(7):1868–78. https://doi.org/10.1111/ajt.14187.

23. Wolf JS Jr, Tchetgen MB, Merion RM. Hand-assisted laparoscopic live donor nephrectomy. Urology. 1998;52(5):885–7. https://doi.org/10.1016/s0090-4295(98)00389-6.

24. Kokkinos C, Nanidis T, Antcliffe D, Darzi AW, Tekkis P, Papalois V. Comparison of laparoscopic versus hand-assisted live donor nephrectomy. Transplantation. 2007;83(1):41–7. https://doi.org/10.1097/01.tp.0000248761.56724.9c.

25. Gershbein AB, Fuchs GJ. Hand-assisted and conventional laparoscopic live donor nephrectomy: a comparison of two contemporary techniques. J Endourol. 2002;16(7):509–13. https://doi.org/10.1089/089277902760367476.

26. Choi SW, Kim KS, Kim S, Choi YS, Bae WJ, Hong SH, et al. Hand-assisted and pure laparoscopic living donor nephrectomy: a matched-cohort comparison over 10 yr at a single institute. Clin Transpl. 2014;28(11):1287–93. https://doi.org/10.1111/ctr.12462.

27. Kortram K, Ijzermans JN, Dor FJ. Perioperative events and complications in minimally invasive live donor nephrectomy: a systematic review and meta-analysis. Transplantation. 2016;100(11):2264–75. https://doi.org/10.1097/TP.0000000000001327.

28. Horgan S, Vanuno D, Sileri P, Cicalese L, Benedetti E. Robotic-assisted laparoscopic donor nephrectomy for kidney transplantation. Transplantation. 2002;73(9):1474–9. https://doi.org/10.1097/00007890-200205150-00018.

29. Bhattu AS, Ganpule A, Sabnis RB, Murali V, Mishra S, Desai M. Robot-assisted laparoscopic donor nephrectomy vs standard laparoscopic donor nephrectomy: a prospective randomized comparative study. J Endourol. 2015;29(12):1334–40. https://doi.org/10.1089/end.2015.0213.

30. Rizvi S.J. MPR. Retroperitoneoscopic donor nephrectomy. Desai M. GA, editor. Singapore: Springer; 2017.

31. Barth RN, Phelan MW, Goldschen L, Munivenkatappa RB, Jacobs SC, Bartlett ST, et al. Single-port donor nephrectomy provides improved patient satisfaction and equivalent outcomes. Ann Surg. 2013;257(3):527–33. https://doi.org/10.1097/SLA.0b013e318262ddd6.

32. Stamatakis L, Mercado MA, Choi JM, Sanchez EJ, Gaber AO, Knight RJ, et al. Comparison of laparoendoscopic single site (LESS) and conventional laparoscopic donor nephrectomy at a single institution. BJU Int. 2013;112(2):198–206. https://doi.org/10.1111/j.1464-410X.2012.11763.x.

33. Desai M. Single-port surgery for donor nephrectomy: a new era in laparoscopic surgery? Nat Clin Pract Urol. 2009;6(1):1. https://doi.org/10.1038/ncpuro1278.

34. Pietrabissa A, Abelli M, Spinillo A, Alessiani M, Zonta S, Ticozzelli E, et al. Robotic-assisted laparoscopic donor nephrectomy with transvaginal extraction of the kidney. Am J Transplant. 2010;10(12):2708–11. https://doi.org/10.1111/j.1600-6143.2010.03305.x.

35. Segev DL, Muzaale AD, Caffo BS, Mehta SH, Singer AL, Taranto SE, et al. Perioperative mortality and long-term survival following live kidney donation. JAMA. 2010;303(10):959–66. .

36. Nanidis TG, Antcliffe D, Kokkinos C, Borysiewicz CA, Darzi AW, Tekkis PP, et al. Laparoscopic versus open live donor nephrectomy in renal transplantation: a meta-analysis. Ann Surg. 2008;247(1):58–70. https://doi.org/10.1097/SLA.0b013e318153fd13.
37. Wilson CH, Sanni A, Rix DA, Soomro NA. Laparoscopic versus open nephrectomy for live kidney donors. Cochrane Database Syst Rev. 2011;(11):CD006124. https://doi.org/10.1002/14651858.CD006124.pub2.
38. Yuan H, Liu L, Zheng S, Yang L, Pu C, Wei Q, et al. The safety and efficacy of laparoscopic donor nephrectomy for renal transplantation: an updated meta-analysis. Transplant Proc. 2013;45(1):65–76. https://doi.org/10.1016/j.transproceed.2012.07.152.
39. Dols LF, Kok NF, d'Ancona FC, Klop KW, Tran TC, Langenhuijsen JF, et al. Randomized controlled trial comparing hand-assisted retroperitoneoscopic versus standard laparoscopic donor nephrectomy. Transplantation. 2014;97(2):161–7. https://doi.org/10.1097/TP.0b013e3182a902bd.
40. Klop KW, Kok NF, Dols LF, Dor FJ, Tran KT, Terkivatan T, et al. Can right-sided hand-assisted retroperitoneoscopic donor nephrectomy be advocated above standard laparoscopic donor nephrectomy: a randomized pilot study. Transpl Int. 2014;27(2):162–9. https://doi.org/10.1111/tri.12226.
41. Wang H, Chen R, Li T, Peng L. Robot-assisted laparoscopic vs laparoscopic donor nephrectomy in renal transplantation: a meta-analysis. Clin Transpl. 2019;33(1):e13451. https://doi.org/10.1111/ctr.13451.

Follow-Up Care after Living Kidney Donation

14

Jane Long, Krista L. Lentine, and Macey L. Henderson

Introduction

Based on data collected by the Global Observatory on Donation and Transplantation (GODT), in 2018, more than 34,000 living donor kidney transplantations took place worldwide [1]. According to the Organ Procurement and Transplantation Network (OPTN)/United Network for Organ Sharing (UNOS), more than 160,000 living persons in the United States have donated a kidney since 1988 to help a family member, a friend, or even a stranger [2]. The substantial benefits of living kidney donation from the perspective of the recipient's health are well-established. Living donor (LD) transplantation provides patients with end-stage kidney disease (ESKD) with the best chance of dialysis-free survival compared to dialysis or deceased donor transplantation, at lowest costs to the healthcare system [3–7]. Based on such data, LD transplantation is endorsed as the best treatment option for most patients with chronic kidney failure [8]. Living donors derive no medical benefit from donation, nor do they expect to. However, LDs do deserve robust commitment to high-quality care across all phases of donation including, careful assessment, transparent risk disclosure, and follow-up and support to help ensure optimal long-term post-donation health.

The risks of living donation, in carefully selected candidates, have been accepted to be low enough to justify its practice. However, much of the available evidence has

J. Long · M. L. Henderson (✉)
Division of Transplantation, Department of Surgery, Johns Hopkins School of Medicine, Baltimore, MD, USA
e-mail: jlong32@jhmi.edu; macey@jhmi.edu

K. L. Lentine
Center for Abdominal Transplantation, Division of Nephrology, Saint Louis University School of Medicine, St. Louis, MO, USA
e-mail: krista.lentine@health.slu.edu

© Springer Nature Switzerland AG 2021
K. L. Lentine et al. (eds.), *Living Kidney Donation*,
https://doi.org/10.1007/978-3-030-53618-3_14

303

been limited by issues such as short observation periods, high proportion of donors lost to follow-up, missing or unreported data, insufficient power to quantify rare events, and limited racial diversity [9–11]. Moreover, until recently, most outcomes studies compared donors to the general population who are not screened for donation [12]. Follow-up information on donors' health is critical for understanding the risks and consequences of LD kidney donation [13], supporting donor selection, and providing informed consent and care using the best available information [12, 14]. Importantly, patient-centered engagement in follow-up, risk assessment, and disclosure is also vital to maintaining and supporting trust in the process of living donation and transplantation [13].

A 2011 consensus conference on "Living kidney donor follow-up: state-of-the-art and future directions" articulated the fundamental ethical principles and clinical needs that ground the role of follow-up in supporting the practice of living donation, including: [14]

- The need to provide accurate outcomes information to donor candidates and their recipients as a basis for informed consent, especially regarding trends in outcomes and incremental hazards that may be associated with race/ethnicity, baseline comorbidity, changes in surgical approaches and management strategies.

1. The need to acquire more robust outcomes data to improve the evaluation process and to provide reliable counseling for donor candidates tailored for demographic and health profile.
2. The possibility of identification of individual donor clinical problems through surveillance at a time when intervention is possible.
3. Provision of program-specific feedback to guide quality assurance and performance improvement.
4. Recognition of the professional obligation of the transplant community to continue to collect and monitor information on living donor outcomes.

Elements of Living Donor Follow-up

Medical

Historically, long-term donor morbidity and mortality inferences were drawn from single-center studies with survival estimates based on comparisons to the general population. In the United States, this was in part due to the fact that living donor follow-up (LDF) reporting to the national registry, through the mechanism of the OPTN, was limited in scope and duration. Furthermore, international long-term donor registries were uncommon. Recent advances in acquiring follow-up information through data linkages, recognition of these deficiencies in donor outcomes data, and the vital need to address them, have prompted a growing body of research over the past decade that has helped advance understanding of donor risks [15]. The study methodologies include construction of multicenter cohorts

[16, 17], integration of national donor registries with other data sources to acquire longer-term information for a broader spectrum of outcomes [5, 18–26], and importantly, assembly of healthy nondonor controls for estimation of donation-attributable risks [27–32]. The resulting evidence from these changes suggests small donation-related increases in the risk of kidney failure that have impacted policy requirements and guidelines for informed consent, care, and follow-up of LDs [33, 34].

Upon reviewing physiologic and epidemiologic studies, Cheng and colleagues [35] put forth a "multiple hit" hypothesis that attributes additional insults as the precipitants of elevated risk of kidney disease after donation, in the context of benign course in most kidney donors (Fig. 14.1). Although post-donation kidney disease is uncommon, it likely arises due to either a "first hit" from birth (i.e., Apolipoprotein L1 genotype, low birthweight, etc.) or a "second hit" acquired later in life (i.e., diabetes). Living kidney donation puts donors at higher risk for developing end-stage renal disease compared to similarly healthy nondonors [35]. A modest decrease in glomerular filtration rate (GFR) and greater propensity toward arterial hypertension and albuminuria are the main adverse effects of donation.

Risk differences based on race and gender are also being recognized, and are highly relevant to counseling, care, and follow-up. Higher risks of ESKD and pre-end stage kidney complications in black compared to white donors may be due to

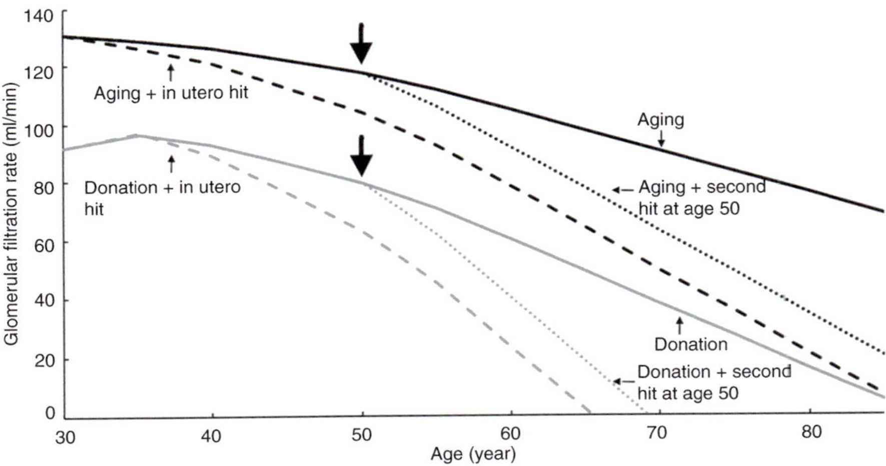

Fig. 14.1 A schematic presentation of the multiple-hit hypothesis of kidney disease progression in LDs. A hypothetical 30-year-old candidate contemplates kidney donation with three possible scenarios: (1) Without donation and with perfect health, glomerular filtration rate (GFR) declines gradually with age (black solid line, adopted from 35). With donation, adaptive compensation keeps GFR at 70% of binephric level (grey solid line). (2) A first hit exists (low birth weight or genetic predisposition), and baseline GFR decline worsens significantly after donation (hashed lines). (3) A medical risk factor develops at age 40 and causes a significant increase in the baseline GFR decline (dotted lines). In scenarios (2) and (3), the donor's time advanced kidney failure (horizontal line) is significant shortened by donation. (From Cheng et al. [35])

incidence of hypertension and diabetes, access to care, and other environmental or genetic factors [5, 18]. Modest rises in uric acid levels early post-donation and a small increase in 8-year incidence of gout have also been reported in donors compared to healthy nondonors [31], and this risk appears higher in black donors [31]. Living donation may also accelerate the rise in blood pressure and need for antihypertensive treatment compared to those who have not donated, especially among black donors with high normal blood pressure readings prior to donating [5, 18, 22, 36, 37]. Donation may also increase the risk of gestational hypertension or pre-eclampsia in post-donation pregnancies [8].

Supported by the "multiple hit hypothesis," all LDs should receive long-term clinical care after donation that focuses on detection, prevention, and management of conditions that are considered a "second hit." These conditions, such as arterial hypertension, diabetes mellitus, and obesity [35] could diminish nephron reserve and increase risks of developing ESKD. As such, follow-up data collected should also include intermediate outcomes such as albuminuria, "second hit" conditions that could affect GFR decline after donation, and terminal endpoints such as death due to ESKD. Over half of surveyed transplant centers agreed that blood pressure, serum creatinine, the development of hypertension, urine protein, and urinalysis are parameters that should be tracked for living kidney donors [13].

Psychosocial and Socioeconomic

Current post-donation follow-up focuses on medical data; however, there is an increased recognition that living donation can have important emotional and psychosocial impacts that should be monitored, and that resources should be developed to support donors with psychosocial complications [38]. A multicenter survey of 231 transplantation programs found that the majority of programs felt that donors' psychologic well-being, disability and employment status, and insurance status should be monitored [13], despite challenges in implementation given the limited scope and duration of current donor follow-up in most jurisdictions. A 2006 systematic review by Clemens et al. [39] combined data for more than 5000 LDs and estimated that 5–23% of donors are affected by depression at an average of 4 years after nephrectomy. Increased rates of depression and exacerbation of preexisting depression have also been reported [40, 41]. In a privately insured group, Lentine et al. [20] found that recipient death and graft loss predict increased depression risk. Post-donation care should consider the impact of recipient outcomes on the psychological health of the donor, and efforts should be made to assess and support the donor after recipient complications. Another factor that should be considered in LDF is the financial implications to LDs, particularly in healthcare systems without national insurance. Currently in the United States, the 6-month, 1-year, and 2-year follow-up required by the OPTN are not allowable as organ acquisition costs on the Medicare Cost Report cannot be billed to the recipient's health insurance claim number [42]. Cost concerns such as lack of insurance is one of the financial barriers reported for limited follow-up [43].

Follow-Up Processes

United States: Policy and Practice

In the United States, more than 5500 individuals become living kidney donors each year. The OPTN maintains a national registry of all organ donors, transplant candidates and recipients in the United States, which includes baseline information on all LDs. In 1999, the OPTN implemented Living Donor Follow-up (LDF) Forms in order to collect 6-month and 1-year follow-up information from LD recovery programs on their LDs. However, the policy did not establish requirements for data completeness [44], which resulted in poor follow-up reporting for many donors. In February 2013, the OPTN/UNOS responded to a Health Resources and Services Administration (HRSA) directive to develop policies regarding LD care [45] that included mandated thresholds for collecting and reporting clinical and laboratory data for LDs at 6 months, 1 year, and 2 years following donation. US transplant programs are now required to report clinical data for at least 80% and laboratory data for 70% of LDs [46]. There is allowance for some missed follow-up to avoid penalties in cases of donors who decline to participate despite the program's efforts. Under the 2013 policy, the LDF forms collect data on nine clinical components (Table 14.1): patient status, income, loss of medical insurance due to donation, recent hospitalizations, kidney-related complications, dialysis, hypertension requiring treatment, diabetes, and cause of death (if applicable) and two laboratory components: serum creatinine and urine protein levels. Donor data must be collected within 60 days of the reporting periods to be considered timely [46].

As recognition of follow-up as part of the donation process, the 2017 Kidney Disease Improving Global Outcomes (KDIGO) Living Donor Guideline recommends that a personalized post-donation care plan be provided before donation to clearly describe recommendations for follow-up care, who the providers of care will be, and how often (Table 14.2) [34]. The KDIGO guidelines also recommend the following be performed at least annually post-donation: blood pressure measurement, body mass index (BMI) measurement, serum creatinine, GFR estimation, and albuminuria measurement. In addition, the guidelines recommend review and promotion of healthy lifestyle including regular exercise, healthy diet, and abstinence from tobacco as well as review and support of psychosocial health and well-being. Acknowledging that donors in many countries report regular follow-up with a primary provider, the guideline notes that donor follow-up and care may be appropriately performed by a primary care provider to preserve convenience for the donor. However, communication of follow-up information back to the transplant program is necessary for centers to be aware of the health status of their donors, to comply with reporting mandates (when applicable), and to direct additional care if needed [34]. Standardized follow-up at serial time points may contribute to more regular follow-up. The guidelines also stress the importance of continued donor education on "health promoting practices" as they recover and age.

According to the guidelines, donors should receive age-appropriate healthcare maintenance. Their clinical conditions and health risk factors should be managed

Table 14.1 Content of post-donation follow-up information collected in existing living donor registries

Registry, Content and Timing of Follow-up

OPTN LDF Form [46]	EULID Registry Data Recommendations [49, 87]	SOL-DHR [55]	ANZADATA Long Term Follow-Up (Yearly)Form [60]	Scandiatransplant Follow-Up Form [59]
Transplant Program Reporting 6 months, 1 year, and 2 years post-donation	• Annual checkups arranged by the donor • 2014 LIDOBS [88] recommendation: short- and long-term donor medical follow-up post-donation • 2014 LIDOBS [88] recommendation: Psychosocial follow-up is mandatory in the short term; long-term follow up for donors with high medical or psychological stress levels	• Follow-up reporting and biennial follow-up questionnaire completed by local family physicians, nephrologist, or transplant center • SF-8 form and social-status questionnaire completed by donor • Lifelong follow-up after donation at 1, 3, 5, 7, and 10 years and then biennially after	• Reporting by the transplant hospital or current treating nephrologist • Annual follow-up	• Transplant program reporting • Lifelong follow-up after donation at 1, 3, 5, 7, and 10 years and then biennially after
Kidney Donor Status and Clinical Information				
Patient status	Date of follow-up, patient status, weight, and height[a]	Body weight	Date of follow-up	Donor number, name, birth number, date of consultation, next follow-up/lost to follow-up, telephone surgery, weeks out of work due to donation, economic loss due to donation
Working for income, and if not working, reason for not working	Blood pressure	Sitting blood pressure (3×)	Follow-up physician	Restitution (overall positive/ negative effect of donation, pain relating to donation)
Loss of medical (health, life) insurance due to donation	GFR	Nephrectomy scar	Vital status	• Complications (late complications or readmissions related to donation, significant intercurrent disease, pregnancy) • Date of death

Has the donor been readmitted since last LDR or LDF form was submitted?	Surgical reintervention	Interim medical history (includes questions on pain and serious health problems, i.e., stroke, diabetes, malignancies)	Date of death	Clinical parameters (height, weight, cholesterol, triglycerides, p-HDL/LDL, anti-lipid drugs, smoking, blood pressure, anti-hypertensive drugs)
Kidney complications	Pain requiring treatment	All drugs currently taken	Cause of death (if applicable)	• Kidney function (laboratory values, eGFR, microalbuminuria) • Diabetes diagnosis
Maintenance dialysis	Would complications requiring treatment	SF-8 Questionnaire +3 supplemental questions (collected every 5 years post-donation)	Medical results: Blood pressure and lab values (see below)	
Donor developed hypertension requiring medication	Psychological complications requiring treatment		Comorbidities at follow-up: • Hypertension • Number of drugs taken • Cigarette smoking • Diabetes • Renal problems • Vascular event	
Diabetes	Hypertension requiring treatment		Pregnancy	
• Cause of death, if applicable and known	• Required transplantation			
Kidney Laboratory Values				
• Serum creatinin • Urine protein	• Serum creatinine • Urine protein	• Urine dipstick • Blood and urine samples	• Serum creatinine • Protein-to-creatinine ratio	• Serum creatinine • Cystatin C

(continued)

Table 14.1 (Continued)

Registry, Content and Timing of Follow-up				
OPTN LDF Form [46]	EULID Registry Data Recommendations [49, 87]	SOL-DHR [55]	ANZADATA Long Term Follow-Up (Yearly)Form [60]	Scandiatransplant Follow-Up Form [59]
				• Urine protein • Urine albumin
Social Status Questionnaire				
		• Professional activity • Working capacity • Efficiency and physical fitness of donor • Open-ended questions (a) Drawbacks because of donation (i.e., financial, insurance, pension, or professional disadvantages) (b) Donor's suggestions for possible improvement of SOL-DHR activities (What can SOL-DHR do better for you?)		

[a]In addition: patient initials, gender, year of birth, donor country of residence, recipient nationality and country of residence, relationship of donor to recipient, and type of donation; *Abbreviations: ANZDATA* Australia and New Zealand Dialysis and Transplant Living Kidney Donor Registry, *eGFR* estimated glomerular filtration rate, *EULID* European Living Donation and Public Health, *LDR* living donor registration, *LDF* living donor follow-up, *OPTN* Organ Procurement and Transplantation Network, *p-HDL* plasma high-density lipoproteins, *p-LDL* plasma low-density lipoproteins, *SF-8* 8-Item Short Form Survey, *SOL-DHR* Swiss Organ Living Donor Health Registry

Table 14.2 Recommendations for routine kidney donor follow-up based on the 2017 KDIGO Living Donor Guideline [34]

Roles and responsibilities
- Transplant societies should publish guidelines to outline clearly the roles and responsibilities of transplant programs and primary care physicians.
- Aim to establish relationship between transplant program and the donor's primary care physician prior to donation and clearly outline each other's roles and responsibilities in follow-up.
- The transplant program should be available as a resource for the donor's primary care physician.
- A personalized follow-up plan should be developed prior to donation for each donor and clearly communicated to the donor and his/her primary care physician.

Follow-up schedule
- Kidney donors should undergo at least annual medical follow-up.
- Personalized follow-up should account for the donor's unique risk profile.
- Female donors who become pregnant should have close follow-up with obstetrics with nephrology involvement, as needed.

Management guidelines
- Adhere to 2012 KDIGO blood pressure guidelines for management of hypertension post-donation.
- Adhere to 2012 KDIGO CKD guidelines for diagnosis and management of decreased eGFR after donation.
- Emphasize prevention and treatment of metabolic risk factors, especially diabetes mellitus and obesity.

Abbreviations: CKD Chronic kidney disease, *eGFR* estimated glomerular filtration rate, *KDIGO* Kidney Disease Improving Global Outcomes

according to clinical practice guidelines for the regional population. Donors should be monitored for chronic kidney disease and those who meet criteria for chronic kidney disease based on estimated GFR should be managed according to the 2012 KDIGO Clinical Practice Guideline for the Evaluation and Management of Chronic Kidney Disease (Fig. 14.2) [34, 47]. Psychosocial metrics such as health-related quality of life (HRQoL) have been recommended to monitor general well-being and to help transplant centers identify donors at risk for poor psychosocial outcomes and could be based on existing test standards (i.e., scores below 0.50 standard deviation of the normative mean of the "Short Form" class of measure, SF-36, 12, or 8) [34]. The 2017 guidelines also stress the importance that the data collected at regular time points should be pertinent, attainable, and not overly burdensome to the donor or transplant center.

International Models of Donor Follow-Up

Long-term follow-up of LDs is successfully achieved in some countries. Over the past two decades, the European Union has funded several projects on living donation. The European Living Donation and Public Health (EULID) project began as an assessment of living donation practices in 11 European nations (Cyprus, France, Italy, Norway, Poland, Portugal, Romania, Slovenia, Spain, Sweden, and the UK) in

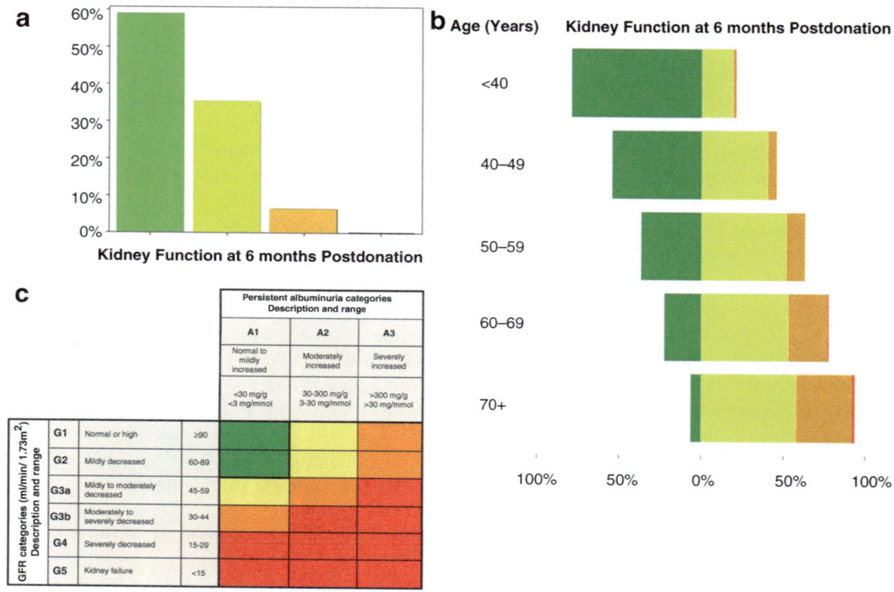

Fig. 14.2 Application of estimated glomerular filtration rate (eGFR)-based chronic kidney disease (CKD) classification to the 6-month serum-creatinine derived eGFR in 25,595 living kidney donors in Scientific Registry Transplant Recipients, without (**a**) and with (**b**) stratification by age at time of donation. The Kidney Disease Improving Global Outcomes classification 2012 is included (**c**) for reference. (From Cheng et al. [35])

regard to legal, ethical, protection and registration in order to create standards and recommendations for LD health and safety. EULID's main objective is to guarantee the health and safety of LDs. The project was co-funded by the European Union (EU) in the framework of the EU Health Programme 2003–2008. Twelve partners from 11 nations worked for 30 months to reach an agreement on statements for protection of LDs [48]. Among the final recommendations included mandatory registration and follow-up data collection [49] for all LDs through a centralized donor database system (Table 14.1), in addition to mandatory regulatory audits at the national and institutional level [50]. Between 2009 and 2012, the European Living Donor Psychosocial Follow-up (ELIPSY) study, co-funded by the European Union (EU) in the framework of the EU Health Programme 2009–2015 [51] and the Executive Agency for Health and Consumers (EAHC), was conducted in seven European countries (Cyprus, France, Germany, Portugal, Spain, Sweden, and Turkey). The study aimed to develop a tools and a common method for all European Union countries to monitor donor long-term psychosocial well-being and quality of life follow-up [14] and used data from the EULID registry of over 1400 registered LDs [51].

Living Donor Observatory (LIDOBS) is a group composed of transplant coordinators, nephrologists, hepatologists, transplant surgeons, physicians, and nurses working in LD focused on improving living donation. The group arose from a EULID project research group and [52] aims to establish a consensus among professions on ethical, legislation, and protection practices of living donation to create a common Living Donor Assessment model [53]. They work to promote an international online LD registry, assess safety of LDs through follow-up surveys, and capture new issues and dilemmas regarding LD [52]. LIDOBS allows for the continuity and application of LD assessment and follow-up surveys developed through EULID and ELIPSY that focus on psychological well-being, quality of life, and social impact. As of 2014, the online database registry had over 1700 LDs with mandatory data from 19 centers in 13 countries from the European Union [53].

The Swiss Organ Living Donor Health Registry (SOL-DHR) was established in 1993 as an integrated care system for monitoring short and long-term donor health and wellness. Six transplant centers have joined SOL-DHR since 1993. The SOL-DHR organizes lifelong follow-up after donation at 1, 3, 5, 7, and 10 years and then biennially after [54]. Living donors are examined by their local family physicians, a nephrologist, or a transplant center [55]. Prior to each follow-up visit, the SOL-DHR center sends the donor a package reminding them to make an appointment with the physician of their choice. The package also contains brief information for the donor and the physician, a health questionnaire, sample tubes for blood and urine, and a prepaid envelope for sending the samples at room temperature to the central laboratory. The basic biennial follow-up questionnaire is completed by the family physician and every 5 years (Table 14.1), the donor completes the additional Eight-Item Short-Form (SF-8) and social-status questionnaire [55]. If there is no response from the donor within 2 months after the follow-up material was sent out, SOL-DHR initiates a search for the donor where they contact the recipient, the donor's health insurance and the public registries to identify whether the donor has died and, if applicable, cause of death. Blood and urine analysis results are sent to the family physician and cohort manager at SOL-DHR [55]. Lifelong follow-up of LDs' health by transplant centers is required by the Swiss Transplant Law. Although donors may choose to stop participating, compliance is promoted by informing donors about the aims of the protocol and the registry before their donation.

Similarly, in Norway, donor follow-up begins at week 3–4, then at month 3, followed by yearly monitoring for 5 years, and then lifelong follow-up every fifth year afterwards. Clinical assessment of donors includes blood pressure, blood tests, and urinalysis examinations performed by local county hospitals. At 1, 5, 10, and 15 years follow-up, 99, 95, 84, and 77% of donors are still seen by local nephrologists, respectively [34, 56].

Follow-up registries of LDs for Denmark, Finland, Iceland, Norway, Sweden, and Estonia is maintained and operated by Scandiatransplant, a collaborative non-profit organ exchange organization. The organization was founded in 1969 and is owned and managed by member transplant hospitals [57]. Follow-up data is collected at 3 months after donation, 1 year after donation, and then every 5 years after donation. The donor consents to these follow-ups and can withdraw at any time [58]. Data is collected on donors' basic information, restitution, complications, risk factors, and kidney function (Table 14.1) [59].

Another program that has collected long-term data on LDs is the Australia and New Zealand Dialysis and Transplant Living Kidney Donor Registry (ANZDATA), which was established in 1977 through the merging of separate dialysis and transplant registries. Since 2004, the ANZDATA Living Kidney Donor Registry has collected data on living kidney donors across Australia and New Zealand [60]. Data are collected via forms for pre-donation assessment, operative data, and annual donor follow-up. Data are collected at baseline and then annually after donation. Baseline data are reported by the transplant hospital and follow-up data are reported either by the transplant hospital or the current treating nephrologist, depending on local practice [61]. Living kidney donor coordinators perform data entry through a web-enabled data entry system [62]. The ANZDATA long-term donor follow-up form collects the following information: date of follow-up; follow-up physician; vital status; date and cause of death, if applicable; blood pressure; renal labs (serum creatinine, protein creatinine ratio, albumin creatinine ratio, other protein measure); comorbidities (hypertension and number of drugs taken, cigarette smoking, diabetes, renal problems, vascular events); and pregnancy (Table 14.1) [60]. In 2020 (through September), 19 transplanting centers reported data on LDs [63].

Challenges To Living Donor Follow-Up

Post-donation follow-up presents logistical and financial challenges for donors as well as transplant programs [13, 43]. Based on US data collected in 2008–2018, prior the 2013 OPTN/UNOS policy revision, Schold [64] and colleagues reported that complete follow-up at 6, 12, and 24 months was 67%, 60%, and 50% for clinical data and 51%, 40%, and 30% for laboratory data; however, follow-up was improving over time. From their model, 30–40% of missing data was explained at the center level, suggesting that the processes and protocols of transplant programs are strongly associated with the success of LDF [64].

Recent data by Henderson et al. in 2017 found that the proportion of living kidney donors with complete and timely 2-year LDF increased from 33% to 54% after the 2013 OPTN/UNOS LDF policy was implemented, and the odds of 2 year complete follow-up increased by 22% per year pre-policy and 23% per year post-policy in an adjusted model [65]. Despite yearly improvements, more than 50% of transplant programs did not meet all policy requirements for 2013 LDs [65].

Some donor characteristics are associated with higher risk of loss to follow-up. Missing or incomplete follow-up data are more common among donors who are younger, of black ethnicity, without health insurance, have lower educational attainment, reside further distances from transplant centers [64], and are unmarried [66]. Nondirected donors, who have no previous connection to their recipient, did not differ from donors with established recipient relationships in likelihood of follow-up. Notably, amongst subgroups of LDs who are at increased risk for loss to follow-up based on sociodemographic traits, nondirected donors are *more* likely to complete follow-up. This may be related to their sense of preparation for donation, connectedness with the medical community, or sense of urgency or commitment regarding their decision to donate, which leads to continued engagement with one's own health and the transplant center post-donation [67]. Non-US citizen/non-US residents who come to the United States for living donation (international donors) are at particularly high risk for loss-to-follow-up [68] and require careful consideration and support to achieve follow-up after return to their home country. These observations can help direct efforts to support and increase LDF, particularly among groups most vulnerable to loss-to-follow-up [66].

Successfully achieving LDF requires planning, commitment, communication, and resources. One of the most commonly reported barriers to LDF is difficulty for donors to return to the transplant centers for medical tests [13, 43]. An early multicenter survey also reported that donors oftentimes did not find a need for follow-up because their health was good (based on reporting by program staff) [43]. Another multicenter survey found that the most common barriers to LDF were the inconvenience of returning for tests and outdated contact information [13]. It may be that some programs failed to utilize strategies to maximize the likelihood of reaching donors at required follow-up time points. More importantly, however, the OPTN/UNOS policy does not specify the location of follow-up, and coordination through a primary care provider can be a useful strategy to preserve donor convenience, especially for donors who live remotely from the transplant center. However, this strategy requires planning and communication in order to be successful. Other reported barriers to LDF include staff resources. Programs cited lack of staff time to follow-up with or locate LDs to conduct ongoing medical assessments of LDs or complete OPTN forms.

Lack of reimbursements to programs for follow-up costs, as well as lack of reimbursement to donors for costs of follow-up testing and additional subsequent medical testing, have also been identified as barriers to LDF in the United States [13]. Although the majority of programs inform potential donors of OPTN/UNOS follow-up requirements, fewer programs have discussions regarding who will be responsible for associated costs or develop plans with donors to achieve follow-up [13].

In April 2016, Centers for Medicare & Medicaid Services (CMS) revised the Provider Reimbursement Manual to specifically exclude the costs of the OPTN/UNOS mandated donor follow-up at 6 months, 1 year, and 2 years from organ acquisition and to disallow billing these services to the recipient's insurance [42]. Recovering the costs of mandated follow-up is complicated and likely varies by transplant program. Currently, there is no formal mechanism to reimburse donors or programs for the costs of complying with this follow-up mandate. Variation in practice across programs regarding interpretation and use of the CMS cost report, as well as access to other resources, can dramatically impact costs passed on to donors [69, 70]. Although donor follow-up and care may be appropriately performed by a primary care provider for the convenience of the donor, this generally requires donors to use their own insurance (which may incur copayments). Thus, options for covering the costs of follow-up include: [71]

1. Billing the non-Medicare beneficiary recipient's insurance. These costs can also be included in the fee that is charged to commercial payers if not explicitly excluded by contract.
2. Covering the costs with institutional or charitable funds at the transplant program [72]. For example, the Yale Center of Living Organ Donors recently described their new integrated follow-up initiative that partners with their hospital to pay the costs of a complete metabolic panel and spot urine protein ($14 per donor) [73].
3. Allowancing donor costs at the transplant program level and deeming them "uncollectable or un-reimbursable" but necessary expenses to comply with a regulatory mandate.
4. Billing the donor or donor's insurance (for service either at the program or with a primary care physician). Notably, even since the passage of the Affordable Care Act, approximately 9% of US living kidney donors lack health insurance. As such, some donors may be paying full costs for this follow-up or simply not complying [74].

LDF might be improved if mechanisms were developed for systematic reimbursement of costs for all donors, regardless of recipient or donor insurance status [13].

International models aiming to address long-term LDF also face limitations to long-term participation, with cited barriers including distance and expense. SOL-HR has, thus far, been a successful program that has provided data on post-donation incidence of hypertension and microalbuminuria [75]. With government-mandated coverage of biennial medical follow-up testing, as well as a funded central donor registry, 10 year follow-up data were complete only for 74% of LDs. Missing follow-up data was attributed to donors frequently living far from transplant center or donors who regarded themselves as healthy without needing regular medical checkups. Similar to challenges faced by some other registries, completeness in the ANZDATA registry is limited by lack of formal audit mechanism to reinforce data collection [60].

Additional Considerations

Though there is consensus on the importance of program compliance with LDF, the impact of these mandates should also be considered [64] and examined to avoid unintended consequences [76–80] due to regulatory oversight. For instance, a potential consequence may be the generation of disincentives for programs to accept donors that are at higher risk of loss to follow-up [64]. However, beyond concern for mandates, programs may be genuinely concerned for the well-being of a donor who they anticipate will be difficult to follow. Respect for donor autonomy in the case of informed decisions to discontinue follow-up is debated [64], but importantly, the OPTN/UNOS follow-up thresholds were established at less than 100% to recognize that some donors may choose not to participate despite appropriate efforts by the transplant program.

Ongoing Efforts and Strategies

The KDIGO 2017 Clinical Practice Guideline on the Evaluation and Care of Living Kidney Donors [34] provided the following research recommendations:

- Develop communication and integrated care models to:
  1. Examine electronic tools such as websites or portals to maintain contact with donors, facilitate data collection, and provide messaging to disseminate educational information to donors [43].
  2. Formulate strategies for using interinstitution-compatible electronic medical records to facilitate transmission of donor follow-up information, such as clinical data from care encounters, directly to national registries [9].
  3. Formulate and assess the outcomes of center-based initiatives to provide long-term donor follow-up and support through integrated laboratory and clinical monitoring, expansion of preventive health strategies, and fostering of peer education through social support networks between past, current, and future donors [73].

- Establish, improve, and integrate national/international donor registries to facilitate capture and analysis of long-term outcomes information for large representative samples of LDs to:
  1. Address knowledge gaps related to the long-term consequences of donation
  2. Provide data to inform donor selection criteria
  3. Support quality assurance and program improvement at transplant centers
  4. Sustain and strengthen public confidence in the practice of living donation [9, 14].

- Develop HRQoL metric thresholds to identify the presence of impairment in post-donation psychosocial well-being, warranting closer attention by the clinician.
- Improve and assess the efficacy of educational resources to promote sustained healthy lifestyle choices and behaviors, and participation in regular post-donation follow-up and care, such as via newsletters, links to transplant center health recommendations, or national guideline website documents.
- Develop and assess strategies for communicating new information that differs from what a donor was told before donation, to past donors and their physicians.

Currently, there are numerous ongoing collaborative efforts and strategies amongst donors, transplant centers, primary care providers and family physicians, as well as policy makers to improve LDF.

Living Donor Collective

Under contract with the HRSA, the Scientific Registry of Transplant Recipients (SRTR) is piloting a national Scientific Registry for Living Donors where participating transplant programs register all potential LD candidates evaluated at their center [81]. For the pilot, SRTR recruited 16 (10 kidney and 6 liver) transplant programs, with the ultimate aim of including all transplant programs in the United States [82]. After registration by the center, the SRTR plans to perform lifelong follow-up in several areas including medical health, labs, as well as measure of psychosocial well-being (e.g., quality of life, insurance problems). Mechanism of data collection will include direct donor contacts for administration of a brief survey instrument approximately 1 year after donation or after determination of non-donation and approximately every 1–2 years afterwards, as well as data linkages. Focused surveys will address specific complications of interest such as preeclampsia [82]. The pilot will allow SRTR exploring the logistics of enrolling LD candidates, regardless of whether they donate, and a transition from program-based follow-up reporting to a national registry accomplished through government funding [81]. Once the pilot phase is completed by the end of 2020, additional centers will be added over the subsequent 2 years [83].

Novel Technological Strategies for Patient Reporting

Novel smartphone-based mobile health (mHealth) technologies are also being developed that may help reduce the burden of living kidney donor follow-up for both follow-up centers as well as donors. These technologies may help transplant programs meet federal data collection and reporting requirements. A single-center survey study by Eno et al. [84] found that smartphone ownership was high among LDs and that more than 70% of surveyed smartphone-owning donors felt it would be useful to complete their required follow-up with an mHealth tool. These findings of high interest in mHealth technology among LDs was consistent with prior single-center studies of transplant recipients and candidates that found positive attitudes toward mHealth for monitoring and managing medical regimens [85] and increasing physical activity [86].

Currently, mHealth is being applied to LDF in a pilot randomized control trial of the mKidney system® (Fig. 14.3) that was developed by researchers at Johns Hopkins University. This pilot trial will evaluate the impact of the mKidney system® on rates of living kidney donor (LKD) and hospital compliance with OPTN-mandated LKD follow-up at a large volume living kidney donor program (the Texas Transplant Institute in San Antonio, Texas). The results of the trial will provide valuable information on strategies for implementing such a system in a clinical setting and inform effect sizes for future RCT sample size calculations. Should a system such as mKidney® be deemed useful to donors and transplant centers, it could vastly improve the ability for submission and reporting of LDF data.

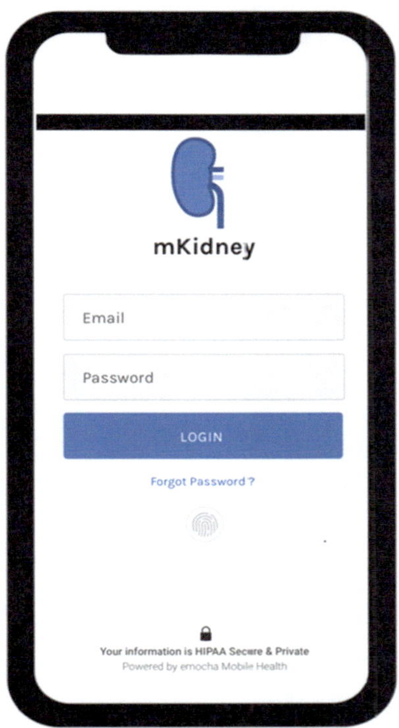

Fig. 14.3 Homescreen for mKidney system,® an mHealth technology developed by researchers at Johns Hopkins University to facilitate compliance with OPTN-mandated donor follow-up. The results of the mKidney pilot trial will provide valuable information on strategies for implementing such a system in the clinical setting and inform effect sizes for future RCT sample size calculations. Should a system such as mKidney® be deemed useful to donors and transplant centers, it could improve the ability for submission and reporting of LDF data

Transplant Center-Based Initiatives

Center-based initiatives that provide long-term donor follow-up and support through integrated laboratory and clinical monitoring, expansion of preventive health strategies, and social networks between past, current, and future donors are currently being piloted [73]. A single-center study suggests that initiatives with dedicated resources towards improving transplant program reporting compliance as well patient compliance with post-donation follow-up, associated factors, and overall financial costs of the transplant, is financially feasible and leads to more accurate and complete follow-up [72].

The Living Donor initiative developed by the Yale-New Haven Hospital was founded on a joint recognition by their transplant team and hospital leadership regarding the importance of supporting the long-term welfare of LDs in order to expand LD transplantation. The priorities of the program include: (1) providing long-term follow-up and monitoring for living organ donors to facilitate preventive health measures; (2) addressing and preempting any unanticipated clinical and

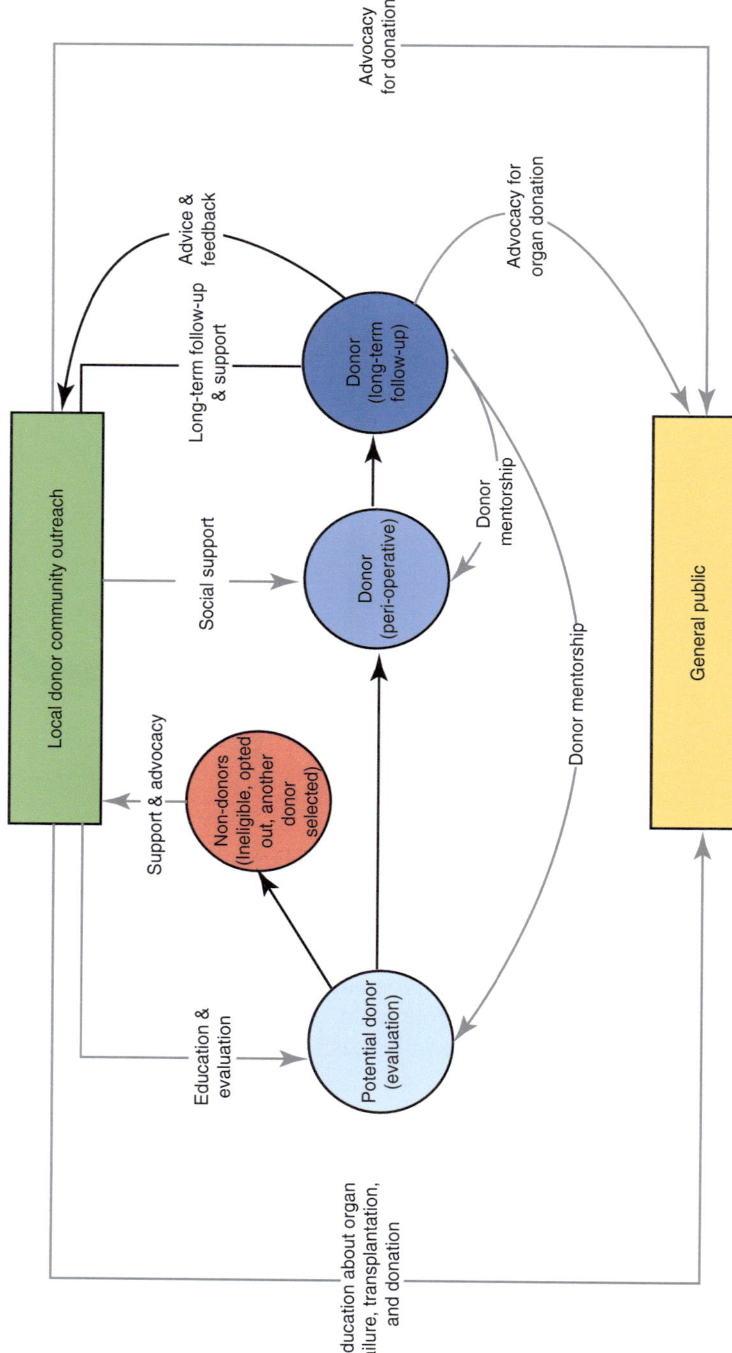

Fig. 14.4 Schematic representation of donor outreach and donor community development. Engagement through local outreach efforts is the basis for providing long-term donor follow-up, peer support, and community-based education on the importance and realities of living donation. (From Kulkarni et al. [73])

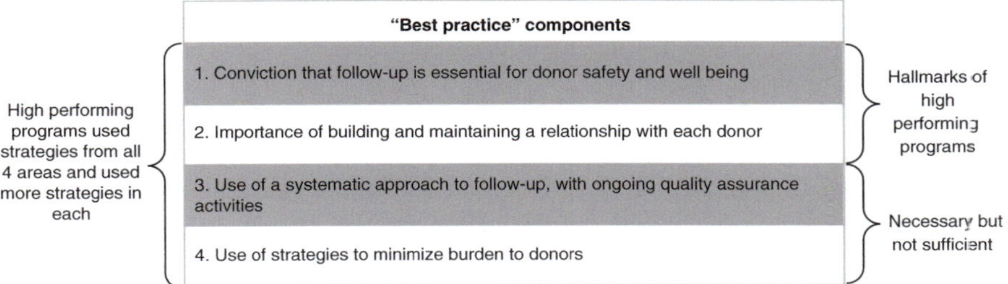

Fig. 14.5 Categories of best practice factors for LDF, based on the OPTN's "best practices" components [44]. Although the specific strategies utilized by any given program vary, all high-performing programs had developed and implemented core activities that reflect all four of the components

psychological risks associated with living organ donation; (3) engaging living organ donors in the creation of a social architecture that will support prior and future LDs; and (4) raising local public awareness of the importance and realities of living organ donation directed at potential new donors. The initiative also aims to address donor and center factors that contribute to lack of long-term follow-up. Their ultimate goal is to develop local LD community networks through social engagement, which will serve as a platform for greater population education on the importance of living donation (Fig. 14.4) [73].

OPTN/UNOS "Toolbox" Recommendations

To help LD programs succeed in achieving LDF, the OPTN/UNOS Living Donor Committee has developed a "toolbox" of recommendations to assist programs in attaining higher rates of successful follow-up with their LDs. The resource consists of suggestions intended for transplant programs' voluntary use and is meant to help programs to review, discuss, and generate ideas to develop their own strategies for follow-up. Key themes were identified based on semi-structured interviews with staff at 50 transplant programs [44], including those with high and low success rates in achieving LDF. Foundation of "best practice" at high-performing programs included: (1) conviction that follow-up is essential for donor safety and well-being; (2) importance of building and maintaining a relationship with each donor; (3) use of a systematic approach to follow-up, with ongoing quality assurance activities; (4) use of strategies to minimize burden to donors (Fig. 14.5).

Conclusions

Understanding the long-term medical outcomes as well as the psychosocial and socioeconomic impact of living donation is critical to ensuring the health and safety of current and future LDs. There have been mandates and recommendations made in the United States, as well as internationally, to improve LD follow-up practices that have achieved varying levels of success in terms of completeness of data collected. To improve LD follow-up, it is necessary to understand and address the logistical and financial challenges and barriers that donors and transplant centers face in trying to achieve long-term follow-up. Ongoing efforts and strategies to reduce the burden of LD follow-up for centers and donors in addition to strategies and center-based initiatives that prioritize and dedicate resources to LD follow-up may lead to more accurate and complete follow-up.

References

1. World Health Organization (WHO)- Organización Nacional de Trasplantes (ONT). Global Observatory on Donation and Transplantation (GODT). Available at: http://www.transplant-observatory.org/. Accessed: 7 Sept 2020.
2. Organ Procurement and Transplantation Network (OPTN). Transplants by Donor Type. National Data. Available at: https://optn.transplant.hrsa.gov/data/view-data-reports/national-data/#. Accessed: 7 Sept 2020.
3. Hart A, Lentine KL, Smith JM, Miller JM, Skeans MA, Prentice M, et al. OPTN/SRTR 2019 Annual Data Report: Kidney. Am J Transplant. 2021;21(Suppl 2):21–137. https://doi.org/10.1111/ajt.16502.
4. United States Renal Data System (USRDS) 2018 Annual Data Report. End-stage Renal Disease (ESRD) in the United States. Chapter 6. Transplantation. Available at: https://www.usrds.org/annual-data-report/. Accessed: 7 Sept 2020.
5. Lentine KL, Schnitzler MA, Xiao H, Axelrod D, Garg AX, Tuttle-Newhall JE, et al. Consistency of racial variation in medical outcomes among publicly and privately insured living kidney donors. Transplantation. 2014;97(3):316–24. https://doi.org/10.1097/01.TP.0000436731.23554.5e.
6. Chang P, Gill J, Dong J, Rose C, Yan H, Landsbeg D, et al. Living donor age and kidney allograft half-life: implications for living donor paired exchange programs. Clin J Am Soc Nephrol. 2012;7(5):835–41. https://doi.org/10.2215/cjn.09990911.
7. Axelrod DA, Schnitzler MA, Xiao H, Irish W, Tuttle-Newhall E, Chang SH, et al. An economic assessment of contemporary kidney transplant practice. Am J Transplant. 2018;18(5):1168–76. https://doi.org/10.1111/ajt.14702.
8. Lapointe Rudow D, Hays R, Baliga P, Cohen DJ, Cooper M, Danovitch GM, et al. Consensus conference on best practices in live kidney donation: recommendations to optimize education, access, and care. Am J Transplant. 2015;15(4):914–22. https://doi.org/10.1111/ajt.13173.
9. Ommen ES, LaPointe Rudow D, Medapalli RK, Schröppel B, Murphy B. When good intentions are not enough: obtaining follow-up data in living kidney donors. Am J Transplant. 2011;11(12):2575–81. https://doi.org/10.1111/j.1600-6143.2011.03815.x.
10. Lentine KL, Patel A. Risks and outcomes of living donation. Adv Chronic Kidney Dis. 2012;19(4):220–8. https://doi.org/10.1053/j.ackd.2011.09.005.
11. Lentine KL, Segev DL. Health outcomes among non-Caucasian living kidney donors: knowns and unknowns. Transpl Int. 2013;26(9):853–64. https://doi.org/10.1111/tri.12088.
12. Davis CL. Living kidney Donor follow-up: state-of-the-art and future directions. Adv Chronic Kidney Dis. 2012;19(4):207–11. https://doi.org/10.1053/j.ackd.2012.03.002.
13. Waterman AD, Dew MA, Davis CL, McCabe M, Wainright JL, Forland CL, et al. Living-donor follow-up attitudes and practices in U.S. kidney and liver donor programs. Transplantation. 2013;95(6):883–8. https://doi.org/10.1097/tp.0b013e31828279fd.
14. Leichtman A, Abecassis M, Barr M, Charlton M, Cohen D, Confer D, et al. Living kidney donor follow-up: state-of-the-art and future directions, conference summary and recommendations. Am J Transplant. 2011;11(12):2561–8. https://doi.org/10.1111/j.1600-6143.2011.03816.x.
15. Lentine KL, Segev DL. Understanding and communicating medical risks for living kidney donors: a matter of perspective. J Am Soc Nephrol. 2017;28(1):12–24. https://doi.org/10.1681/asn.2016050571.

16. Gross CR, Messersmith EE, Hong BA, Jowsey SG, Jacobs C, Gillespie BW, et al. Health-related quality of life in kidney donors from the last five decades: results from the RELIVE study. Am J Transplant. 2013;13(11):2924–34. https://doi.org/10.1111/ajt.12434.
17. Clemens K, Boudville N, Dew MA, Geddes C, Gill JS, Jassal V, et al. The long-term quality of life of living kidney donors: a multicenter cohort study. Am J Transplant. 2011;11(3):463–9. https://doi.org/10.1111/j.1600-6143.2010.03424.x.
18. Lentine KL, Schnitzler MA, Xiao H, Saab G, Salvalaggio PR, Axelrod D, et al. Racial variation in medical outcomes among living kidney donors. N Engl J Med. 2010;363(8):724–32. https://doi.org/10.1056/nejmoa1000950.
19. Lentine KL, Schnitzler MA, Xiao H, Davis CL, Axelrod D, Abbott KC, et al. Associations of recipient illness history with hypertension and diabetes after living kidney donation. Transplantation. 2011;91(11):1227–32. https://doi.org/10.1097/tp.0b013e31821a1ae2.
20. Lentine KL, Schnitzler MA, Xiao H, Axelrod D, Davis CL, McCabe M, et al. Depression diagnoses after living kidney donation. Transp J. 2012;94(1):77–83. https://doi.org/10.1097/tp.0b013e318253f1bc.
21. Lentine KL, Vijayan A, Xiao H, Schnitzler MA, Davis CL, Garg AX, et al. Cancer diagnoses after living kidney donation: linking U.S. Registry data and administrative claims. Transplantation. 2012;94(2):139–44. https://doi.org/10.1097/tp.0b013e318254757d.
22. Lentine KL, Schnitzler MA, Garg AX, Xiao H, Axelrod D, Tuttle-Newhall JE, et al. Understanding antihypertensive medication use after living kidney donation through linked national registry and pharmacy claims data. Am J Nephrol. 2014;40(2):174–83. https://doi.org/10.1159/000365157.
23. Lentine KL, Lam NN, Schnitzler MA, Garg AX, Xiao H, Leander SE, et al. Gender differences in use of prescription narcotic medications among living kidney donors. Clin Transpl. 2015;29(10):927–37. https://doi.org/10.1111/ctr.12599.
24. Lentine KL, Schnitzler MA, Garg AX, Xiao H, Axelrod D, Tuttle-Newhall JE, et al. Race, relationship and renal diagnoses after living kidney donation. Transplantation. 2015;99(8):1723–9. https://doi.org/10.1097/tp.0000000000000733.
25. Lentine KL, Lam NN, Axelrod D, Schnitzler MA, Garg AX, Xiao H, et al. Perioperative complications after living kidney donation: a National Study. Am J Transplant. 2016;16(6):1848–57. https://doi.org/10.1111/ajt.13687.
26. Lentine KL, Lam NN, Schnitzler MA, Hess GP, Kasiske BL, Xiao H, et al. Predonation prescription opioid use: a novel risk factor for readmission after living kidney donation. Am J Transplant. 2017;17(3):744–53. https://doi.org/10.1111/ajt.14033.
27. Segev DK, Muzaale AD, Caffo BS, Mehta SH, Singer AI, Taranto SE, et al. Perioperative mortality and long-term survival following live kidney donation. JAMA J Am Med Assoc. 2010;303(10):959–66. https://doi.org/10.1001/jama.2010.237.
28. Muzaale AD, Massie AB, Wang M-C, Montgomery RA, McBride MA, Wainright JL, et al. Risk of end-stage renal disease following live kidney donation. JAMA. 2014;311(6):579–86. https://doi.org/10.1001/jama.2013.285141.
29. Mjøen G, Hallan S, Hartmann A, Foss A, Midtvedt K, Øyen O, et al. Long-term risks for kidney donors. N Engl J MED. 2014;86(1):162–7. https://doi.org/10.1038/ki.2013.460.
30. Garg AX, McArthur E, Lentine KL. Gestational hypertension and preeclampsia in living kidney donors. N Engl J MED. 2015;372(15);1469–70. https://doi.org/10.1056/nejmc1501450.
31. Lam NN, McArthur E, Kim SJ, Prasad GVR, Lentine KL, Reese PP, et al. Gout after living kidney donation: a matched cohort study. Am J Kidney Dis. 2015;65(6):925–32. https://doi.org/10.1053/j.ajkd.2015.01.017.
32. Lam N, Huang A, Feldman LS, Gill JS, Karpinski M, Kim J, et al. Acute dialysis risk in living kidney donors. Nephrol Dial Transplant. 2012;27(8):3291–5. https://doi.org/10.1093/ndt/gfr802.
33. Organ Procurement and Transplantation Network (OPTN) / United Network for Organ Sharing (UNOS). Policy 14: Living Donation. Available at: https://optn.transplant.hrsa.gov/governance/policies/. Accessed: 7 Sept 2020.
34. Lentine KL, Kasiske BL, Levey AS, Adams PL, Alberú J, Bakr MA, et al. KDIGO clinical practice guideline on the evaluation and care of living kidney donors. Transplantation. 2017;101(8S Suppl 1):S1–S109. https://doi.org/10.1097/TP.0000000000001769.

35. Cheng XS, Glassock RJ, Lentine KL, Chertow GM, Tan JC. Donation, not disease! A multiple-hit hypothesis on development of post-donation kidney disease. Curr Trans Rep. 2017;4(4):320–6. https://doi.org/10.1007/s40472-017-0171-8.
36. Boudville N , Ramesh Prasad GV, Knoll G, et al. Meta-analysis: risk for hypertension in living kidney donors. Ann Intern Med. 2006;145(3):185–96. https://doi.org/10.7326/0003-4819-145-3-200608010-00006.
37. Garg AX, Meirambayeva A, Huang A, Kim J, Prasad GVR, Knoll G, et al. Cardiovascular disease in kidney donors: matched cohort study. BMJ. 2012;344;e1203. https://doi.org/10.1136/bmj.e1203.
38. Allen MB, Abt PL, Reese PP. What are the harms of refusing to allow living kidney donation? An expanded view of risks and benefits. Am J Transplant. 2014;14(3):531–7. https://doi.org/10.1111/ajt.12599.
39. Clemens KK, Thiessen-Philbrook H, Parikh CR, Yang RC, Karley ML, Boudville N, et al. Psychosocial health of living kidney donors: a systematic review. Am J Transplant. 2006;6(12):2965–77. https://doi.org/10.1111/j.1600-6143.2006.01567.x.
40. Hassanzadeh J, Hashiani AA, Ragaeefard A, Salahi H, Khedmati E, Kakaei F, et al. Long-term survival of living donor renal transplants: a single center study. Indian J Nephrol. 2010;20(4):179–84. https://doi.org/10.4103/0971-4065.73439.
41. Minz M, Udgiri N, Sharma A, Heer MK, Kashyap R, Nehra R, et al. Prospective psychosocial evaluation of related kidney donors: Indian perspective. Transplant Proc. 2005;37(5):2001–3. https://doi.org/10.1016/j.transproceed.2005.03.110.
42. Center for Medicare & Medicaid Studies (CMS). Provider Reimbursement Manual (PRM). CMS Pub. 15–1, Chapter 31: Section 3106. Available at: https://www.cms.gov/Regulations-and-Guidance/Guidance/Manuals/Paper-Based-Manuals-Items/CMS021929.html Accessed: 7 Sept 2020.
43. Mandelbrot DA, Pavlakis M, Karp SJ, Johnson SR, Hanto DW, Rodrigue JR. Practices and barriers in long-term living kidney donor follow-up: a survey of U.S. transplant centers. Transplantation. 2009;88(7):855–60. https://doi.org/10.1097/tp.0b013e3181b6dfb9.
44. Organ Procurement and Transplantation Network (OPTN). Procedures to collect post-donation follow-up data from living donors. Available at: https://optn.transplant.hrsa.gov/resources/guidance/procedures-to-collect-post-donation-follow-up-data-from-living-donors/. Accessed: 7 Sept 2020.
45. Department of Health and Human Resources. Response to Solicitation on Organ Procurement and Transplantation Network (OPTN) Living Donor Guidelines. In: Federal Register, vol. 71(116): Government Publishing Office; 2006. p. 34946–8.
46. Organ Procurement and Transplantation Network (OPTN) / United Network for Organ Sharing (UNOS). Policy 18: Data Submission Requirements. Available at: https://optn.transplant.hrsa.gov/governance/policies/. Accessed: 7 Sept 2020.
47. Kidney Disease: Improving Global Outcomes (KDIGO) CKD Work Group. KDIGO 2012 Clinical Practice Guideline for the Evaluation and Management of Chronic Kidney Disease. Kidney Int Suppl. 2013;3(1):1–150.
48. Euro Living Donor (EULID). What is Eulid? Available at: https://www.eulivingdonor.eu/eulid/what-is-eulid.html. Accessed: 7 Sept 2020.
49. Euro Living Donor (EULID). Informative Leaflet to the Public About Living Donation. Available at: http://www.eulivingdonor.eu/media/upload/arxius/eulid-leaflet/Leaflet%20eng.pdf. Accessed: 7 Sept 2020.
50. Manyalich M, et al. EULID project: European living donation and public health. Transplant Proc. 2009;41:2021–4.
51. Euro Living Donor Psychosocial Follow-Up (ELIPSY). Available at: http://www.eulivingdonor.eu/elipsy/. Accessed: 7 Sept 2020.
52. Living Donor Observatory (LIDOBS): Background and motivation. Available at: http://www.eulivingdonor.eu/lidobs/background-motivation.html. Accessed: 7 Sept 2020.
53. Vidal MM, et al. Living Donor Observatory: LIDOBS Community.- Abstract #B1225. Transplantation. 2014;98:835.

54. Thiel GT, Nolte C, Tsinalis D. The Swiss Living Donor Health Registry (SOL-DHR). Ther Umschau. 2005;62(7):449–57. https://doi.org/10.1024/0040-5930.62.7.449.
55. Thiel GT, Nolte C, Tsinalis D. Prospective Swiss cohort study of living-kidney donors: study protocol. BMJ Open. 2011;1(2);e000202. https://doi.org/10.1136/bmjopen-2011-000202.
56. Lentine KL, Vella J. Kidney transplantation in adults: Evaluation of the living kidney donor candidate. Follow-up after kidney donation. Available at: http://www.UptoDate.com. Accessed: 7 Sept 2020.
57. Scandiatransplant. Articles of Association for Foreningen Scandiatransplant. Available at: http://www.scandiatransplant.org/about-scandiatransplant/organisation/ARTICLESOFASSOCIATION_amended9.May2019Aarhus.pdf. Accessed: 7 Sept 2020.
58. Jørgensen K. A. Personal Correspondence: Kaj Anker Jørgensen, MD. 2019
59. Scandiatransplant. Living Donor Database. Available at: http://www.scandiatransplant.org/organ-allocation/LD_kidney_jan_2018.pdf. Accessed: 7 Sept 2020.
60. Australia and New Zealand Dialysis and Transplant Registry (ANZDATA). Data definitions. Available at: https://www.anzdata.org.au/anzdata/services/data-management/data-definitions/. Accessed: 7 Sept 2020.
61. Clayton PA, Saunders JR, McDonald SP, Allen RDM, Pilmore H, Saunder A, et al. Risk-factor profile of living kidney donors: The Australia and New Zealand dialysis and transplant living kidney donor registry 2004–2012. Transplantation. 2016;100(6):1278–83. https://doi.org/10.1097/tp.0000000000000877.
62. Australia and New Zealand Dialysis and Transplant Registry (ANZDATA). Living Kidney Donation: Data Collection. Available at: https://www.anzdata.org.au/anzlkd/data-collection/. Accessed: 7 Sept 2020.
63. Australia and New Zealand Dialysis and Transplant Registry (ANZDATA). Monthly Report on Living Kidney Donation in Australia: Available at: https://www.anzdata.org.au/report/anzlkd-monthly-activity-report-july-2020-australia/. Accessed: 7 Sept 2020.
64. Schold JD, Buccini LD, Rodrrigue JR, Mandelbrot D, Goldfarb DA, Flechner SM, et al. Critical factors associated with missing follow-up data for living kidney donors in the United States. Am J Transplant. 2015;15(9):2394–403. https://doi.org/10.1111/ajt.13282.
65. Henderson ML, Thomas AG, Shaffer A, Massie AB, Luo X, Holscher CM, et al. The national landscape of living kidney donor follow-up in the United States. Am J Transplant. 2017;17(12):3131–40. https://doi.org/10.1111/ajt.14356.
66. Reed RD, Shelton BA, Maclennan PA, Sawinski DL, Locke JE. Living kidney donor pheno-type and likelihood of postdonation follow-up. Transplantation. 2018;102(1):135–9. https://doi.org/10.1097/tp.0000000000001881.
67. Tong A, Craig JC, Wong G, Morton J, Armstrong S, Schollum J, et al. 'It was just an unconditional gift.' Self reflections of non-directed living kidney donors. Clin Transpl. 2012;26(4):589–99. https://doi.org/10.1111/j.1399-0012.2011.01578.x.
68. Al Ammary F, Thomas AG, Massie AB, Muzaale AD, Shaffer AA, Koons B, et al. The landscape of international living kidney donation in the United States. Am J Transplant. 2019;19(7);2009–19. https://doi.org/10.1111/ajt.15256.
69. LaPointe Rudow D, Cohen D. Practical approaches to mitigating economic barriers to living kidney donation for patients and programs. Curr Trans Rep. 2017;4:24–31.
70. Tushla L, Rudow DL, Milton J, Rodrigue JR, Schold JD, Hays R. Living-donor kidney transplantation: reducing financial barriers to live kidney donation— recommendations from a consensus conference. Clin J Am Soc Nephrol. 2015;10(9):1696–702. https://doi.org/10.2215/cjn.01000115.
71. Tietjen A, Hays R, McNatt G, Howey R, Lebron-Banks U, Thomas CP, et al. Billing for living donor care: balancing cost recovery, regulatory compliance, and minimized donor burden. Curr Trans Rep. 2019:6(2);155–66. https://doi.org/10.1007/s40472-019-00239-0.
72. Keshvani N, Feurer ID, Rumbaugh E, Dreher A, Zavala E, Stanley M, et al. Evaluating the impact of performance improvement initiatives on transplant center reporting compliance and patient follow-up after living kidney donation. Am J Transplant. 2015;15(8):2126–35. https://doi.org/10.1111/ajt.13265.

73. Kulkarni S, Thiessen C, Formica RN, Schilsky M, Mulligan D, D'Aquila R. The long-term follow-up and support for living organ donors: a center-based initiative founded on developing a community of living donors. Am J Transplant. 2016;16(12):3385–91. https://doi.org/10.1111/ajt.14005.
74. Rodrigue JR, Fleishman A. Health insurance trends in United States living kidney donors (2004 to 2015). Am J Transplant. 2016;16(12):3504–11. https://doi.org/10.1111/ajt.13827.
75. Thiel GT, Nolte C, Tsinalis D, Steiger J, Bachmann LM. Investigating kidney donation as a risk factor for hypertension and microalbuminuria: findings from the swiss prospective follow-up of living kidney donors. BMJ Open. 2016;6(3):e010869. https://doi.org/10.1136/bmjopen-2015-010869.
76. Abecassis MM, Burke R, Klintmalm GB, Matas AJ, Merion RM, Millman D, et al. American Society of Transplant Surgeons Transplant Center outcomes requirements – a threat to innovation. Am J Transplant. 2009;9(6):1279–86. https://doi.org/10.1111/j.1600-6143.2009.02606.x.
77. Axelrod DA. Balancing accountable care with risk aversion: transplantation as a model. Am J Transplant. 2013;13(1):7–8. https://doi.org/10.1111/j.1600-6143.2012.04346.x.
78. Schold J, Arrington C, Levine G. Significant alterations in reported clinical practice associated with increased oversight of organ transplant center performance. Prog Transplant. 2010;20(3):279–87. https://doi.org/10.7182/prtr.20.3.bj6mh237p6912251.
79. Schold JD, Buccini LD, Srinivas TR, Srinivas RT, Poggio ED, Flechner SM, et al. The association of center performance evaluations and kidney transplant volume in the United States. Am J Transplant. 2013;13(1):67–75. https://doi.org/10.1111/j.1600-6143.2012.04345.x.
80. White SL, Zinsser DM, Paul M, Levine GN, Shearon T, Ashby VB, et al. Patient selection and volume in the era surrounding implementation of medicare conditions of participation for transplant programs. Health Serv Res. 2015;50(2):330–50. https://doi.org/10.1111/1475-6773.12188.
81. Scientific Registry of Transplant Recipients (SRTR). The Living Donor Collective: SRTR to Launch a Pilot Project to Create a Registry of Living Donors. Press Releases & Announcements. Posted: 21 Dec 2016. Available at: https://www.srtr.org/news-media/news/news-items/news#ldc. Accessed: 7 Sept 2020.
82. Kasiske BL, Asrani SK, Dew MA, Henderson ML, Henrich C, Humar A, et al. The living donor collective: a scientific registry for living donors. Am J Transplant. 2017;17(12):3040–8. https://doi.org/10.1111/ajt.14365.
83. Living Donor Collective. About us: pilot program. Living donor collective. 2019.
84. Eno AK, Thomas AG, Ruck JM, Rasmussen SEVP, Halpern SE, Waldram MM, et al. Assessing the attitudes and perceptions regarding the use of mobile health technologies for living kidney donor follow-up: survey study. J Med Internet Res. 2018;6(10):e11192. https://doi.org/10.2196/11192.
85. Mcgillicuddy JW, Weiland AK, Frenzel RM, Mueller M, Brunner-Jackson BM, Taber DJ, et al. Patient attitudes toward mobile phone-based health monitoring: questionnaire study among kidney transplant recipients. J Med Internet Res. 2013;15(1):1–10. https://doi.org/10.2196/jmir.2284.
86. Sieverdes JC, Raynor PA, Armstrong T, Jenkins CH, Sox LR, Treiber FA. Attitudes and perceptions of patients on the kidney transplant waiting list toward mobile health-delivered physical activity programs. Prog Transplant. 2015;25(1):26–34. https://doi.org/10.7182/pit2015884.
87. Euro Living Donor (EULID). Results. Available at: http://www.eulivingdonor.eu/eulid/results.html. Accessed: 7 Sept 2020.
88. Living Donor LIDOBS Observatory. Available at: http://www.eulivingdonor.eu/lidobs/index.html. Accessed: 7 Sept 2020.

Ethical and Policy Considerations in Living Kidney Donor Evaluation and Care

15

Jed Adam Gross and Marie-Chantal Fortin

The Ethics of Living Donor Transplantation: Values and Principles

Given current constraints on the availability of deceased donor kidneys for transplantation and comparative recipient outcomes data, living donor kidney transplantation (LDKT) is the preferred strategy for many patients with end-stage kidney disease (ESKD). Bypassing the need to wait for a deceased donor organ, LDKT offers timelier access to transplantation and greater scheduling flexibility. LDKT is associated with better recipient and allograft survival [1] and is cost-saving for the healthcare system [2, 3]. In studies, living donors have reported good psychosocial outcomes after donation; some report psychosocial benefits including increased quality of life related to helping their recipient or, in the case of donation to a family member, reduced caregiver burden [4–7].

Despite such benefits, living donation is ethically fraught because it strains the general system of norms governing clinical practice, which focus on singular patients as highly individualized beings. In typical surgical cases, a successful procedure will respect or enhance a patient's autonomy, improve the patient's physiological functioning, and be conducive to human flourishing in a broader sense. Even

J. A. Gross (✉)
Bioethics Program, University Health Network, Toronto, ON, Canada

Canadian Donation and Transplantation Research Program, Edmonton, AB, Canada
e-mail: Jed.Gross@uhn.ca

M.-C. Fortin
Canadian Donation and Transplantation Research Program, Edmonton, AB, Canada

Centre de recherche du CHUM, Montreal, Canada

Deparatment of Medicine, Université de Montréal, Montreal, Canada
e-mail: marie-chantal.fortin.chum@ssss.gouv.qc.ca

if there are some tradeoffs among these objectives (e.g., a procedure is likely to prolong a patient's life with a diminished quality of life), the implications of proceeding can be balanced against each other in the relatively well-organized context of a discrete individual's values, goals, and preferences.

Transplantation from a living donor complicates this idealized picture because it involves two individuals, a donor and a recipient, whose surgical outcomes are interconnected, if only by the transplant itself. Before LDKT was available, the individuals who now express interest in donation would not have had indications for nephrectomy. Today, some literature characterizes denying interested persons the opportunity to donate as potentially harmful to these individuals [8].

Moreover, evolving capabilities continue to redefine the criteria for participation as a living donor. On the one hand, advances in immunology have enabled a wider range of plausible donor-recipient pairings. Whereas donation and LDKT were initially limited to close biological relatives, today a pre-existing relationship is no longer necessary for good outcomes. Donors and recipients may find each other through an online appeal or be paired by a registry organizing a chain of transplants across time and geography [9, 10]. On the other hand, increasingly precise information about lifetime health risks, such as the association between certain variants of the apolipoprotein L1 *(APOL1)* gene and chronic kidney disease, has raised new questions about who should donate and the optimal timing of donation [11]. In scenarios involving a multiplicity of stakeholders with diverse stakes, familiar ethical concepts such as informed consent and equitable access can take on new complexities.

This chapter reviews the professional values and commitments implicated in living donation and LDKT and then addresses emergent ethical challenges in the field. As some of these questions are unsettled, we believe there is value in simply describing them and identifying possible management strategies. Empirically, what constitutes an ethical problem or an acceptable solution can vary across time and place, reflecting different understandings of the relationships among individuals, society, and biomedical expertise. Nonetheless, transplant professionals have formed transnational communities of practice, with common reference points such as studies, guidelines, classification schemes, and consensus statements. Thus, we can outline the contours of an ethical framework around living donation, without denying the existence of unresolved questions, diversity of opinion, and local nuances.

Why Living Donation and LDKT Are Ethically Challenging

The ethics of organ replacement emerged in response to a set of clinical and administrative dilemmas in the twentieth century, as technical innovations disrupted traditional understandings of how we can help one another. Advances in hemodialysis and LDKT (initially between identical twins) enabled innovative programs to achieve compelling outcomes for patients with failing kidneys, as measured by ordinary medical criteria. Resource scarcity and uncertainty about outcomes, however, prompted questions of when to offer such treatments and how to allocate access [12–14].

Living donation in the absence of any direct physiological benefit to the donor was not entirely new; volunteers had occasionally lined up to give swatches of skin to burn victims [15]. But the more invasive nature of kidney retrieval posed pressing questions in an era of increased sensitivity to human rights. If helping a loved one recover from kidney failure would be psychologically gratifying for the donor, albeit physically taxing, might facilitating donation be consistent with medicine's ideal of beneficence with respect to the donor's health? If an ostensible donor and recipient were minor siblings, not legally capable of making choices on their own behalf, what would be the roles of parents, children, clinicians, and courts?

Although the ethical challenges of LDKT have evolved with improved access to dialysis, histocompatibility testing, and immunosuppression, the professional values implicated in navigating these early dilemmas remain fundamental. Among these values are human health, individual bodily autonomy, distributive justice, accountability, and trust. With experience, clinicians and policymakers have developed some pragmatic scaffolds for equilibrating and operationalizing these values in the practice of living donation.

> **Key Ethical Values and Principles Underpinning Living Donation and LDKT**
> - **Autonomy and respect for persons**
>   (reflected in the doctrine of informed consent)
> - **Anticipated benefit and justifiable risk**
>   (embodied in the concept of double equipoise)
> - **Procedural justice and equity**
> - **Trust and trustworthiness**
> - **Non-abandonment**

Informed Consent

When individuals are able to exercise autonomy over their bodies and lives, respect for this autonomy is a cornerstone of biomedical ethics. Thus, a capable adult may decline a procedure necessary to prevent certain death, even if the procedure's physical risks are negligible, because it would violate the individual's religious or philosophical convictions. Diverse schools of thought regard autonomy as a good in itself or emphasize its close connection to other ideals such as respect for persons, moral or intellectual development, non-coercion, and epistemic humility [16–18]. Without definitive resolution of these theoretical differences, the core value of patient autonomy can do important work in clinical scenarios [19]. Respecting medical decisions, the emphasis on *bodily* autonomy draws force from the close nexus between bodies and persons. We live embodied lives, and, although a person may donate a kidney without losing one's sense of self, we cannot seamlessly replace or swap bodies at will [20].

The norm of informed consent plays a critical role in ensuring the autonomy of capable persons in research and clinical interactions. In some jurisdictions, statutes and judicial opinions spell out what informed consent requires as a matter of law and implications of its breach. Given information asymmetries between specialized clinicians and capable lay people, a robust ethical commitment to informed consent will entail actively pursuing opportunities to enhance patients' abilities to make treatment decisions consistent with their own values, goals, and preferences. Hence, it can be helpful to think of informed consent as the sum of an interactive process involving communications tailored to individual participants in light of their circumstances [21]. "The signature on a surgical consent form is merely the culmination and formalization of [the] proceeding consent discussion and agreement" [22].

What elements are integral to this process? Intrinsic to the idea of "informed" consent is a sufficient *understanding* to make an informed decision about the proposed intervention. In jurisdictions where the physician-patient relationship is characterized by fiduciary duties, informational requirements articulated by courts have increasingly centered on what is material for patients (individually or generally), rather than intra-professional norms [23, 24]. In broad strokes, the discussion should encompass a description of the proposed treatment, its risks, its anticipated benefits, as well as information about reasonable alternatives, including no active treatment. While the level of detail that individual patients desire may vary, withholding information of interest, ostensibly for the patient's own good, is not defensible in this post-paternalistic paradigm, absent extraordinary circumstances (unlikely to occur in donor assessment) such as an immediate risk of grievous self-harm [25].

To fulfill its purposes, consent to a medical procedure must be *voluntary*. In a culture committed to autonomy, where individuals are free to direct their own lives—or charged with this responsibility—the choice to undergo elective surgery must, in some recognizable way, be adopted by the patient as their own [26, 27]. At a minimum, the clinical team should take care to ascertain that individuals presenting for donor evaluation are not acting under coercion or passively acquiescing to another person's will. Whether a perceived lack of acceptable alternatives can negate voluntariness is a contentious question [28]; some scholars regard voluntariness as a continuum consisting of degrees of freedom [29]. Consistently, donor education and assessment strategies should be structured to maintain space for intentional action by candidates, including changing their minds and pausing the process.

Further, legal and philosophical conceptions of informed consent imply the *capacity* to process the relevant information. While the art and science of capacity assessment are beyond the scope of this chapter, a few points are worth noting. In contrast to holistic, persistent categorizations of patients' conditions or legal status, medical decision-making capacity is time- and situation-specific [30]. Hence, while capacity assessment tools and neuropsychiatric consultations may be helpful in assessing an individual's capacity to consent to elective surgery, this cannot be reduced to a test result or the presence or absence of a specific psychiatric diagnosis [31]. The technical complexity of organ donation and transplantation, the absence of direct physiological benefit to the donor, and longstanding feelings of obligation between donors and recipients may warrant especially searching evaluation before proceeding with living donation. In particular, when assessing how donor candidates process information, clinicians should be attentive to reasons why these individuals may be inclined to engage in impression management [32, 33]. Clinicians should also be mindful of any procedure-specific regulatory considerations. For example, an Ontario statute effectively precludes alternative means of authorizing living donation on behalf of an individual who is unable to give first-person consent, even if such substitute decision-making would be adequate for other procedures [34].

Additionally, some idealized accounts of medical decision-making, rooted in notions of autonomy or beneficence, emphasize *rationality* [35, 36]. To the extent that this means engaging in logical reasoning, and not simply landing on a reasonable decision, the rationality requirement stands in tension with many donors' reports that their decision to donate was spontaneous, even instinctual [37]. Nonetheless, clinicians engaged in donor assessment can insist that candidates reflect on their willingness and explain how they weigh relevant considerations, such as the implications of clinical complications and the availability of deceased donor transplantation. Persons interested in living donation may be offered an opportunity to explore the ins and outs of donation with a prior donor who is willing to share experiential insights. Further, requiring a degree of certainty and stability before acting on an expressed willingness to donate may help to ensure that this choice is consistent with the values of an authentic self [38]. Please see Chap. 2 for additional discussion of informed consent and a framework for donor care.

Balancing Anticipated Benefits and Potential Harms

The crucial need for informed consent does not mean that the ethics of living donation and LDKT reduce to carrying out donor and recipient candidates' informed wishes when these wishes (e.g., to proceed with a highly risky donation and transplant) overlap. Transplant clinicians are not passive conduits in the movement of organs, but moral agents who have taken up a professionalized calling [39]. Beneficence is a canonical value of clinical ethics as is autonomy [16]. What does the former commitment entail with respect to living donor assessment and follow-up?

Anticipated donor benefit has historically been salient, albeit not uncontroversial, in the ethical analysis of living donation, including historic cases involving legal minors or other candidates without full decisional capacity [40, 41]. While there is ample reason to believe that living donors often do benefit from donation, clinicians' assessments of capable candidates' interests are inherently problematic for at least two reasons. First, as critics of paternalism have long appreciated, individuals are likely in a better position to assess whether an act, such as living donation, is in their interest than are third parties (with their own interests), such as clinicians [17]. Additionally, the philosophy of medicine has not yet arrived at a consistent position regarding how narrowly or expansively physicians ought to be gauging benefits and burdens beyond the direct physiological effects (e.g., anticipated financial and lifestyle impacts) within these professionals' respective subject matter expertise [42]. For these reasons, accurate and respectful consideration of whether donation is in a candidate's interest will be advanced through shared decision-making.

Highly valued in clinical relationships, the shared model of medical decision-making calls for dialogue between patient and healthcare professionals with the aim of reaching agreement on the best option for the patient based on their values and situation. Although analytically distinguishable from consent requirements, shared decision-making is likewise supportive of autonomy in that the shared approach involves empowering patients to make an informed decision [43–45]. In the context of living kidney donation and transplantation, anticipated benefits, burdens, and risks should be individualized to the donor and to potential recipients. Once a clinician has been engaged in the decision process, the risks of rejecting a potential donor should also be considered [46].

One potentially constructive way of engaging patients in decisions about surgical procedures, proposed by Bester, aims to integrate the clinician's objective physiological knowledge with the patient's broader conception of their own good to arrive at a balanced understanding of benefit or well-being [47]. Regardless of *exactly* how benefit is construed, or how much weight is assigned to beneficence in relation to autonomy, however, there is broad agreement that a surgeon may—indeed should—decline to perform a desired procedure if, in the surgeon's judgment, the objective risk of harm is too great to proceed as a conscientious professional. A clarifying framework for assessing this risk in the unique context of living donor transplantation has been laid out by Siegler and colleagues. Consistent with the theory of "double equipoise," the clinical team should proceed only if the anticipated benefit to the recipient exceeds the anticipated risk to the donor and the risk of harm to the donor is acceptable in light of the local medicolegal culture (Fig. 15.1) [48]. A variation on this framework, developed in the context of liver transplantation, emphasizes that what is an acceptable risk may also depend on recipient need, as shaped by the

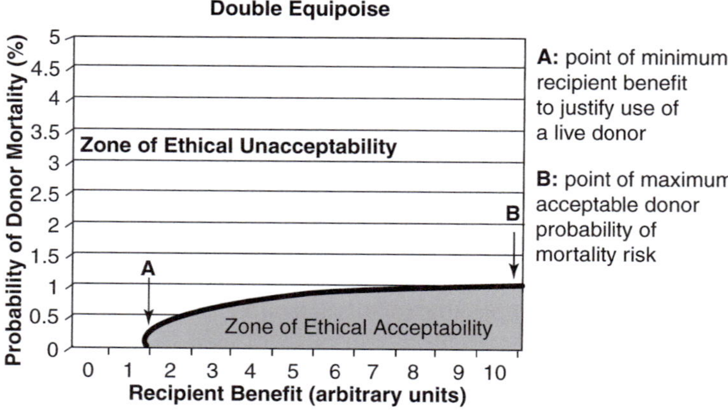

Fig. 15.1 Double equipoise, the interdependent relationship between donor risk and recipient benefit. (From Siegler et al. [48])

relative availability or unavailability of suitable deceased donor organs [49]. Similarly, if a patient in need of a kidney is fortunate enough to have multiple candidates volunteering for living donation, risk minimization is likely to be an important consideration in the choice of donor. Finally, the value of beneficence in the clinician-patient relationship does not end with living donation and LDKT; it also provides a normative basis for follow-up care, especially with respect to complications stemming from donation and transplantation.

Considerations of Fairness

Justice—in its manifold and contested specifications—is also a central concern of the bioethics literature [50]. Because living donor transplantation is often highly personal (e.g., in the case of a pre-existing emotional relationship) or regarded as beyond what we owe each other (e.g., in the case of anonymous, nondirected donation), there is no centralized system specifically designed for distributing living donor organs, so questions of distributive justice are less prominent than in the context of allocating deceased donor organs. Living donor programs should adhere to the basic expectations of fairness that apply to healthcare generally, for example, the avoidance of favoring one patient or another if speaking to the media about the need for more living donors [51]. Differences in rates of living donation (e.g., women are more likely to be donors than men) are widely reported though the underlying reasons may be complex, unclear, or reflect socioeconomic inequalities in the larger society [52]. While researchers seek a better understanding of these disparities, transplant professionals should be careful to avoid reinforcing them through assumptions about who is socially best positioned to donate.

With the expansion of kidney paired donation, questions of distributive justice across candidates and transplant patients have begun to play a larger part in discussion of living donation and LDKT. A major system design challenge, subject to intensive deliberation, is defining and striking the optimal balance between helping more people and not further disadvantaging those whose access is worse [53]. Additionally, transplant professionals may choose to advocate for better societal support for donors, e.g., just compensation of expenses related to donation so it will be a financial neutral act for all [54, 55].

Other Ethical Values Bearing on LDKT

Although *trust* is essential to the relationships between donor candidates and the clinical team, transplant programs perhaps best engender this trust by aiming for *trustworthiness*. This characteristic can be thought of as the sum of structural and personal factors such as honesty, competency, and reliability [56]. In the context of living donation and LDKT, an especially salient design choice is the distribution of resources between the care of donor candidates and recipients. Consensus recommendations for donor assessment and care include the involvement of professionals who are sufficiently removed from the recipient and procedural supports for voluntary decision-making [57]. Even if the interests of donors and recipients are psychologically intertwined, there is a societal expectation that their needs and concerns will be addressed individually. A robust process of communication and assessment that minimizes actual or perceived conflicts of interest can help satisfy this expectation [58]. Finally, professional fidelity to donors does not necessarily end with the act of donation or discharge from the hospital. Following up on their health periodically and attending to any complications arising from living donation can demonstrate a commitment to *non-abandonment*, consistent with notions of compensatory justice, beneficence, and care.

Current Ethical Challenges in Living Donor Kidney Transplantation

This section examines three emerging trends in living kidney donation that have given rise to ethical questions and considers strategies for navigating these challenges. Namely, these scenarios involve the participation of compatible donor-recipient pairs in kidney paired donation (KPD); the use of donor genetic testing, as illustrated by testing for *APOL1* in African ancestry living donor candidates; and public appeals for living kidney donation in an era of widespread access to communication platforms.

Representative Ethical Challenges in Living Donation and LDKT
- **System design choices**
  (participation of compatible pairs in kidney paired donation)
- **Predictive genetic testing**
  (*APOL1* genotyping for patients of African ancestry)
- Supporting all patients while harnessing energy exerted on behalf of individual patients (public solicitation of living donors)

Participation of Compatible Pairs in Kidney Paired Donation

Kidney paired donation (KPD) is a strategy for increasing the number of LDKTs by swapping biologically incompatible donors to create compatible combinations. In KPD, the donor in pair A is willing to donate but is biologically incompatible with recipient A based on blood type of pre-existing donor-specific antibodies in the intended recipient. The donor in pair B is willing to donate but is incompatible with recipient B. The KPD program identifies that donor A is compatible with recipient B and donor B is compatible with recipient A, enabling a crosswise exchange between the pairs as they originally presented themselves. Several pairs may be involved in a closed "chain." A nondirected donor (willing donor without an intended paired recipient) has the powerful potential to initiate a chain of donations, with the final donor in the chain either donating to an unpaired individual on the deceased donor waitlist or initiating a new KPD chain [9].

Although most pairs participating in KPD are biologically incompatible, there have been reports of compatible pairs participating, for the rationale of, for example, obtaining a transplant from a better matched or younger donor [59–61]. Participation of compatible pairs has been advanced as a way of addressing unequal access to KPD, which faces continued difficulties extending its benefits to recipients who are highly sensitized or have type O blood. More generally, the participation of compatible pairs would increase the chances of finding a match for all pairs participating in KPD [62–65].

Several ethical challenges have been identified relating to the participation of compatible pairs in KPD [66]. One set of questions stems from the potentially unbalanced nature of the exchange. Commentators have widely (but not universally) condemned offering material consideration for human organs on a variety of grounds, including concerns about undue influence, the distribution of burdens and benefits, and expressive significance [67]. Although KPD in some sense entails such consideration, these concerns are greatly attenuated because of the roughly equivalent nature of what is given and received. Measured against the alternative of remaining on the waitlist for a deceased donor transplant, utilizing KPD can be viewed as a reciprocal exchange of a "gift of life" that reduces the inequality between compatible and incompatible pairs [68]. The reality that not all kidneys offer recipients a *precisely* equal prospect of posttransplant allograft function (e.g., because of differences in the quality of the organ, the tissue match, or the recipient's condition) is a small detail in comparison.

Conversely, if a compatible pair is going to participate in KPD, remaining on the waitlist is not the only viable alternative; there is also the possibility of a more straightforward living donation and LDKT within the pair. The kidney that donor A can provide directly to recipient A may present a different quality or risk profile in various respects (e.g., donor age, immunological match) than the kidney available to recipient A through KPD [65]. In such circumstances, clinicians caring for donor may experience tensions among what they believe to be in each individual's physiological interest, what aligns most closely with each individual's values, and the organizational goal of expanding access to transplantation. One influential scholar posits that offering a compatible pair the opportunity to participate in KPD is only acceptable if the recipient will receive an organ as good as or better than the organ they would have received from the intended donor [69]. In practice, however, there may be substantial uncertainty as to what is a "better" quality organ. Further complicating ethical decision-making, to the extent that members of the transplant program will be key in assessing what are reasonable alternatives, these professionals are not necessarily disinterested since they may, for various reasons, desire to increase the volume of LDKT through KPD.

The process of developing guidelines around compatible pairs' participation in KPD, in conversation with stakeholders, is ongoing. A 2014 qualitative study conducted among Canadian transplant professionals generated actionable recommendations regarding the terms and conditions of compatible pairs' participation in KPD [70]. The results of this exercise underscored possible tension between enabling KPD and protecting individual patients' physiological well-being. Respondents supported providing compatible pairs with complete and neutral information about the possibility of KPD. At the same time, the group took the position that, if a compatible pair is to participate in KPD, the intended recipient in the pair should receive an organ of equal or better quality that would be available within the pair. Participants also stated that there should be agreement within the medical team about the participation of a compatible pair in KPD. Some reported that they would disagree with the participation of HLA identical compatible pairs in KPD. The Canadian study was noteworthy for its attention to logistics. Consistent with the principle of not disadvantaging compatible pairs, recommendations included a short timeline for finding a KPD match and shipping organs or reimbursing travel expenses to minimize burdens on participating pairs. Study participants also suggested a designated provincial program to manage the participation of compatible pairs, adequate resources for KPD, anonymity between pairs, and research to better understand the impact of compatible pairs' participation on donors, recipients, and the transplant system.

The initial emphasis within the transplant community on fair exchange and individual patients' physiological outcomes is consistent with commonly understood professional roles. Other potentially relevant values, however, should not be left out of the discussion. These considerations include the patients' own goals, values, and preferences, perhaps especially when they would be conducive to extending the benefits of transplantation to more people. Patients choosing among treatments sometimes place substantial weight on values other than maximizing anticipated objective physiological well-being, such as cost or convenience or appearance. One respectful approach to the underlying problem of defining beneficence is to structure medical decision-making so that the clinician focuses on promoting the patient's physiological well-being and avoiding physiological harm, while the patient has latitude to pursue a fuller set of considered interests [47]. Indeed, outside the KPD context, psychosocial interests have historically been central to the ethics of living donation [40].

What, in this light, do members of compatible pairs think about the option to participate in KPD? Empirical findings to date have been mixed. Two Canadian studies, one survey-based and one interview-based, showed different results. A survey of prospective compatible transplant candidates with their potential living donors showed that compatible pairs are willing to participate in KPD: 77.3% of transplant candidates and 63.3% of potential living donors were willing to participate in KPD. Receiving a better matched kidney, advantages for the recipient, prioritization for a match in KPD, facilitating more than one transplant, reimbursement of travel expenses for the donor and a companion, and reimbursement of donor income are factors increasing the willingness to participate. Also, offering a priority for a deceased donor kidney in case of graft failure of the recipient of the compatible pair increased the willingness to participate in KPD. In contrast, a delay of more than 6 months associated with participation in KPD decreased the willingness to participate [71]. In the interview-based study, few potential donors were willing to participate in KPD (2/18 potential living kidney donors), while almost half of transplant candidates were willing to participate (8/17). The major reasons evoked for being unwilling to participate were the personal relationship between the donor and the recipient and not knowing the donor and the recipient personally. The principal reason for participating in KPD was altruism and helping another person. Delay in transplantation, risks of chain break and donor reneging, donors' travel, and the quality of the organ were major concerns expressed by participants [72]. A US study described the characteristics of 11 compatible pairs who participated in KPD at a single center. The pairs took part in ten exchanges, facilitating 33 living donor kidney transplants. Reasons for participating included obtaining a younger kidney for the recipient (63.6%), a size mismatch in the compatible pair (18.2%), and altruistic motives (18.2%) [60].

One modifiable factor that did appear to influence compatible pairs' willingness to participate in KPD was the incentive of offering recipients in compatible pairs who participate priority for a deceased donor kidney in the event of graft failure at any time after transplantation [71]. Mathematical simulation indicates that offering a priority for a deceased donor kidney transplantation for the recipient of a compatible pair could significantly increase the total number of LDKT [73]. However, these gains would come at a cost of further stratifying access to transplantation. Presumably, recipients of living donor kidneys who did not participate in KPD and recipients who presented in incompatible pairs would not be accorded the same priority for a deceased donor kidney transplantation when they suffer graft failure [74]. While the former group may have made an informed choice between direct transplantation and KPD (along with their compatible donors), the latter population did not have the same choice as members of compatible pairs. Additionally, prioritizing KPD recipients who may be better off in various respects—and at greater risk of adverse outcomes—over patients on the waitlist without living donors seems likely to disadvantage patients who are already relatively disadvantaged in the allocation system, violating Rawlsian principles of justice [75]. At the least, the implications of this strategy for modifying allocation priority in exchange for participation of compatible pars in KPD would need to be examined closely, and its acceptability would have to be gauged in relation to public understandings of the social contract around transplant medicine.

Genetic Testing: The Case of *APOL1*

In the last decade, the presence of two renal risk variants (RRVs) in the *APOL1* gene has been identified as a genetic marker of increased risk of ESKD and chronic kidney disease (CKD) among persons of African ancestry (AA) [76]. Approximately 39% of all AA individuals carry one increased risk variant of *APOL1*, and 13% carry a higher risk genotype comprised by two *APOL1* variants. Extrapolating from current data, about 20% of this latter population might be anticipated to develop ESKD [77]. Outside the context of living kidney donation, the risk of developing ESKD among carriers of two *APOL1* variants has been estimated as three times that of individuals with 0 or 1 RRVs [76]. The same findings, however, mean that most carriers of even the higher-risk genotype do not develop ESKD. A "second-hit" hypothesis has been proposed to explain why carriers have a higher incidence of ESKD. Of special relevance to our discussion, it has been hypothesized that living kidney donation could constitute such a "hit" among individuals with the high-risk genotype [78, 79].

Kidneys from deceased donors carrying a high-risk *APOL1* genotype have been shown to have a higher incidence of allograft failure and shorter graft survival than kidneys from deceased donors with 0 or 1 *APOL1* RRVs [80]. A recipient's *APOL1* genotype, on the other hand, does not appear to have a substantial impact on graft survival [80]. Among living donors with a high-risk genotype, there are reported cases of living kidney donors developing ESKD after donation [81, 82]. One of these donors developed ESKD with nephrotic syndrome 7 years after donating to her brother. Renal biopsy showed focal and global segmental sclerosis [81]. In another case, an identical twin donated a kidney to his brother at the age of 21 years and developed CKD and nephrotic syndrome 7 years after the donation [82]. A recent study has also shown that, among past living kidney donors, the rate of decline in glomerular filtration rate was greater in those with a high-risk genotype than in donors with 0 or 1 *APOL1* RRVs [83].

The discovery of the association of *APOL1* genotype with CKD has prompted questions around whether living kidney donor candidates should be tested for *APOL1* and in what circumstances [84, 85]. There is currently no consensus in the literature or across transplant professionals. In 2017, an American Society of Transplantation work group published consensus-based recommendations on *APOL1* testing and living donation and recommended that all AA donor candidates be informed about the association between *APOL1* and the increased risk of CKD and ESKD, the availability of the test and impossibility of predicting precise individual risk, and the potential anxiety associated with testing [86]. The work group concluded that *APOL1* testing should be offered to all AA donor candidates who wish to know their genotype [86]. A 2017 Kidney Disease: Improving Global Outcomes (KDIGO) guideline on the evaluation and care of living kidney donors similarly recommended offering screening for *APOL1* to potential living kidney donors with ancestors from sub-Saharan Africa and informing them of the increased risk of CKD and ESKD among those with two RRVs [57]. The KDIGO guideline nevertheless acknowledged the uncertainty in predicting the precise individual risk of ESKD related to the *APOL1* genotype. In contrast, the British Transplantation Society's guidelines on LDKT state that there is not sufficient data to support *APOL1* genetic testing, but recommends counseling black living donors about their increased statistical risk of CKD and ESRD, particularly if the potential donor is young [87].

What stakeholders' perspectives can inform approaches to *APOL1* genetic testing in the setting of living kidney donor education and assessment? Gordon and colleagues surveyed AA prior donors, transplant nephrologists, and surgeons on *APOL1* genetic testing [88, 89]. During qualitative interviews with AA prior living kidney donors, participants supported offering *APOL1* genetic testing to all AA potential living kidney donors, and, if this opportunity for testing had been available at the time of donation, 87% would have been willing to be tested before donation. The presence of a high-risk genotype was not regarded as an absolute barrier to donation for participants: 61% would still have donated if they had such a genotype. Rather, participants considered *APOL1* testing information a means for making an informed decision and modifying lifestyle habits with hopes of decreasing the risk of CKD and ESKD. Psychological distress associated with testing, the costs of the test, insurance coverage, and the possibility that *APOL1* testing could worsen existing discrimination against the AA population were the major concerns identified [88]. For nephrologists and transplant surgeons, *APOL1* genetic testing was also considered to be information that could improve informed consent of potential living kidney donors about the long-term risk of ESKD. At the time of the study, 4% of nephrologists reported using *APOL1* genetic testing in the evaluation of all AA living kidney donors, and 14% were using it on a case-by-case basis. Participants who had previously used *APOL1* genetic testing reported discouraging AA potential living kidney donors carrying the two RRVs from proceeding with donation. An absence of professional guidelines and the lack of prospective data and randomized controlled trials were identified as barriers for using genetic testing [89]. The *APOL1* Long-term Kidney Transplantation Outcomes (APOLLO) and Living Donor Extended Time Outcomes (LETO) studies in the United States aim to generate prospective data on the impact of *APOL1* in deceased donor kidney transplantation, living donation, and LDKT and will likely help transplant physicians and surgeons to counsel their patients in the future [90].

The model of shared medical decision-making, mentioned above, is well-suited to decisions about *APOL1* genetic testing in connection with living kidney donation, which implicate evolving statistical data and donor candidates' values, goals, and preferences. While the nature of clinician-patient conversations should be tailored to individual patients and their circumstances, these conversations could be expected to involve counseling about genetic testing and offering genotyping for interested potential living kidney donors during their evaluation. Culturally and ethically sensitive educational materials can be critical to proper counseling [91].

Public Solicitation of Living Donors

Some patients in need of kidney have sought donors through public solicitation. This term is used to refer to search activity conducted by a transplant candidate or their representative to enlist a potential organ donor from among the general public or a large swathe of the public [92]. The strategy has often been employed to find compatible hematopoietic stem cell donors. In 2004, a website, *Matchingdonors. com*, was launched to allow potential living organ donors to connect with transplant candidates. More recently, several high-profile instances of public solicitation have resulted in notable media coverage [93–97].

In a relatively small but notable study, Pronk and colleagues reported on the motives and experiences of 20 kidney transplant candidates who engaged in public solicitation for organ donors [98]. Candidates reported a variety of reasons for engaging in solicitation, including the difficulty of discussing living organ donation within their social network, reluctance to accept an organ from a loved ones, moral objections to payment for organ donation, the ease of using social media, the urge to take action, encouragement from others, and the ends as justification for the means. Although the patients mostly characterized their experience with public solicitation as a positive one, they reported that they had to act as screeners and educators; that the process was draining in terms of time, energy, and emotions; and that they had limited cooperation from transplant professionals. At the time of the interview, four of the 20 had received a kidney transplantation with a living donor through public solicitation.

Even before *Matchingdonors.com* went live, efforts by enterprising individuals to find donors for identified patients via media such as billboards and television news drew and attracted critical scrutiny, provoking concerns about unequal access and the integrity of the donor assessment process [99]. Against the backdrop of an organ allocation system commitment to equitable access based on medical criteria, campaigns focused on individual patients can be predicted to favor those with the most appealing story, or the most visually appealing pictures will attract more potential living kidney donors [100]. Other concerns that have been raised include the possibility that permitting public solicitation will heighten the risk of covert organ trafficking [100] and donation based on false or misleading representations by recipients. Finally, to the extent that members of the public perceive public solicitation as unfair, suspect, or even "jumping the queue," such perceptions may undermine critical support for donation and transplantation [101].

Nonetheless, public solicitation has several points in its favor. For patients who do not have a compatible living donor with their immediate social network, public solicitation offers a strategy for easing disadvantages to donor identification, such as for those who are socially isolated, highly sensitized, or O blood group. Further, in a society where living donation is unusual, LDKT is unlikely to be zero-sum phenomenon, where directing a kidney to one recipient deprives another recipient of something they would otherwise have received [102]. Rather, public solicitation can potentially increase awareness of the need for donated organs, the possibilities of living organ donation, and organ donation generally, benefiting patients who are waiting as well as those who are actively seeking a donor from among the general public [103, 104]. In political cultures that are broadly supportive of self-help and freedom of association, the burden of persuasion would seem to fall on those intent on restricting this activity [105]. A survey of US kidney transplant patients published in 2016 found that 11.6% of this population used social media to share their need for living kidney donation or to ask for a living kidney donor [106]. Concerns about exploitation might be weighed against the possibility that the availability of regulated channels for actively finding a donor will diminish motives for candidates to seek transplants through more problematic "underground" means.

The reality of public solicitation has created opportunities for researchers to sharpen understanding empirically by engaging with patients. In one of the first formal studies of the topic in 2013, Chang and colleagues analyzed 91 Facebook pages seeking living donors for specific individuals [107]. Seventy-five percent of the pages included recipient's pictures and some personal information. Few mentioned the risks and associated costs of living kidney donation. In 10% of pages, there were invitations to sign donors' cards or to register as an organ donor. With respect to outcomes, 32% of pages mentioned having donors tested and 13 pages reported a kidney transplantation: three from deceased donors, nine from living donors, and one from an unspecified donor. Pages reporting donor testing shared more recipient and transplantation information and had higher traffic. In 3% of pages, however, there were offers for organ selling. A team from John Hopkins University developed a Facebook app to help kidney and liver transplant candidates find living kidney donors and evaluated the tool in a prospective study with 54 liver and kidney transplant candidates [108, 109]. Compared to controls, patients who used the Facebook app had six times more chances of finding a potential living donor who began evaluation [108].

Clearly, several ethical and logistical challenges are associated with public solicitation. These include managing privacy/publicity and the implications of one-sided anonymity, which are compounded if the intended recipient is a legal minor [110]. Ensuring that donor candidates receive appropriate education and are in a position to grant informed consent is also an apparent challenge [111]. Communications with a potential recipient will not necessarily provide potential donors with an accurate, comprehensive understanding of all the risks associated with the donation (medical, psychological, financial, etc.) and alternatives to LDKT availability to the transplant candidate (e.g., hemodialysis). The potential donor may not know all the living kidney donation options, such as participating in a KPD program or donating to someone on the deceased donor waiting list. Another complexity involves resource commitments and prioritization [110]. "Successful" public appeals may stimulate a surge of individuals who express interest in living donation. Transplant programs should be prepared to respond to these inquiries without unduly disadvantaging candidates undergoing donor assessment and other transplant candidates.

In 2017, the Canadian Society of Transplantation (CST) published a position statement on public solicitation to offer guidance to transplant professionals facing cases of public solicitation [110]. This document affirmed the acceptability of engaging with individuals who come forward in response to public solicitation as potential living donors. At the same time, CST acknowledged that transplant professionals and transplant programs might have conscientious objections and endorsed referral as a means of navigating this tension. CST also recommended that both transplant candidates and potential living donors be informed about issues of privacy and one-sided anonymity, as well as the full range of clinical options. Other recommendations included the use of standard criteria in donor and transplant candidate assessments and having a surge plan to manage any sudden influx of potential donors. To minimize potential conflicts of interest, the guidance cautions that transplant professionals should not be involved in public solicitation on behalf of individual patients. Finally, CST called for research aimed at gathering data that will elucidate the impact of public solicitation for donors, recipients, the public, and the organ donation system [57].

Separately, Pronk and colleagues have formulated recommendations for patients considering public solicitation for organ donors [98]. These recommendations advise that transplant candidates discuss their search for a living donor with their transplant team, inform themselves about their transplant programs' policies on public solicitation, and consider in advance how they would handle requests for information on living donation. They further suggest that the candidates define their own personal boundaries, such as what they want to share on social media and what their expectations of relationships with strangers are. Transplant candidates must anticipate they may receive living kidney offers for illegal monetary payment and should have a plan to decline such offers. Finally, the authors caution that transplant candidates should be given realistic information about their likelihood of finding a suitable donor while acknowledging that engaging in public solicitation itself could generate positive feelings. Transplant programs can help interested patients manage possible offers by working together to see that these are seamlessly referred to the transplant center.

Conclusion

Since their inception, living kidney donation and LDKT have raised numerous ethical questions directly bearing on clinical practice. Many of these challenges stem from the unique ways in which a kidney offered by a healthy living donor can be used to improve the health of another person. Living donation entails both known medical risks and documented potential psychosocial benefits for donors.

Even as broad ethical principles governing living donation and LDKT have been established, innovative allied activities have forced us to clarify these principles. The possibility of matching pairs to increase the number of LDKTs raises an issue of whether compatible pairs should be invited to participate in KPD and, if so, in what circumstances. Developments in living donor evaluation, such as genetic testing, complicate our understanding of the risk-benefit balance for donor candidates and, by extension, their informed consent. Public solicitation and the use of social media to appeal for living donors have also spurred members of the transplant community to revisit expectations and practices relating to living donation.

These are only a few examples of contemporary ethical quandaries in the field of living kidney donation and transplantation. Thoughtful reflection on these challenges and lessons learned will help the transplant community to address new and emerging issues in living donation and LDKT as the field continues to evolve.

References

1. Gjertson DW, Cecka JM. Living unrelated donor kidney transplantation. Kidney Int. 2000;58:491–9. https://doi.org/10.1046/j.1523-1755.2000.00195.x.
2. Rabaux Y. Étude sur l'économique de l'insuffisance rénale. La Fondation canadienne du rein - Division Québec; 2012. https://doi.org/10.1186/2054-3581-1-2.

3. Axelrod D, Schnitzler M, Xiao H, Irish W, Tuttle-Newhall E, Chang S, et al. An economic assessment of contemporary kidney transplant practice. Am J Transplant. 2013;18(5):1168–76. https://doi.org/10.1111/ajt.14702.

4. Van Pilsum Rasmussen S, Henderson M, Kahn J, Segev D. Considering tangible benefit for interdependent donors: extending a risk-benefit framework in donor selection. Am J Transplant. 2017;17(10):2567–71. https://doi.org/10.1111/ajt.14319.

5. Li T, Dokus M, Kelly K, Ugoeke N, Rogers J, Asham G, et al. Survey of living organ donors' experience and directions for process improvement. Prog Transplant. 2017;27(3):232–9. https://doi.org/10.1177/1526924817715467.

6. Kisch A, Forsberg A, Fridh I, Almgren M, Lundmark M, Lovén C, et al. The meaning of being a living kidney, liver or stem cell donor - a meta-ethnography. Transplantation. 2018;102(5):744–56. https://doi.org/10.1097/tp.0000000000002073.

7. Isotani S, Fujisawa M, Ichikawa Y, Ishimura T, Matsumoto O, Hamami G, et al. Quality of life of living kidney donors: the short-form 36-item health questionnaire survey. Urology. 2002;60(4):588–92. https://doi.org/10.1016/s0090-4295(02)01865-4.

8. Allen MB, Abt PL, Reese PP. What are the harms of refusing to allow living kidney donation? An expanded view of risks and benefits. Am J Transplant. 2014;14(3):531–7. https://doi.org/10.1111/ajt.12599.

9. Ashlagi I, Gilchrist DS, Roth AE, Rees MA. Nonsimultaneous chains and dominos in kidney- paired donation-revisited. Am J Transplant. 2011;11(5):984–94. https://doi.org/10.1111/j.1600-6143.2011.03481.x.

10. Rees MA, Kopke JE, Pelletier RP, Segev DL, Rutter ME, Fabrega AJ, et al. A nonsimultaneous, extended, altruistic-donor chain. N Engl J Med. 2009;360(11):1095–101. https://doi.org/10.1056/NEJMoa0803645.

11. Vallée-Guignard V, Fortin M-C. Emerging ethical challenges in living kidney donation. Curr Transplant Rep. 2019.

12. Rothman DJ. Strangers at the bedside : a history of how law and bioethics transformed medical decision making. New York, NY: Basic Books; 1991. xi, 303 p. p

13. Peitzman SJ. Dropsy, dialysis, transplant : a short history of failing kidneys. Baltimore: Johns Hopkins University Press; 2007. xxi, 213 p., 2 p. of plates p

14. Fox RC, Swazey JP. The courage to fail : a social view of organ transplants and dialysis. 2nd ed. Chicago: University of Chicago Press; 1978. p. xx, 437.

15. Lederer SE. Flesh and blood : organ transplantation and blood transfusion in twentieth-century America. Oxford ; New York: Oxford University Press; 2008. xvi, 224 p. p

16. Beauchamp TL, Childress JF. Principles of biomedical ethics. 7th ed. New York: Oxford University Press; 2013. xvi, 459 p.

17. Mill JS, Spitz D. On liberty. 1st ed. New York: Norton; 1975. xi, 260 p. p

18. Mackenzie C. Relational autonomy, normative authority and perfectionism. J Soc Philos. 2008;39(4):512–33. https://doi.org/10.1111/j.1467-9833.2008.00440.x.

19. Gunderson M. Justifying a principle of informed consent: a case study in autonomy-based ethics. Public Aff Q. 1990;4(3):249–65. https://pubmed.ncbi.nlm.nih.gov/11659297/.

20. Dworkin G. The theory and practice of autonomy. Cambridge; New York: Cambridge University Press; 1988. xiii, 173 p.

21. Lidz CW, Appelbaum PS, Meisel A. Two models of implementing informed consent. Arch Intern Med. 1988;148(6):1385–9. https://pubmed.ncbi.nlm.nih.gov/3377623/.

22. Bernat JL, Peterson LM. Patient-centered informed consent in surgical practice. Arch Surg. 2006;141(1):86–92. https://doi.org/10.1001/archsurg.141.1.86.

23. Canterbury v. Spence. 464 F.2d 772 (D.C. Cir.). 1972.

24. Montgomery v. Lanarkshire. 2013. Available at: https://www.supremecourt.uk/cases/docs/uksc-2013-0136-judgment.pdf. Accessed: 7 Sept 2020.

25. Murray B. Informed consent: what must a physician disclose to a patient? Virtual Mentor. 2012;14(7):563–6. https://doi.org/10.1001/virtualmentor.2012.14.7.hlaw1-1207.

26. Korsgaard CM. Self-constitution : agency, identity, and integrity. Oxford; New York: Oxford University Press; 2009. xiv, 230 p. p.

27. O'Shea T. A law of one's own: self-legislation and radical Kantian constructivism. Eur J Philos. 2015;23(4):1153–73. https://doi.org/10.1111/ejop.12044.

28. Buss S, Overton L. Contours of agency : essays on themes from Harry Frankfurt. Cambridge, Mass: MIT Press; 2002. xx, 361 p. p.

29. Feinberg J. Oxford university press. The moral limits of the criminal law volume 3: harm to self. New York: Oxford University Press; 1989. Available at: http://www.oxfordscholarship. com/oso/public/content/philosophy/9780195059236/toc.html. Accessed: 7 Sept 2020.

30. Sessums LL, Zembrzuska H, Jackson JL. Does this patient have medical decision-making capacity? JAMA. 2011;306(4):420–7. https://doi.org/10.1001/jama.2011.1023.

31. Leo RJ. Competency and the capacity to make treatment decisions: a primer for primary care physicians. Prim Care Companion J Clin Psychiatry. 1999;1(5):131–41. https://doi. org/10.4088/pcc.v01n0501.

32. Shippee-Rice RV, Fetzer SJ, Long JV. Gerioperative nursing care : principles and practices of surgical care for the older adult. New York: Springer; 2012. xii, 626 p. p.

33. Hildebrand L, Melchert TP, Anderson RC. Impression management during evaluation and psychological reactions post-donation of living kidney donors. Clin Transpl. 2014;28(8):855–61. https://doi.org/10.1111/ctr.12390.

34. Trillium Gift of Life Network Act, R.S.O. 1990, c. H.20 Government of Ontario. Available at: https://www.ontario.ca/laws/statute/90h20. Accessed: 7 Sept 2020.

35. Savulescu J, Momeyer RW. Should informed consent be based on rational beliefs? J Med Ethics. 1997;23(5):282. https://doi.org/10.1136/jme.23.5.282.

36. Brock DW, Wartman SA. When competent patients make irrational choices. N Engl J Med. 1990;322(22):1595–9. https://doi.org/10.1056/NEJM199005313222209.

37. McGrath P, Pun P, Holewa H. Decision-making for living kidney donors: an instinctual response to suffering and death. Mortality. 2012;17(3):201–20. https://doi.org/10.108 0/13576275.2012.696356.

38. Schelling TC. Ethics, law, and the exercise of self-command. In: Rawls J, McMurrin SM, editors. Liberty, equality, and law: selected Tanner lectures on moral philosophy: University of Utah Press; 1987.

39. Elliott C. Doing harm: living organ donors, clinical research and the tenth man. J Med Ethics. 1995;21(2):91–6. https://doi.org/10.1136/jme.21.2.91.

40. Spital A. Donor benefit is the key to justified living organ donation. Camb Q Healthc Ethics. 2004;13(1):105–9. https://doi.org/10.1017/S0963180104131174.

41. Dwyer J, Vig E. Rethinking transplantation between siblings. Hastings Cent Rep. 1995;25(5):7–12. https://doi.org/10.2307/3562788.

42. Bester JC. Beneficence, interests, and wellbeing in medicine: what it means to provide benefit to patients. Am J Bio: AJOB. 2020;20(3):53–62. https://doi.org/10.1080/15265161.202 0.1714793.

43. Edwards A, Elwyn G. Shared decision-making in health care: achieving evidence-based patient choice. Oxford: Oxford University Press; 2009. p. 414.

44. Whitney SN, McGuire AL, McCullough LB. A typology of shared decision making, informed consent, and simple consent. Ann Intern Med. 2004;140(1):54–9. https://doi. org/10.7326/0003-4819-140-1-200401060-00012.

45. King JS, Moulton BW. Rethinking informed consent: the case for shared medical decision-making. Am J Law Med. 2006;32(4):429–501. https://doi.org/10.1177/009885880603200401.

46. Ralph AF, Chadban SJ, Butow P, Craig JC, Kanellis J, Wong G, et al. The experiences and impact of being deemed ineligible for living kidney donation: semi-structured interview study. Nephrology (Carlton). 2020;25(4):339–50. https://doi.org/10.1111/nep.13628.

47. Bester JC. Beneficence, interests, and wellbeing in medicine: what it means to provide benefit to patients. Am J Bioeth. 2020;20(3):53–62. https://doi.org/10.1080/15265161.202 0.1714793.

48. Siegler M, Simmerling MC, Siegler JH. Cronin DC, 2nd. Recipient deaths during donor surgery: a new ethical problem in living donor liver transplantation (LDLT). Liver Transpl. 2006;12(3):358–60. https://doi.org/10.1002/lt.20670.

49. Miller CM. Ethical dimensions of living donation: experience with living liver donation. Transplant Rev. 2008;22(3):206–9. https://doi.org/10.1016/j.trre.2008.02.001.
50. Callahan D. Is justice enough? Ends and means in bioethics. Hast Cent Rep. 1996;26(6):9–10. https://doi.org/10.2307/3528744.
51. Gillon R. Justice and allocation of medical resources. Br Med J (Clin Res Ed). 1985;291(6490):266–8. https://doi.org/10.1136/bmj.291.6490.266.
52. Gill J, Joffres Y, Rose C, Lesage J, Landsberg D, Kadatz M, et al. The change in living kidney donation in women and men in the United States (2005-2015): a population-based analysis. J Am Soc Nephrol. 2018;29(4):1301–8. https://doi.org/10.1681/asn.2017111160.
53. Tenenbaum EM. Swaps and chains and vouchers, oh my!: evaluating how saving more lives impacts the equitable allocation of live donor kidneys. Am J Law Med. 2018;44(1):67–118. https://doi.org/10.1177/0098858818763812.
54. Gill JS, Delmonico F, Klarenbach S, Capron AM. Providing coverage for the unique lifelong health care needs of living kidney donors within the framework of financial neutrality. Am J Transplant. 2017;17(5):1176–81. https://doi.org/10.1111/ajt.14147.
55. Hays R, Rodrigue J, Cohen D, Danovitch G, Matas A, Schold J, et al. Financial neutrality for living organ donors: reasoning, rationale, definitions, and implementation strategies. Am J Transplant. 2016;16(7):1973–81. https://doi.org/10.1111/ajt.13813.
56. O'Neill O. Linking trust to trustworthiness. Int J Philos Stud. 2018;26(2):293–300. https://doi.org/10.1080/09672559.2018.1454637.
57. Lentine K, Kasiske B, Levey A, Adams P, Alberú J, Bakr M, et al. KDIGO clinical practice guideline on the evaluation and Care of Living Kidney Donors. Transplantation. 2017;101(8S Suppl 1):S1–S109. https://doi.org/10.1097/tp.0000000000001769.
58. Ethics Committee of the Transplantation S. The consensus statement of the Amsterdam Forum on the Care of the Live Kidney Donor. Transplantation. 2004;78(4):491–2. https://doi.org/10.1097/01.tp.0000136654.85459.1e.
59. Ratner LE, Rana A, Ratner ER, Ernst V, Kelly J, Kornfeld D, et al. The altruistic unbalanced paired kidney exchange: proof of concept and survey of potential donor and recipient attitudes. Transplantation. 2010;89(1):15–22. https://doi.org/10.1097/tp.0b013e3181c626e1.
60. Weng FL, Grogan T, Patel AM, Mulgaonkar S, Morgievich MM. Characteristics of compatible pair participants in kidney paired donation at a single center. Clin Transpl. 2017;31(6). https://doi.org/10.1111/ctr.12978.
61. Bingaman AW, Wright FH, Kapturczak M, Shen L, Vick S, Murphey CL. Single-center kidney paired donation: the Methodist San Antonio experience. Am J Transplant. 2012;12(8):2125–32. https://doi.org/10.111/j.1600-6143.2012.04070.x.
62. Segev DL. Innovative strategies in living donor kidney transplantation. Nat Rev Nephrol. 2012;8(6):332–8. https://doi.org/10.1038/nrneph.2012.82.
63. Gentry SE, Segev DL, Simmerling M, Montgomery RA. Expanding kidney paired donation through participation by compatible pairs. Am J Transplant. 2007;7:2361–70. https://doi.org/10.1111/j.1600-6143.2007.01935.x.
64. Glorie KM, de Klerk M, Wagelmans APM, van de Klundert JJ, Zuidema WC, Claas FHJ, et al. Coordinating unspecified living kidney donation and transplantation across the blood-type barrier in kidney exchange. Transplantation. 2013;96(9):814–20. https://doi.org/10.1097/tp.0b013e3182a132b7.
65. Lee LY, Pham TA, Melcher ML. Living kidney donation: strategies to increase the donor pool. Surg Clin North Am. 2019;99(1):37–47. https://doi.org/10.1016/j.suc.2018.09.003.
66. Fortin M-C. Is it ethical to invite compatible pairs to participate in exchange programs? J Med Ethics. 2013;39(12):743–7. https://doi.org/10.1136/medethics-2012-101129.
67. Cohen I. The Price of everything, the value of nothing: reframing the commodification debate. Harv Law Rev. 2003;117:689–710.
68. Morley M. Increasing the supply of organs for transplantation through paired organ exchanges. Yale Law & Policy Review. 2003;21:221–62.
69. Veatch RM. Organ exchanges: fairness to the O-blood group. Am J Transplant. 2006;6:1–2. https://doi.org/10.1111/j.1600-6143.2005.01164.x.

70. Durand C, Duplantie A, Fortin M-C. Transplant professionals' proposals for the implementation of an altruistic unbalanced paired kidney exchange program. Transplantation. 2014;98(7):754–9. https://doi.org/10.1097/tp.0000000000000127.
71. Gill J, Gill J, Ballesteros F, Fortin M-C. Transplant candidates and potential living kidney donors are supportive of reciprocity for transplant candidates who participate in kidney paired donation with a compatible donor. Am J Transplant. 2018;18(S4):528–9.
72. Fortin M-C, Gill J, Ballesteros F, Gill J. Compatible donor and recipient pairs' perspectives on participation in kidney paired donation programs: emotional relationships matter. Transplant Summit. October 16–20; Ottawa. 2018.
73. Gill J, Tinckam K, Fortin M, Rose C, Shick-Makaroff K, Young K, et al. Reciprocity to increase participation of compatible living donor and recipient pairs in kidney paired donation. Am J Transplant. 2017;17(7):1723–8. https://doi.org/10.1111/ajt.14275.
74. Fortin M-C. Is it ethical to offer priority points to compatible pairs participating in kidney exchange programs? In: Massey E, Ambagtsheer F, Weimar W, editors. Ethical, legal and psychosocial aspects of transplantation: global challenges. Lengerich: PABST; 2017. p. 75–81.
75. Tenenbaum EM. Swaps and chains and vouchers, oh my!: evaluating how saving more lives impacts the equitable allocation of live donor kidneys. Am J Law Med. 2018;44(1):67–118. https://doi.org/10.1177/0098858818763812.
76. Foster MC, Coresh J, Fornage M, Astor BC, Grams M, Franceschini N, et al. APOL1 variants associate with increased risk of CKD among African Americans. J Am Soc Nephrol. 2013;24(9):1484–91. https://doi.org/10.1681/asn.2013010113.
77. Tedla FM, Yap E. Apolipoprotein L1 and kidney transplantation. Curr Opin Organ Transplant. 2019;24(1):97–102. https://doi.org/10.1097/mot.0000000000000600.
78. Chang JH, Husain SA, Santoriello D, Stokes MB, Miles CD, Foster KW, et al. Donor's APOL1 risk genotype and "second hits" associated with De novo collapsing Glomerulopathy in deceased donor kidney transplant recipients: a report of 5 cases. Am J Kidney Dis. 2019;73(1):134–9. https://doi.org/10.1053/j.ajkd.2018.05.008.
79. Lentine KL, Mannon RB. Apolipoprotein L1: role in the evaluation of kidney transplant donors. Curr Opin Nephrol Hypertens. 2020.;29(6):645–55. https://doi.org/10.1097/mnh.0000000000000653.
80. Freedman BI, Julian BA, Pastan SO, Israni AK, Schladt D, Gautreaux MD, et al. Apolipoprotein L1 gene variants in deceased organ donors are associated with renal allograft failure. Am J Transplant. 2015;15(6):1615–22. https://doi.org/10.1111/ajt.13223.
81. Zwang NA, Shetty A, Sustento-Reodica N, Gordon EJ, Leventhal J, Gallon L, et al. APOL1-associated end-stage renal disease in a living kidney transplant donor. Am J Transplant. 2016;16(12):3568–72. https://doi.org/10.1111/ajt.14035.
82. Kofman T, Audard V, Narjoz C, Gribouval O, Matignon M, Leibler C, et al. APOL1 polymorphisms and development of CKD in an identical twin donor and recipient pair. Am J Kidney Dis. 2014;63(5):816–9. https://doi.org/10.1053/j.ajkd.2013.12.014.
83. Doshi MD, Ortigosa-Goggins M, Garg AX, Li L, Poggio ED, Winkler CA, et al. APOL1 genotype and renal function of black living donors. J Am Soc Nephrol: JASN. 2018;29(4):1309–16. https://doi.org/10.1681/ASN.2017060658.
84. Mena-Gutierrez AM, Reeves-Daniel AM, Jay CL, Freedman BI. Practical considerations for APOL1 genotyping in the living kidney donor evaluation. Transplantation. 2020;104(1):27–32. https://doi.org/10.1097/tp.0000000000002933.
85. McIntosh T, Mohan S, Sawinski D, Iltis A, DuBois JM. Variation of ApoL1 testing practices for living kidney donors. Prog Transplant. 2020;30(1):22–8. https://doi.org/10.1177/1526924819892917.
86. Newell KA, Formica RN, Gill JS, Schold JD, Allan JS, Covington SH, et al. Integrating APOL1 gene variants into renal transplantation: considerations arising from the American Society of Transplantation expert conference. Am J Transplant. 2017;17(4):901–11. https://doi.org/10.1111/ajt.14173.

87. British Transplantation Society (BTS). Guidelines for living donor kidney transplantation. 2018. Available at: https://bts.org.uk/wp-content/uploads/2018/07/FINAL_LDKT-guidelines_June-2018.pdf. Accessed: 7 Sept 2020.

88. Gordon EJ, Amomicronrtegui D, Blancas I, Wicklund C, Friedewald J, Sharp RR. African American living Donors' attitudes about APOL1 genetic testing: a mixed methods study. Am J Kidney Dis. 2018;72(6):819–33. https://doi.org/10.1053/j.ajkd.2018.07.017.

89. Gordon EJ, Wicklund C, Lee J, Sharp RR, Friedewald J. A National Survey of transplant surgeons and nephrologists on implementing Apolipoprotein L1 (APOL1) genetic testing into clinical practice. Prog Transplant. 2018:1526924818817048. https://doi.org/10.1177/1526924818817048.

90. Freedman B, Moxey-Mims M, Alexander A, Astor B, Birdwell K, Bowden D, et al. APOL1 long-term kidney transplantation outcomes network (APOLLO): Design and rationale. Kidney Int Rep. 2020(5):278–88. https://doi.org/10.1016/j.ekir.2019.11.022.

91. Ross LF, Thistlethwaite JR Jr. Introducing genetic tests with uncertain implications in living donor kidney transplantation: ApoL1 as a case study. Prog Transplant. 2016;26(3):203–6. https://doi.org/10.1177/1526924816654608.

92. Wright L, Buchman D, Chandler J, Schultz K, Fortin M-C, Greenberg R, et al. Fast facts: public solicitation for solid organs and hematopoietic stem cells from living donors. 2015. Available at: http://media.wix.com/ugd/5a805e_be3abb0f072144698ded27047d221e70.pdf. Accessed: 7 Sept 2020.

93. CBC News. Eugene Melnyk, Ottawa Senators owner, needs urgent liver transplant. Posted: 14 May 2015. Available at: http://www.cbc.ca/news/canada/ottawa/eugene-melnyk-ottawa-senators-owner-needs-urgent-liver-transplant-1.3074658. Accessed: 7 Sept 2020.

94. Coyle J. 'The rich do better': ethics and Eugene Melnyk's new liver. The Star. Posted: 23 May 2015. Available at: https://www.thestar.com/news/canada/2015/05/23/the-rich-do-better-ethics-and-eugene-melnyks-new-liver.html. Accessed: 7 Sept 2020.

95. Friscolanti M. The miracle twins. Available at: https://site.macleans.ca/longform/miracle-twins/index.html. Accessed: 7 Sept 2020.

96. Goldberg A. Advertising for organs.Virtual Mentor. 2005;7(9):virtualmentor.2005.7.9.msoc2-0509. https://doi.org/10.1001/virtualmentor.2005.7.9.msoc2-0509.

97. Miller AM. Please give me your kidney: how to crowdsource for an organ. Posted: 30 June 2016. Available at: https://health.usnews.com/health-news/patient-advice/articles/2016-06-30/please-give-me-your-kidney-how-to-crowdsource-for-an-organ. Accessed: 7 Sept 2020.

98. Pronk M, Slaats D, Zuidema W, Hilhorst M, Dor F, Betjes M, et al. "what if this is my chance to save my life?" a semistructured interview study on the motives and experiences of end-stage renal disease patients who engaged in public solicitation of a living kidney donor. Transpl Int. 2017. https://doi.org/10.1111/tri.13095.

99. Rossi E. C-reactive protein and progressive atherosclerosis. Lancet. 2002;360(9344):1436–7. https://doi.org/10.1016/s0140-6736(02)11486-3.

100. Neidich EM, Neidich AB, Coober JT, Bramstedtd KA. The ethical complexities of online organ solicitation via donor–patient websites: avoiding the "beauty contest". Am J Transplant. 2012;12(1):43–7. https://doi.org/10.1111/j.1600-6143.2011.03765.x.

101. Marcon AR, Caulfield T, Toews M. Public solicitation and the Canadian media: two cases of living liver donation, two different stories. Transplant Direct. 2019;5(12). https://doi.org/10.1097/txd.0000000000000950.

102. Robertson C. Who is really hurt anyway? The problem of soliciting designated organ donations. Am J Bioethics : AJOB. 2005;5(4):16–7. https://doi.org/10.1080/15265160500194493.

103. Frunza M, Van Assche K, Lennerling A, Sterckx S, Citterio F, Mamode N, et al. Dealing with public solicitation of organs from living donors—an ELPAT view. Transplantation. 2015;99(10):2210–4. https://doi.org/10.1097/tp.0000000000000669.

104. Hanto DW. Ethical challenges posed by the solicitation of deceased and living organ donors. N Engl J Med. 2007;356(10):1062–6. https://doi.org/10.1056/nejmsb062319.
105. Glazier AK, Sasjack S. Should it be illicit to solicit? A legal analysis of policy options to regulate solicitation of organs for transplant. Health Matrix (Cleveland, Ohio : 1991). 2007;17(1):63–99. https://pubmed.ncbi.nlm.nih.gov/17849817/.
106. Kazley AS, Hamidi B, Balliet W, Baliga P. Social media use among living kidney donors and recipients: survey on current practice and potential. J Med Internet Res. 2016;18(12):e328. https://doi.org/10.2196/jmir.6176.
107. Chang A, Anderson EE, Turner HT, Shoham D, Hou SH, Grams M. Identifying potential kidney donors using social networking web sites. Clin Transpl. 2013;27(3):E320–6. https://doi.org/10.1111/ctr.12122.
108. Kumar K, King EA, Muzaale AD, Konel JM, Bramstedt KA, Massie AB, et al. A smartphone app for increasing live organ donation. Am J Transplant. 2016;16(12):3548–53. https://doi.org/10.1111/ajt.13961.
109. Bramstedtd KA, Cameron AM. Beyond the billboard: the Facebook-based application, donor, and its guided approach to facilitating living organ donation. Am J Transplant. 2016;
110. Fortin M, Buchman D, Wright L, Chandler J, Delaney S, Fairhead T, et al. Public solicitation of anonymous organ donors: a position paper by the Canadian Society of Transplantation. Transplantation. 2017;101(1):17–20. https://doi.org/10.1097/tp.0000000000001514.
111. Shanker RR, Anthony SJ, Wright L. A scoping review of the literature on public solicitations for living organ and hematopoietic stem cell donations. Prog Transplant. 2018;28(3):288–95. https://doi.org/10.1177/1526924818781578

Living Donor Transplant Program Growth, Innovation and Sustainability

16

David A. Axelrod, David Serur, Matthew Abramson, and Dianne LaPointe Rudow

Barriers to Increased Rates of Living Donation

The well-recognized shortage of kidneys donors contributes to excessive death on the kidney transplantation waiting list. Unfortunately, living donation rates declined beginning in 2004 despite the growing need for organs. Happily, in 2018 we have witnessed an increase in LDKT for the first time in many years. The etiology of this reduction in donation rates is likely multifactorial and disproportionately impacted racial/ethnic minorities, persons with lower socioeconomic status (SES), and older individuals. Unfortunately, the disparity in LDKT access appears to be increasing, based on national data. Purnell et al. demonstrated a progressive decline in access to LDKT for black, Hispanic, and Asian transplant candidates [1]. Among patients listed between 1995 and 99, the adjusted subhazard ratio (aHR) of receiving a LDKT for blacks compared to whites was 0.45 (95% confidence interval [CI] 0.42–0.48). In 2010–14, the aHR decreased further to 0.27 (95% CI 0.26–0.28). While some of this racial disparity is due to differences in the prevalence of medical conditions that preclude safe donation including diabetes mellitus [DM], obesity, hypertension, and genetic predisposition to renal insufficiency (e.g., Apolipoprotein L1 [APOL1]), studies suggest that potentially modifiable risk factors contribute to the growing gap in access [1].

D. A. Axelrod
Department of Surgery, University of Iowa, Iowa City, IA, USA
e-mail: david-axelrod@uiowa.edu

D. Serur · M. Abramson
Transplant Nephrology, New York Presbyterian Hospital/Weill Cornell, New York, NY, USA
e-mail: dserur@nyp.org

D. LaPointe Rudow (✉)
Recanati Miller Transplantation Institute, Mount Sinai Hospital, New York, NY, USA
e-mail: Dianne.LaPointeRudow@mountsinai.org

© Springer Nature Switzerland AG 2021
K. L. Lentine et al. (eds.), *Living Kidney Donation*,
https://doi.org/10.1007/978-3-030-53618-3_16

Population-based analyses of living donation rates demonstrate that access to LDKT is strongly correlated with demographic differences in populations served by transplant programs. Locke et al. correlated living donation rates with population health characteristics drawn from the CDC Behavioral Risk Factor surveillance system [2]. The proportion of LDKT was negatively correlated with the prevalence of racial and ethnic minority populations and low SES. Transplant centers in regions with both low SES and high minority populations had a 10.7% absolute reduction in LDKT rates compared to more affluent communities with predominantly Caucasian populations. In a multivariate analysis, high minority population centers reported 7.1% fewer LDKT compared to those serving predominantly Caucasian populations while low SES regions performed 7.3% fewer compared to transplant centers in high SES regions.

Our understanding of the etiology of the profound differences in access to LDKT appears to be evolving. While there are no direct costs to the living donor/donor candidate for evaluation, surgery, and post-operative care, the process of living donation frequently results in significant economic costs for candidates and donors. Donor candidates often miss time from work for evaluation visits and testing, and those who donate are unable to work for a period of 4–6 weeks after surgery, depending on the nature of their employment. Lost income differentially impacts low SES donors, who more often work in positions that require significant physical labor and may have less options for paid leave through their employers. In the RELIVE study of 2455 prior living donors, Jacobs et al. report that 20% of donors felt that donation was a financial burden and 5% reported that they had difficulty with monthly bills after surgery [3]. It was not surprising that recipients with living donors who were older (odds ratio [OR] 0.62 [95% CI 0.51–0.75]) or had higher SES (OR 0.58 [95% CI 0.46–0.73]) reported fewer financial concerns. Average time to recovery was also impacted, as white donors and donors with higher SES reported shorter recovery periods than minority and low SES patients undergoing donor nephrectomy.

The absolute magnitude of the economic burden of living donation has been estimated in several prospective studies. A prospective evaluation of 912 Canadian living donors reported a median total cost of donation of $2217 CAD including both out-of-pocket costs and lost productivity [4]. For these donors, the donation process was associated with $1254 CAD in out-of-pocket costs, largely for transportation, accommodations, and post-donation prescriptions. US estimates of the direct economic costs of donation average $5000 [5]. This cost represents a substantial economic barrier to donation, which may contribute to the marked reduction in donation rates among the population with low SES overall, and racial and ethnic minorities specifically.

Barriers to broader acceptance of living donation among kidney failure patients with low SES include more than simply the financial aspects of living donation. End-stage renal disease (ESRD) patients with low SES have been shown to have a greater incidence of maladaptive interactions with the healthcare system. Bailey et al. reported on a qualitative study of recipients of deceased donor organs in the United Kingdom to identify factors that prevented access to LDKT among otherwise acceptable candidates [6]. This population was chosen as it ensured that patients were, in fact, medically cleared for kidney transplant which is paid for by the National Health Service. Through structured interviews, patients with high socioeconomic deprivation scores displayed greater passivity, reported feeling disempowered, lacked social support, and maintained a "short-term" focus on health-related issues. These behaviors limited patients' ability to act as their own advocates. For example, passivity and disempowerment manifested as patients' decision not to discuss LDKT with providers, assuming that they were not candidates. Lack of social support limited patients' ability to successfully solicit potential living donors. Interestingly, the issue of the cost of transplant and location of potential donors were only identified in discussions with patients with less socioeconomic deprivation. This research suggests the need to tailor interventions designed to increase LDKT by focusing on strategies that build knowledge and empower lower SES patients to actively seek living donors, in addition to direct financial subsidies to removal financial burdens to living donors.

Institutional Culture to Promote Living Donor Transplantation

The first step in providing safe and available LDKT to all potential recipients is to embrace the importance of donation and LDKT. Transplant programs have a responsibility to develop programs with sufficient expertise to evaluate, care for, and follow all living donors, including those with complex medical and surgical conditions. To develop a culture of living donation at the transplant center, program leadership should incorporate the recommendations from the 2014 American Society of Transplantation (AST) Consensus Conference on Best Practices in Live Kidney Donation [7]. The primary recommendation of the consensus statement was that transplant programs, healthcare professionals, and support staff serving patients with chronic kidney disease (CKD) utilize a philosophical approach that emphasizes LDKT as the best treatment option for most patients with kidney failure. Without a culture that prioritizes living donation, centers and kidney care providers will fail to address existing multicultural, financial, and medical barriers; and innovative practice will lag. Developing this culture can be challenging if clinicians have bias against living donation or their belief system conflicts with this principle. Tong et al. surveyed nephrologists and surgeons at transplant programs across the world and found that providers faced challenges in defining acceptable risk to the donor, burden of responsibility for decision making, medical protectiveness, respecting donor autonomy, and driving ideologies/ pressures [8]. Transplant programs need to address these concerns directly to ensure that patients and families receive accurate and appropriate counseling in regard to living donation and LDKT. This counseling needs to ensure risks are accurately communicated in a way that is honest but does not inadvertently discourage donation. Additional programmatic components needed to ensure a culture that supports and promotes LDKT are shown in Table 16.1 and are described below. We include the necessary medical, surgical, financial, psychosocial supports described in the 2014 Consensus Conference report [7]. As the medical and surgical aspects of living donation are addressed elsewhere in this textbook, this chapter focuses on the programmatic resources and other interventions that can be employed to support and improve the practice of living donation and LDKT.

Table 16.1 Programmatic components needed to ensure a culture that promotes LDKT. (Adapted from LaPointe Rudow et al. [7])

- Programmatic components needed to ensure a culture that promotes LDKT
- Resources and expertise to provide culturally tailored LDKT education to racial/ethnic minority patients
- Provide patients and their caregivers with training about how to identify and approach potential living donors
- Ensure systems and personnel are in place to respond immediately and thoroughly to living donor inquiries
- Create an expedited process for transplant candidates with potential living donors who are at lower risk/lower morbidity or who may be able to receive a transplant pre-emptively
- Provide expertise to evaluate medically and surgically complex donors
- Collect and systematically review living donor metrics to measure efficiencies
- Create a quality improvement program to ensure ongoing evaluation and improvement of transplant candidate and living donor education about LDKT

Interventions to Reduce the Financial Burden of Living Donation

As noted, financial barriers to living donation are widely perceived as dominant forces limiting donation. In direct evidence of this link is the correlation between living donation rates and community SES. In the United States, the National Living Donor Assistance Center (NLDAC) was initially funded in 2006 under the Organ Donation and Recovery Improvement Act (P.L. 108–216) which granted authority to the US Secretary of Health and Human Services to create a program to provide direct financial assistance to living donors [9]. These funds were designed to eliminate financial disincentives resulting from the cost of travel, housing, and non-medical expenses. The funds do not replace lost income, although a White House Executive Order issued July 10, 2019 seeks to provide lost wage reimbursement through NLDAC [10]. Implementation of NLDAC funding was accomplished via a request for proposals which led to the awarding of the contract to the American Society of Transplant Surgeons (ASTS) which currently administers the program. NLDAC funds are limited to donors who are giving to recipients of limited means (< 300% of the US federal poverty level but this may be expanded to higher income levels). NLDAC is designated as the payer of last resort. Therefore, donors are restricted from receiving assistance if they may access state-based programs or private insurance stipends. Notably, non-directed donors are eligible for NLDAC once a recipient is identified.

In 2018, Mathur et al. analyzed the outcomes of NLDAC applications received between 2012 and 15 [11]. During this period, 2425 applications were approved, leading to 1330 living donors. The average award was $2071, and the median income of recipients whose donor received assistance was $42,510. The authors then considered the return on investment (ROI) achieved through this modest level of support. By facilitating earlier transplantation and limited spending on dialysis, NLDAC was estimated to have saved $256 million in direct costs at 5 years (a 28.2-fold ROI). The program continues to grow; and, to date, more than 4855 living donors have received assistance which now covers travel, meals, lodging, and other out-of-pocket expenses. Other foundation resources to offset the cost of donation include the American Transplant Foundation, which assists low-income patients with income replacement. However, these funds are limited to $700.

Private insurers have also recognized the significant clinical and financial benefits which accrue from living donation. United Health Care/OPTUM announced, at the American Transplant Congress in 2016, that donors would be eligible for up to $5000 travel-related expense reimbursement to offset the cost of living donation [12]. Similar assistance may be offered from other private payers, based on contractual agreements. Several states have programs that offer support for living donor expenses.

Transplant program billing practices to minimize financial consequences of evaluation, surgical, and follow-up care to living donor candidates and donors have also recently been articulated in recommendations from an AST Live Donor Community of Practice workgroup. Some recommendations made were to utilize a standard acquisition charge with all payers, place all donor charges as a kidney acquisition cost on the Medicare Cost Report, reduce donor travel burden, verify a coverage plan for donor complications prior to donation, and encourage recipients to obtain Medicare Part A and B to ensure coverage for donor complications [13].

Interventions to Increase Living Donor Transplantation among Racial and Ethnic Minorities

Lack of engagement and empowerment of living donors from underrepresented minority communities remains a significant barrier to LKDT for minority transplant candidates. The first step in improving access to LDKT is empowering recipients and their social network. Various programs have been developed and evaluated to accomplish this goal [14, 15]. Garonzik-Wang et al. reported on the Living Donor Champion program in 2012 [16]. In this program, individuals within a transplant candidate's social network received training in sharing about transplant, donation, and the kidney patient's need for an organ donor with their social network. In a pilot trial of 15 patients, 25 potential donors came forward, 4 patients were transplanted, and another 3 had donors in evaluation. In comparison, a matched control group of waitlist patients had no living donor transplants. A similar program, the Kidney Coach Program, was recently reported from Mount Sinai, NY [17]. In this program, an advocate for the potential recipient was trained to seek out potential donors. Candidates with at least one donor inquiry increased from 37% in the control group to 80% in the intervention arm ($p = 0.001$).

An alternative strategy was proposed by Rodrigue et al. in 2008 [18]. In their "House Calls" intervention, a culturally sensitive program of in-home outreach was developed for African American kidney patients. The program provides an in-home education session for the transplant candidate and invited members of their social network. This includes a brief video and a one-hour interactive session with a representative from the transplant program. Assessed in a formal randomized controlled trial, the House Calls intervention increased living donor inquiries markedly for minority recipients when compared to the clinic-based education. Compared with historical controls, the study increased the percent of patients with a living donor inquiry (77.4% vs. 51.7%), a donor evaluated (48.4% vs. 17.2%), and a LDKT (45.2% vs. 13.8%). The program was also successful in the Caucasian population [18].

Unfortunately, withdrawal of donor candidates who contact the center for evaluation continues to be a significant issue, particularly among African American potential donors. Kumar et al. recently compared outcomes of 911 prospective donors at Johns Hopkins, 27% of whom self-identified as African American [19]. There was a marked reduction in progression to donation by 2 years on the basis of race (20% AA vs. 36%, non-AA; HR 0.41, $p < 0.001$). Among the 74% of AAs who did not donate, 42% did not progress due to medical factors including hypertension, obesity, and kidney abnormalities. Other reasons for non-donation included social (10%), personal (18%), or other. By comparison, while 73% of the non-AAs also did not progress to donation, medical conditions were responsible for only 26% of the declines. AAs were significantly less likely to progress from initial medical screening to formal evaluation (aHR 0.62, $P = 0.02$) and from final clearance to donation (aHR 0.51, $P = 0.02$). The authors conclude that the barriers for AAs in reaching medical clearance include a higher incidence of medical comorbidities in biologically related donors and extended time to complete required evaluations despite living geographically closer to the center. The authors suggest the need to provide additional support for donor candidates with limited social networks to assist with the completion of the living donor evaluation process, such as donor navigators or peer support.

Living donation rates have also been disproportionately low for Hispanic patients, despite higher rates of ESRD [20]. Waitlisted Hispanic transplant candidates are less likely to receive any transplant (17.8% vs. 25.1%) and specifically a LDKT (4.6% vs. 10.5%) when compared to non-Hispanic white transplant candidates. To address this disparity, the transplant program at Northwestern Memorial Hospital has developed a culturally sensitive "Hispanic Transplant Program." This comprehensive program provides education, medical care, and care coordination by Spanish-speaking professionals. The transplant recipient educational program is taught by bilingual medical professionals and specifically addresses "Hispanic cultural and religious concerns and myths" to encourage donation. The program has led to a 70% expansion in the number of LDKT in Hispanic patients. This program is now being evaluated at two additional institutions [21].

Role of Technology in Advancing Living Donation

The need for accurate, accessible, and culturally sensitive decision tools to promote living donation has never been greater. Patients increasingly turn to on-line sources for basic knowledge about the risks and benefits of living donation. Unlike the

Northwestern Memorial Hospital program referenced above for Hispanics, the majority of websites providing information on living donation and LDKT do not provide content that is written within guidelines for reading level and comprehension. Rodrigue et al. examined 21 websites that provide information to potential donors in the United States [22]. Among these sources, 62% where classified as difficult to read and all were above the sixth grade reading level. Content analysis revealed that the average website presented only 62% of 30 recommended elements of donor information. Missing data included information on complications beyond death, infection, or pain. Similarly, while most websites reported that donors may experience out-of-pocket costs, most websites were not specific and only 62% suggested possible resources for assistance. Other key factors that were not highlighted included preferential placement on the kidney list for living donors who develop ESRD (38% of websites), privacy protections for donor health information (33%), waiting times for deceased donor transplant (33%), and the benefit of pre-emptive transplant (19%). Furthermore, while many websites included racially diverse photographs, very few explicitly mentioned race (29%), provided non-English text (24%), or included minority patients in videos (10%). Finally, the unique risks of living donation in at-risk minority populations were not mentioned in more than 90% of websites. Many of the online sources on donation and transplantations are at a reading level too high for many potential kidney recipients [23].

These data suggest the need to develop and promote culturally sensitive interactive and web-based tools. Web-based or mobile applications represent an important tool to increase knowledge and acceptance of living donation, if done correctly. Gander et al. reviewed available decision aids that can be used to increase LDKT, particularly among underserved minorities [24]. These websites provide appropriate, culturally competent information for recipients and potential donors.

Providing Resources to Enhance African American Patients' Readiness to Make Decisions about Kidney Disease (Prepared) [25]. This is a video- and text-based program developed to inform AA patients about options for kidney disease including LDKT. The effectiveness of this program is currently being assessed in a clinical trial.

The Big Ask, The Big Give [26]. This campaign was launched by the National Kidney Foundation (NKF) in 2014 in response to community requests. The program includes patient outreach information and a website designed to increase interest in living donation. The core of the program is half-day workshops, held with support of transplant programs, to educate kidney patients and family and/or friends about transplantation, living donation, and strategies for sharing the patient's need with their social network. The impact of this program has not been prospectively evaluated.

Living about Choices in Transplant and Sharing (Living ACTS) [27]. This is a video- and text-based educational program designed specifically to educate AAs about living donation. The program provides culturally sensitive education about donation and treatment options while acknowledging the role of families in health decisions in the AA community. In a randomized trial involving 268 transplant candidates, the Living ACTS program increased knowledge and willingness to purse LDKT.

Infórmate: Inform Yourself about Living Kidney Donation for Hispanic/ Latinos [28]. This resource is a Spanish language web-based intervention targeted to Hispanics. The site combines bilingual education about transplantation and living donation, recognizing cultural norms within the Hispanic community. The site increases engagement through interactive graphics, testimonials, and telenovelas. Randomized prospective evaluation of the intervention demonstrated increased knowledge immediately following the program which was sustained over the subsequent 3 weeks.

The UNOS Kidney Learning Center (KTLC) [29]. This is an online national clearinghouse of public educational resources about kidney transplant and living donation for patients, families, and potential living donors. The KTLC collected and collated information developed by national leaders in the design of transplant education; these programs were unified and then revised for health literacy, resulting in an easy to understand, navigate, and use website. Although the content of the individual programs have been studied for efficacy, the clearinghouse has not.

American Society for Transplantation Live Donor Tool Kit [30]. This resource is a free-standing website with centralized, standardized, data driven, neutral, high-quality living donor education used to complement other existing resources. There are provider- and patient-level chapters to provide information about financial risks (military service, cost-estimation worksheet, employment, insurability after donation, fundraising, financial support funds, and tax laws) and medical risks of kidney donation (e.g., kidney failure, hypertension, obesity, Polycystic kidney disease risk, kidney stones, hematuria, kidney paired donation, and metabolic syndromes) as well as psychosocial risks, informed consent, and primary care provider engagement. The chapters are written with health literacy review for middle school comprehension level and available in English and Spanish.

Each of these programs can be combined with the transplant program's internal education to increase awareness of living donation and LDKT. The interventions differ from standard of care by directly involving the patient's social networks, providing culturally sensitive education for diverse communities, and allowing self-directed learning.

Social Media as a Tool to Increase Living Donation

Social media has been successfully used to promote campaigns to reduce alcohol and smoking, as well as to positively reinforce diet and exercise. As social media becomes more pervasive in our daily lives, so has its use in the kidney donation and transplantation landscape. In 2015, Kazley et al. [31] performed a survey-based cross-sectional study of 199 kidney transplant candidates. 52.2% reported using social media (the majority using Facebook), 25.1% posted about health-related activities, 35.7% reported they are willing to share their health information via social media, and 11.6% promoted their need for kidney donation. In 2013, Chang et al. identified 91 publicly available Facebook pages of kidney transplant candidates asking for donation; 64% displayed the patient's blood type, 43% etiology of kidney failure, and 71% location. With regard to impact, 32% reported donors were being tested and 10% received LDKT but the time of publication. Page traffic was found to be significantly associated with undergoing a living kidney transplant [32]. Kumar et al. [33] developed a Facebook application which allowed transplant candidates to post about their own experiences with kidney disease and their need for a kidney. Compared to controls, those who posted to Facebook using this application were 6.6 times more likely to have a potential live donor come forward. Moorlock [34] explains two distinct strategies using social media: awareness-raising (using population statistics) and personalized approaches (using case studies) to promoting living donation. The authors suggest that case studies with "identifiable victims" appeal toward generation of empathy and an increased tendency toward altruistic living donation. Social media gives transplant candidates the ability to act as the identifiable victim, which would generate empathy, leading to publicly solicited donation. This may lead to a unique opportunity to not only receive the benefits of a transplant, but to take ownership of one's future. Other social media platforms such as Twitter are being used to communicate and share information about transplant and living donation across the public, patients, and providers [35].

In the contact of expanded use of social media related to donation and transplantation, the ethics of using social media to increase an individual's odds of receiving a kidney transplant is also being discussed and debated. First, unsuccessful transplant candidates may develop a sense of abandonment while others using the same tactics were successful. Second, social inequalities may limit access to social media, further exacerbating racial and ethnic differences. Third, there is an ethical conundrum of choosing recipients based on non-medical criteria such as a compelling story or a good marketing campaign as opposed to the person most at need. Lastly, significant programmatic resources are consumed with numerous inquiries for donation but few serious candidates, especially from unrelated social media only contacts. Programmatic guidelines for responsible social media utilization and fiduciary use of program resources and manpower can assist in ethically responsible solicitation for kidney donation using these tools. The Organ Procurement and Transplantation Network (OPTN) Living Donor Committee formed a workgroup in Spring 2019 focused on developing guidance for transplant centers in the appropriate use of social media related to living donation [36].

Social media groups have developed tools to assist with standardized requests for an organ donor. In collaboration with the Johns Hopkins transplant team in 2012, Facebook added an "Organ Donor" option to a user's profile. This provided a link to the state donor registry website and a notification to friends of the profile addition. After the first day of implementation, dubbed the "Facebook Effect," there was a

21-times increase in deceased donor registrations, ranging from 6.9-fold increase in Michigan to 108.9-fold increase in Georgia, and these gains were sustained for 12 days [37]. It is unclear if the organ donor indication will result in higher rates of living donors. "Donor," a free Facebook application, was devised as a non-coercive low-pressure solution for transplant candidate outreach, while at the same time mitigating concerns of unethical solicitation of living donation [38]. The application provides an easy-to-follow template which guides patients to construct as accurate and structured narratives as possible. The patients decide which of their "friends" will have access to this narrative. The patient's living donor champion is also involved in the application, allowing them to expand the posted narrative.

Institutional Strategies and Resources Needed to Increase Living Donation

Identifying and recruiting additional donors is not sufficient to maximize living donor potential. High functioning centers require institutional commitment for optimal program structure and sufficient financial resources to support all of the components of the living donor program. These include oversight to ensure that the program complies with the complex regulations surrounding living donation, sufficient surgical skill and redundancy to ensure coverage for all dates, medical expertise in living donation, psychosocial assessment which encourages and support donation, and programmatic leadership to ensure collaboration [39]. Suggested programmatic structure, education, evaluation, and care processes to optimize successful living donation and LDKT are summarized in Fig. 16.1.

Leadership and Staffing

The program should have significant staffing resources devoted primarily or exclusively to the living donor team; specifically, the program should have at least one living donor coordinator and a dedicated physician champion [7]. The team needs experienced clinical leadership in order to work efficiently to educate, screen, evaluate, and care for potential and actual living donors throughout the process. The physician champion often serves in the role as leader; however, nurses have also been utilized as they may be able to devote more time to the processes and policies needed to maintain efficiency in the living donor team [31]. In contemporary practice, living donor candidates are often less straightforward than in the past, and may have complex medical, surgical, and psychosocial conditions that warrant expert evaluation including nephrology, psychology, and anesthesia.

Because transplant candidate medical issues can derail the LDKT and result in delays and waste resources, a parallel process for expedited evaluation of recipients has been found to improve communication and result in increased LDKT [32]. This process can be facilitated by assigning a coordinator specifically to focus on transplant candidates with potential living donors. Additional administrative staff are

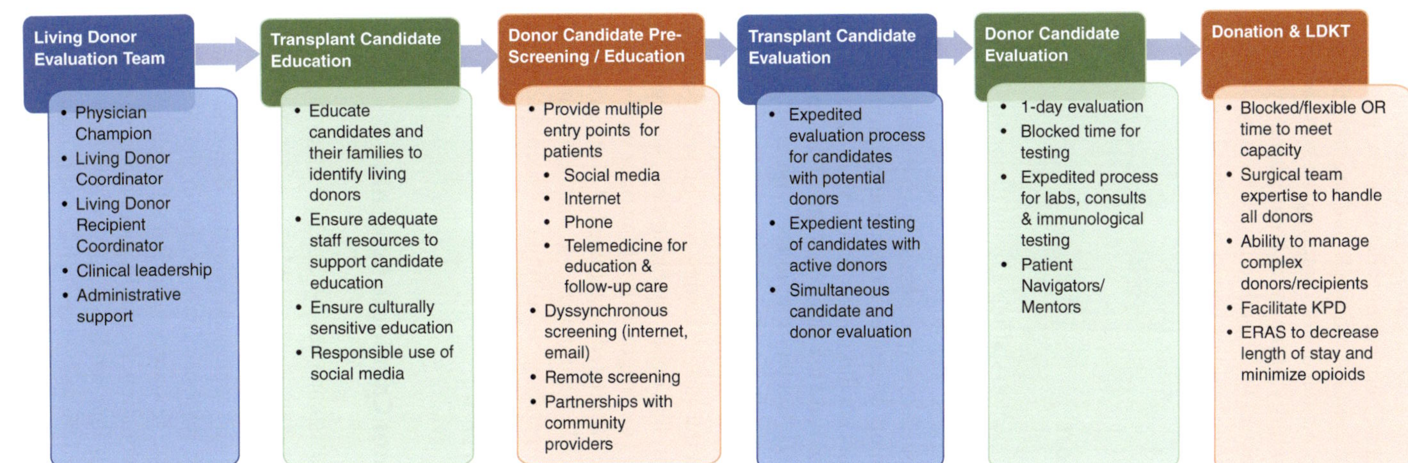

Fig. 16.1 Programmatic structure, education, evaluation, and care processes to optimize successful living donation and LDKT. *Abbreviations: ERAS* enhanced recovery after surgery, *KPD* kidney paired donation, *LDKT* living donor kidney transplant, *OR* operating room

essential to respond promptly to inquiries, gather medical records and assist with scheduling of appointments, help patients navigate the process, and coordinate the pre-, peri-, and postoperative care required. Staffing models should be determined based on the number of potential donors entering the system rather than the number of LDKT since only a minority of potential donors actually donate [40]. Any delay in care can result in a lost LDKT opportunity. Adequate staffing and coordinated communication with routine huddles between medical, surgical, psychosocial, and support staff can improve collaboration and problem solving to address delays and barriers to LDKT [41].

Programmatic Support

In additional to a commitment to staffing a living donor program sufficiently, hospital resources are needed to ensure that the program has capacity to handle the volume of screenings, evaluations, and surgeries anticipated with growth. In one study, potential living donors cited multiple center level barriers to completing a living donor evaluation. The donors described the evaluation process as inefficient and too long, resulting in transplant candidates becoming too sick for transplant or potential donors becoming frustrated and backing out, both of which contribute to the reduction the rate of LDKT [42]. Centers should focus on addressing inefficiencies [43, 44, 45]. This includes providing ample clinic time to offer living donor appointments in a designated clinic with multiple convenient times during the week. There should be blocked time at the various testing sites including radiology, electrocardiography, and laboratory so that donor candidates can be accommodated in a timely and coordinated fashion. The program should partner with common consultants so that appointments can be facilitated when needed. Turnaround times for specialty labs and immunology should be minimized so that delays are avoided. The hospital should provide blocked operating room times to accommodate cleared pairs and prevent a backlog of cases. Living donors should be able to go from referral to donation in less than 3 months [40].

Electronic Living Donor Candidate Screening

Most potential living donors enter the system by calling the transplant program to begin the evaluation process or attending a face-to-face meeting at the center. This can be a barrier, as programs tend to have 9–5 weekday available for phone and in-person contact, requiring any interested potential donor to utilize time away from work or other caretaking responsibilities to begin the process. Additionally, the transplant team staff utilize resources to screen all inquiries, even those with absolute contraindications to donation. Recently, there has been increasing success with web-based screening tools that can be completed any time of day, making it more accessible to the end user [46–48]. Such web-based software platforms have intuitive algorithms, making them user-friendly and able to identify unacceptable donors early in the process, prior to utilization of valuable staff resources. These systems improve convenience for the potential donor and save staff resources to efficiently process appropriate potential donor candidates. One center reported an increase in donor self-referrals from 61 to 116 per month [46]. The electronic screening system significantly expedited initial review of the referral, improved communication, reduced labor costs, and increased living donor referrals.

Education of Transplant and Donor Candidates

Successful living donor programs need to ensure that clinicians caring for transplant candidates and potential donors have the tools and time to devote to living donation and LDKT education. The evidence-based education programs discussed in the previous section can be successful but require staff resources above and beyond general listing practices and medical management. Many educational interventions need to be repeated on more than one occasion and can be challenging, especially among patients with low healthy literacy or cultural barriers. Use of staff designated to provide such education outside the clinic visit has shown success in increasing candidates who try to find potential living donors and living donor inquires [49].

A Timely Evaluation Process for all Donor Candidates

Just as important as a convenient, efficient screening process, transplant programs must have a timely process for the comprehensive donor candidate medical and psychosocial evaluation. Long, tedious living donor evaluation protocols have been attributed to donor drop out of 30% of donors at one program [50]. In contrast, another center reported an 8-fold increase in LDKT when a one-day donor assessment was implemented. Graham and Courtney suggest that streamlining the process can result in more donor candidates progressing to donation [51]. In addition to the efficiently planned day, the donor was assisted by an experienced living donor coordinator who was available for discussions throughout the process. Data suggest that the rapport building during the day contributed to the success of the evaluation process, with 94% of donor candidates expressing satisfaction with the process [52]. The program should perform pre-assessments and education prior to the one-day evaluation to prepare the donor candidate for this expedited process Often the living donor candidate is new to the health care system and navigating their way through the day can be overwhelming. Living donor mentors and patient navigators can also improve support and satisfaction with the process. Having a navigator assist in the evaluation and testing day, getting from one place to another and to explain the purpose of each appointment can relieve any anxiety and improve the experience. Mentors who have gone through the process can explain the process in a very different way than the team who has not experienced living donation first-hand.

It is important to note that not all potential donors can be a candidate for a one-day evaluation. Donors with multiple co-morbidities, ambivalence, or low health literacy may require additional consults and counseling. However, an expedited process can be beneficial for potential donors who are at lower medical or psychosocial risk. Examples include young healthy donors, emotionally close donors and donors with preemptive transplant candidates [7]. If knowledge or ambivalence is the barrier to an expedited evaluation, the center should look into innovative ways to allow donors to avoid additional time away from work due to required travel to the transplant center. Telehealth may be one mechanism to perform preliminary evaluations and education prior to the donor candidate attending the robust face-to-face evaluation or for ongoing supplementation of education and support. There is little information on its utility in living donation; however, published reports in the kidney transplant recipient evaluation have found that telehealth has been associated with reductions in cost and improved satisfaction as a supplement to the standard evaluation [52].

Ensuring Living Donor Follow-Up

Transplant programs must be committed to providing resources to ensure compliance with living donor follow-up. The OPTN requires living donor recovery programs to collect and report clinical and laboratory follow-up data to the OPTN at 6 months, 1 year, and 2 years post-donation within 60 days of follow-up anniversary [53]. Importantly, follow-up can be coordinated though a local primary care provider, but the center is responsible for tracking and reporting the information [53]. This can be labor intensive; and many programs struggle to comply given the financial and logistical barriers that exist including, but not limited to, the assumption that living donors are healthy and do not perceive a need for follow-up, they may not live near the center where they donated, or cost burdens to the donor or program [13]. Despite these barriers, some best practices have been implemented to achieve successful follow-up rates. These included a programmatic conviction that follow-up is essential for donor safety and well-being; embracing the importance of building and maintaining a relationship with each donor; the use of a systematic approach to follow-up, with ongoing quality assurance activities and implementation of strategies to minimize burden to donors [43]. Strategies to minimize the financial impact of follow-up to the donor have also been proposed [13].

One example of an innovative approach is the use of technology to collect living donor follow-up information. Eno et al. surveyed 100 living kidney donors and found that smartphone ownership was high (94.0%), and 79% of smartphone-owning donors felt that it would be useful to complete their required follow-up with a mobile health tool [54]. They found no significant differences by age, sex, or race. These results suggest that living donors would benefit from incorporating a mobile health tool to perform their living donor follow-up. A randomized control trial is underway to determine the impact of the mKidney system (mobile health application) on the transplant program's compliance with OPTN-mandated living donor follow-up at a large transplant hospital. It will provide valuable information on strategies for implementing such a system in a clinical setting [55–56]. Not all living donors, however, would benefit from such electronic communication and may require more personalized attention. Telemedicine may be one mechanism to achieve compliance with follow-up in a personalized manner and avoid travel to the donation center [57].

Mandated OPTN follow-up is only required for 2 years and therefore only captures data on short-term risks to the donor. Until recently there have been no concerted efforts to capture long-term risks to the kidney donor in the United States. There is a need to establish a national living donor registry to prospectively follow donors over their lifetimes. In addition, there is a need to better understand the reasons many potential donors who initially volunteer to donate do not donate and whether the reasons are justified. Therefore, the US Health Resources and Services Administration asked the Scientific Registry of Transplant Recipients to establish a national registry to address these important questions. The Living Donor Collective is a multi-center pilot project underway to determine the feasibility of capturing long-term live donor data through a central location at 10 large, diverse US transplant programs [58]. The project includes living candidates who ultimately do not donate (and may serve as useful controls) and starts at the point of the living donor evaluation. If successful and expanded nationally, this registry should provide valuable information for clinicians and prospective donors during the informed consent process and is aimed at removing data collection burdens from the transplant programs.

Robust Quality Assurance and Performance Improvement Processes

All transplant programs are mandated by the Centers for Medicare & Medicaid Services (CMS) to have a robust Quality Assurance & Performance Improvement (QAPI) program in place to monitor all aspects of the donation and transplant process. For the living donor program, indicators should be process and outcome indicators designed to ensure quality, efficiency, and safety [40]. To ensure that sufficient programmatic and staffing resources are devoted to maximize LDKT potential, the program should collect and systematically review living donor metrics that capture efficiency and productivity (Table 16.2) [7]. Data that is collected should be utilized to modify the program to maximize potential [59].

Living Donor Satisfaction

It is crucial that donors feel that they are supported in the donation process and their donation decision. Up to 96% of donors have reported being "satisfied" with donation. To understand the barriers to living donation, Menjivar et al. studied the factors associated with donor satisfaction [60]. After surveying 332 laparoscopic donors, 21% felt that hospital discharge was premature and 32% reported economic losses due to donation. The least satisfied cluster of donors reported interference with daily activities, pain, and discomfort. Furthermore, up to 25% of recipients who

Table 16.2 Living donor metrics for quality assurance and process improvement

• Living donor metrics for quality assurance and process improvement
• The number of living donor screenings
• The number of living donor evaluations
• The number of living donor kidney transplants
• How potential donors enter the system (in person, by telephone, online screening)
• The length of time in each phase of donation (referral, evaluation, cleared, and waiting for surgery)
• Reasons potential donors are being declined (medical, psychosocial, donor decision, BMI, etc.)
• The number of potential donors who drop out of donation in each phase of the donor process
• Donor demographic characteristics including age, sex, race, and ethnicity
• Recipient characteristics including age, sex, race, ethnicity, time on dialysis, insurance
• Compliance with 6-month, 1-year, and 2-year follow-up
• Accuracy of the clinical and laboratory data collected at OPTN required follow-up

benefitted from donation were dissatisfied with the post-donation care of their donors, leading to dissatisfaction with the transplant process [49]. To improve satisfaction with the evaluation and donation process, living donor programs can improve efficiency, minimize burdens, and tailored education related to the outcomes important to donors [61].

Partnerships with Community Providers to Increase Living Donor Transplantation

Transplant programs should develop partnerships with local dialysis staff and community nephrologists to increase LDKT. Getchell et al. cited a significant systemic level barrier to LDKT resulting from poor and delayed communication between primary providers, nephrologists, dialysis staff, and transplant centers [42]. Community physicians/nephrologists are frontline providers and are in a unique position to offer education about living donation and the benefits of LDKT, and to improve efficiencies in the process. Education for primary nephrologists is needed to ensure that they understand the donor referral and evaluation process, the responsibilities of the transplant program, and the potential role they can play in the process. Transplant programs should strive to engage community nephrologists in living donor education, evaluation, and long-term follow-up [62].

Partnering with Chronic Kidney Disease (CKD) Management Clinics

The transition from early to advanced CKD requires a dramatic change in approach to patient care, with an emphasis on preparation for ESRD. Median time of progression from Stage 5 CKD (glomerular filtration rate <15 mL/min per 1.73 m^2) to

ESRD is 0.6 years [63]. Only 2.6% of patients with advanced CKD will undergo preemptive transplant [64], hospitalization rates are high, and in-hospital initiation of renal replacement continues to be a problem. The low rate of preemptive transplantation is a multifactorial problem including late referral to nephrology and lack of living donors. African Americans and those patients with lower health literacy have a reduced likelihood of referral for transplantation. As such, there has been an increased interest in clinics whose sole purpose is to manage those with advanced CKD, with emphasis on delaying progression as well as education about renal replacement therapy. In 2007, NKF/ Kidney Disease Outcomes Quality Initiative (KDOQI) recognized the need for such clinics specialized in advanced kidney disease, with a goal of increasing preemptive transplantation, and have consequently designed protocols for CKD clinics.

In 2011, the "Healthy Transitions in Late Stage Kidney Disease" intervention was established, with the primary goal of integrating nurse care managers into the preparation phase of ESRD, in order to reduce hospitalizations and improve patient education [65]. The "CKD management clinic" involves an initial nurse manager visit to the patient's home, with focus on discussion regarding renal replacement modality, as well as nutrition education and home assessment. Following the initial visit, the nurse manager devises a patient-centered plan with the nephrologist using an informatics system with an integrated database and protocol. Fishbane et al. [65] compared advanced CKD outcomes in Nassau County, NY between patients in the "Healthy Transitions in Late Stage Kidney Disease" intervention to controls receiving usual care. There were decreased hospitalizations in the intervention group (0.61 per year) compared to control (0.92 per year). There was no difference regarding the time course of reaching ESRD among both groups; 13% of those in intervention group vs 7% in control group received a pre-emptive transplant, although this was not statistically significant [65].

Another example of a CKD clinic is the "Healthy Living Clinic" (HLC) at Northwestern University. The HLC staff includes a physician assistant, 2 registered nurses, and a dietitian, with referral by a Northwestern nephrologist, and follow-up every 4 months. From 2003 to 2005, 67 patients were enrolled into the HLC, 42 were eligible for transplant referral, and 81% of participants, compared to 58% of eligible controls, were referred for transplant [66].

Conclusions

LDKT provides the optimal treatment for patients with ESRD. Nationally, there remains a shortage of available allografts despite a large population of potential donors. Thus, transplant programs and collaborating providers need strategies to increase awareness, reduce unnecessary barriers, and support the courageous donor candidates who do come forward for evaluation. Transplant centers need the institutional support and resources to ensure that potential donors are appropriately evaluated, cared for efficiently and compassionately, and followed longitudinally after their surgery. If approached in a culturally appropriate manner, it is likely that access to LDKT can be significantly increased in a way that is safe, ethical, and cost-effective. Success begins with a partnership with primary nephrologists to ensure timely referral of transplant candidates and accurate information on LKDT at the time of diagnosis of advanced CKD.

References

1. Purnell TS, Luo X, Cooper LA, Massie AB, Kucirka LM, Henderson ML, et al. Association of race and ethnicity with live donor kidney transplantation in the United States from 1995 to 2014. JAMA. 2018;319(1):49–61. https://doi.org/10.1001/jama.2017.19152.
2. Reed RD, Sawinski D, Shelton BA, MacLennan PA, Hanaway M, Kumar V, et al. Population health, ethnicity, and rate of living donor kidney transplantation. Transplantation. 2018;102(12):2080–7. https://doi.org/10.1097/TP.0000000000002286.
3. Jacobs CL, Gross CR, Messersmith EE, Hong BA, Gillespie BW, Hill-Callahan P, et al. Emotional and financial experiences of kidney donors over the past 50 years: the RELIVE study. Clin J Am Soc Nephrol: CJASN. 2015;10(12):2221–31. https://doi.org/10.2215/CJN.07120714.
4. Klarenbach S, Gill JS, Knoll G, Caulfield T, Boudville N, Prasad GVR, et al. Economic consequences incurred by living kidney donors: a Canadian multi-center prospective study. Am J Transplant. 2014;14(4):916–22. https://doi.org/10.1111/ajt.12662.
5. Rodrigue JR, Schold JD, Morrissey P, Whiting J, Vella J, Kayler LK, et al. Direct and indirect costs following living kidney donation: findings from the KDOC study. Am J Transplant. 2016;16(3):869–76. https://doi.org/10.1111/ajt.13591.
6. Bailey PK, Tomson CRV, Macneill S, Marsden A, Cook D, Cooke R, et al. A multicenter cohort study of potential living kidney donors provides predictors of living kidney donation and non-donation. Kidney Int. 2017;92(5):1249–60. https://doi.org/10.1016/j.kint.2017.04.020.
7. Lapointe Rudow D, Hays R, Baliga P, Cohen DJ, Cooper M, Danovitch GM, et al. Consensus conference on best practices in live kidney donation: recommendations to optimize education, access, and care. Am J Transplant. 2015;15(4):914–22. https://doi.org/10.1111/ajt.13173.
8. Tong A, Chapman JR, Wong G, Craig JC. Living kidney donor assessment: challenges, uncertainties and controversies among transplant nephrologists and surgeons. Am J Transplant. 2013;13(11):2912–23. https://doi.org/10.1111/ajt.12411.
9. Mathur AK, Hong B, Ojo A, Merion RM. The National Living Donor Assistance Center perspective on barriers to the use of federal travel grants for living donors. Clin Transpl. 2017;31(7). https://doi.org/10.1111/ctr.12984.
10. Lentine KL, Mannon RB. The Advancing American Kidney Health (AAKH) Executive Order: Promise and Caveats for Expanding Access to Kidney Transplantation. Kidney360. 2020;1(6):557–60. https://doi.org/10.34067/KID.0001172020.
11. Mathur AK, Xing J, Dickinson DM, Warren PH, Gifford KA, Hong BA, et al. Return on investment for financial assistance for living kidney donors in the United States. Clin Transpl. 2018;32(7):e13277. https://doi.org/10.1111/ctr.13277.
12. UnitedHealth Group UnitedHealthcare will reimburse kidney donors' travel expenses, expanding life-saving access to kidney transplants. Date posted: 13 Jun 2016. Available at: https://www.unitedhealthgroup.com/newsroom/2016/0613kidneydonortravelexpenses.html. Accessed: 7 Sept 2020.
13. Tietjen A, Hays R, McNatt G, Howey R, Lebron-Banks U, Thomas CP, et al. Billing for living kidney donor care: balancing cost recovery, regulatory compliance, and minimized donor burden. Curr Transplant Rep. 2019;6(2):155–66. https://doi.org/10.1007/s40472-019-00239-0.
14. Hunt HF, Rodrigue JR, Dew MA, Schaffer RL, Henderson ML, Bloom R, et al. Strategies for increasing knowledge, communication, and access to living donor transplantation: an evidence review to inform patient education. Curr Transplant Rep. 2018;5(1):27–44. https://doi.org/10.1007/s40472-018-0181-1.

15. Lentine KL, Mandelbrot D. Moving from intuition to data: building the evidence to support and increase living donor kidney transplantation. Clinical J Am Soc Nephrol: CJASN. 2017;12(9):1383–5. https://doi.org/10.2215/CJN.07150717.

16. Garonzik-Wang JM, Berger JC, Ros RL, Kucirka LM, Deshpande NA, Boyarsky BJ, et al. Live donor champion: finding live kidney donors by separating the advocate from the patient. Transplantation. 2012;93(11):1147–50. https://doi.org/10.1097/TP.0b013e31824e75a5.

17. Lapointe Rudow D, Geatrakas S, Armenti J, Tomback A, Khaim R, Porcello L, et al. Increasing living donation by implementing the kidney coach program. Clin Transpl. 2019;33(2):e13471. https://doi.org/10.1111/ctr.13471.

18. Rodrigue JR, Pavlakis M, Egbuna O, Paek M, Waterman AD, Mandelbrot DA. The "house calls" trial: a randomized controlled trial to reduce racial disparities in live donor kidney transplantation: rationale and design. Contemp Clin Trials. 2012;33(4):311–8. https://doi.org/10.1016/j.cct.2012.03.015.

19. Kumar K, Tonascia JM, Muzaale AD, Purnell TS, Ottmann SE, Ammary FA, et al. Racial differences in completion of the living kidney donor evaluation process. Clin Transpl. 2018;32(7):e13291. https://doi.org/10.1111/ctr.13291.

20. Gordon EJ, Feinglass J, Carney P, Vera K, Olivero M, Black A, et al. A website intervention to increase knowledge about living kidney donation and transplantation among Hispanic/Latino Dialysis patients. Transplant. 2016;26(1):82–91. https://doi.org/10.1177/1526924816632124.

21. Gordon EJ, Lee J, Kang RH, Caicedo JC, Holl JL, Ladner DP, et al. A complex culturally targeted intervention to reduce Hispanic disparities in living kidney donor transplantation: an effectiveness-implementation hybrid study protocol. BMC Health Serv Res. 2018;18:1. https://doi.org/10.1186/s12913-018-3151-5.

22. Rodrigue JR, Feranil M, Lang J, Fleishman A. Readability, content analysis, and racial/ethnic diversity of online living kidney donation information. Clin Transpl. 2017;31(9). https://doi.org/10.1111/ctr.13039.

23. Zhou EP, Kiwanuka E, Morrissey PE. Online patient resources for deceased donor and live donor kidney recipients: a comparative analysis of readability. Clin Kidney J. 2018;11(4):559–63. https://doi.org/10.1093/ckj/sfx129.

24. Gander J, Gordon E, Patzer R. Decision aids to increase living donor kidney transplantation. Curr Transpl Rep. 2017;4(1):1–12. https://doi.org/10.1007/s40472-017-0133-1.

25. Ephraim PL, Powe NR, Rabb H, Ameling J, Auguste P, Lewis-Boyer L, et al. The providing resources to enhance African American patients' readiness to make decisions about kidney disease (PREPARED) study: protocol of a randomized controlled trial. BMC Nephrol. 2012;13(1):135. https://doi.org/10.1186/1471-2369-13-135.

26. National Kidney Foundation. The Big Ask, The Big Give. Available at: https://www.kidney.org/transplantation/livingdonors. Accessed: 7 Sept 2020.

27. Arriola KRJ, Powell CL, Thompson NJ, Perryman JP, Basu M. Living donor transplant education for African American patients with end-stage renal disease. Prog Transpl. 2014;24(4):362–70. https://doi.org/10.7182/pit2014830.

28. Infórmate: Inform yourself about Living Kidney Donation for Hispanic/Latinos. Available at: http://informate.org/english/. Accessed: 7 Sept 2020.

29. About the Kidney Transplant Learning Center. Available at: https://transplantliving.org/kidney/about-the-kidney-transplant-learning-center/. Accessed: 7 Sept 2020.

30. American Society for Transplantation Live Donor Tool Kit. Available at: https://www.myast.org/patient-information/live-donor-toolkit. Accessed: 7 Sept 2020.

31. Kazley AS, Hamidi B, Balliet W, Baliga P. Social media use among living kidney donors and recipients: survey on current practice and potential. J Med Internet Res. 2016;18(12):e328. https://doi.org/10.2196/jmir.6176.

32. Chang A, Anderson EE, Turner HT, Shoham D, Hou SH, Grams M. Identifying potential kidney donors using social networking web sites. Clin Transpl. 2013;27(3):E320–6. https://doi.org/10.1111/ctr.12122.

33. Kumar K, King EA, Muzaale AD, Konel JM, Bramstedt KA, Massie AB, et al. A smartphone app for increasing live organ donation. Am J Transplant. 2016;16(12):3548–53. https://doi.org/10.1111/ajt.13961.
34. Moorlock G, Draper H. Empathy, social media, and directed altruistic living organ donation. Bioethics. 2018;32(5):289–97. https://doi.org/10.1111/bioe.12438.
35. Ruck JM, Henderson ML, Eno AK, Rasmussen SEVP, DiBrito SR, Thomas AG, et al. Use of twitter in communicating living solid organ donation information to the public: an exploratory study of living donors and transplant professionals. Clin Transpl. 2019;33(1):e13447. https://doi.org/10.1111/ctr.13447.
36. Organ Procurement and Transplantation Network (OPTN). OPTN Living Donor Committee Meeting Minutes. 1 Apr 2019, Chicago, IL. Available at: https://optn.transplant.hrsa.gov/media/2956/20190401_living_donor_meeting_minutes.pdf. Accessed: 7 Sept 2020.
37. Cameron AM, Massie AB, Alexander CE, Stewart B, Montgomery RA, Benavides NR, et al. Social media and organ donor registration: the Facebook effect. Am J Transplant. 2013;13(8):2059–65. https://doi.org/10.1111/ajt.12312.
38. Bramstedt KA, Cameron AM. Beyond the billboard: the Facebook-based application, donor, and its guided approach to facilitating living organ donation. Am J Transplant. 2017;17(2):336–40. https://doi.org/10.1111/ajt.14004.
39. Rudow DL. Development of the center for living donation: incorporating the role of the nurse practitioner as director. Progress Transplant. 2011;21(4):312–6. https://doi.org/10.1177/152692481102100410.
40. Weng FL, Morgievich MM, Kandula P. The evaluation of living kidney donors: how long is too long? Am J Kidney Dis. 2018;72(4):472–4. https://doi.org/10.1053/j.ajkd.2018.07.001.
41. Habbous S, Arnold J, Begen MA, Boudville N, Cooper M, Dipchand C, et al. Duration of living kidney transplant donor evaluations: findings from 2 multicenter cohort studies. Am J Kidney Dis. 2018;72(4):483–98. https://doi.org/10.1053/j.ajkd.2018.01.036.
42. Getchell LE, Mckenzie SQ, Sontrop JM, Hayward JS, Mccallum MK, Garg AX. Increasing the rate of living donor kidney transplantation in Ontario: donor- and recipient-identified barriers and solutions. Can J Kidney Health Dis. 2017;4:2054358117698666. https://doi.org/10.1177/2054358117698666.
43. Habbous S, McArthur E, Sarma S, Begen MA, Lam NN, Manns B, et al. Potential implications of a more timely living kidney donor evaluation. Am J Transplant. 2018;18(11):2719–29. https://doi.org/10.1111/ajt.14732.
44. Habbous S, Sarma S, Barnieh LJ, McArthur E, Larenbach S, Manns B, et al. Healthcare costs for the evaluation, surgery, and follow-up Care of Living Kidney Donors. Transplantation. 2018;102(8):1367–74. https://doi.org/10.1097/TP.0000000000002222.
45. Habbous S, McArthur E, Dixon SN, McKenzie S, Garcia-Ochoa C, Lam NN, et al. Initiating maintenance Dialysis before living kidney donor transplantation when a donor candidate evaluation is well underway. Transplantation. 2018;102(7):e345–53. https://doi.org/10.1097/TP.0000000000002159.
46. Moore DR, Feurer ID, Zavala EY, Shaffer D, Karp S, Hoy H, et al. A web-based application for initial screening of living kidney donors: development, implementation and evaluation. Am J Transplant. 2013;13(2):450–7. https://doi.org/10.1111/j.1600-6143.2012.04340.x.
47. National Kidney Registry. Online living donor screening tool. Available at: https://www.kidneyregistry.org/info/considering-kidney-donation. Accessed: 7 Sept 2020.
48. Breeze web based living donor screening tool. Available at: https://www.medsleuth.com/transplant/. Accessed: 7 Sept 2020.
49. Mount Sinai Hospital Recanati Miller Transplantation Institute. Kidney Coach Playbook. Available at: https://www.mountsinai.org/files/MSHealth/Assets/HS/Care/Transplant/Kidney-Pancreas/KidneyCoachPlaybook17copy%20-%205.22.15.pdf. Accessed: 7 Sept 2020.
50. Shayna LL, Kit SS, Kenneth CD, Kerry MJ, Lucia MG, Lilless SM, et al. Racial disparities in living kidney donation: is there a lack of willing donors or an excess of medically unsuitable candidates? Transplantation. 2006;82(7):876–81. https://doi.org/10.1097/01.tp.0000232693.69773.42.

51. Graham JM, Courtney AE. The adoption of a one-day donor assessment model in a living kidney donor transplant program: a quality improvement project. Am J Kidney Dis. 2018;71(2):209–15. https://doi.org/10.1053/j.ajkd.2017.07.013.

52. Goldfarb DA. Re: A cost comparison for telehealth utilization in the kidney transplant waitlist evaluation process. J Urol. 2017;198(6):1199. https://doi.org/10.1016/j.juro.2017.09.045.

53. Organ Procurement and Transplantation Network (OPTN) / United Network for Organ Sharing (UNOS). Policy 18: Data Submission Requirements. Available at: https://optn.transplant.hrsa.gov/governance/policies/. Accessed: 7 Sept 2020.

54. Procedures to collect post-donation follow-up data from living donors. Available at: https://optn.transplant.hrsa.gov/resources/guidance/procedures-to-collect-post-donation-follow-up-data-from-living-donors/. Accessed: 7 Sept 2020.

55. Eno AK, Thomas AG, Ruck JM, et al. Assessing the attitudes and perceptions regarding the use of mobile health technologies for Living Kidney Donor Follow-up: survey study. JMIR Mhealth Uhealth. 2018;6(10):e11192. https://doi.org/10.2196/11192.

56. Henderson ML, Thomas AG, Eno AK, Waldram MM, Bannon J, Massie AB, et al. The impact of the mKidney mHealth system on live donor follow-up compliance: protocol for a randomized controlled trial. JMIR Research Protocols. 2019;8(1):e11000. https://doi.org/10.2196/11000.

57. Rachel FC, Diane RB, Tommy JB, Angela H-GA, David SA, Douglas HA. A cost comparison for telehealth utilization in the kidney transplant waitlist evaluation process. Transplantation. 2018;102(2):279–83. https://doi.org/10.1097/TP.0000000000001903.

58. Kasiske BL, Asrani SK, Dew MA, Henderson ML, Henrich C, Humar A, et al. The living donor collective: a scientific registry for living donors. Am J Transplant. 2017;17(12):3040–8. https://doi.org/10.1111/ajt.14365.

59. Rodrigue JR, Kazley AS, Mandelbrot DA, Hays R, LaPointe Rudow D, Baliga P. Living donor kidney transplantation: overcoming disparities in live kidney donation in the US—recommendations from a consensus conference. Clin J Am Soc Nephrol. 2015;10(9):1687. https://doi.org/10.2215/CJN.00700115.

60. Menjivar A, Torres X, Paredes D, Avinyo N, Peri JM, Sousa-Amorim ED, et al. Assessment of donor satisfaction as an essential part of living donor kidney transplantation: an eleven-year retrospective study. Transpl Int. 2018;31(12):1332–44. https://doi.org/10.1111/tri.13334.

61. Lentine KL, Lam NN, Segev DL. Risks of living kidney donation: current state of knowledge on outcomes important to donors. Clin J Am Soc Nephrol. 2019;14(4):597–608. https://doi.org/10.2215/CJN.11220918.

62. Moore DR, Serur D, Rudow DL, Rodrigue JR, Hays R, Cooper M. Living donor kidney transplantation: improving efficiencies in live kidney donor evaluation–recommendations from a consensus conference. Clin J Am Soc Nephrol. 2015;10(9):1678–86. https://doi.org/10.2215/CJN.01040115.

63. Wong SPY, Hebert PL, Laundry RJ, Hammond KW, Liu CF, Burrows NR, et al. Decisions about renal replacement therapy in patients with advanced kidney disease in the US Department of veterans affairs, 2000–2011. Clin J Am Soc Nephrol. 2016;11(10):1825–33. https://doi.org/10.2215/CJN.03760416.

64. Wright Nunes JA, Cavanaugh KL, Fagerlin A. An informed and activated patient: addressing barriers in the pathway from education to outcomes. Am J Kidney Dis. 2016;67(1):1–4. https://doi.org/10.1053/j.ajkd.2015.09.017.

65. Fishbane S, Agoritsas S, Bellucci A, Halinski C, Shah HH, Sakhiya V, et al. Augmented nurse care management in CKD stages 4 to 5: a randomized trial. Am J Kidney Dis. 2017;70(4):498–505. https://doi.org/10.1053/j.ajkd.2017.02.366.

66. Khosla N, Gordon E, Nishi L, Ghossein C. Impact of a chronic kidney disease clinic on pre-emptive kidney transplantation and transplant wait times. Prog Transplant. 2010;20(3):216–20. https://doi.org/10.7182/prtr.20.3.m7233h6k776g8003.

Index

A

Albuminuria
    KDIGO recommendation for evaluation, 79
    kidney failure risk
        after kidney donation, 77, 78
        in general population, 75
        lifetime risk for ESRD, 76, 77
        mortality and kidney disease outcomes, 65
    level of, 71
    pathophysiology and measurement, 71
        factors affecting urinary albumin-creatinine ration, 73, 75
        KDIGO CKD recommendations for evaluation, 72
        normal range and variability, 71
    and proteinuria categories, 72, 74
    in US population, 72, 73
Alport nephropathy
    clinical diagnosis, 200
    genes, 200
    phenocopy, 201
    testing living donor candidates, 201
Ambulatory blood pressure monitoring (ABPM), 121–123
American Society of Transplantation (AST), 5
Antibody-mediated rejection (ABMR), 237
Anti-human globulin (AHG)-enhanced CDC crossmatch, 236
APOL1 genotyping
    environmental factor, 207
    frequency, 207
    identification of, 206
    recommended testing, 209
    risk variants
        associated between ESKD and CKD, 207
        copies of, 205
        distribution of, 206
    role in living donor kidney transplantation, 208
    vs. sickle cell disease, 209
Apolipoprotein L1 (*APOL1*) gene
    current recommendations for selection, 152
    measurement, 151
    outcomes data, 152
APOL1 long-term outcomes (APOLLO), 339
Atherosclerotic renal artery disease, 96
Atypical hemolytic uremic syndrome (aHUS)
    clinical manifestations, 203
    genes, 203
    phenocopy, 203
    testing living donor candidates, 204
Australia and New Zealand Dialysis and Transplant Living Kidney Donor Registry (ANZDATA), 314
Autosomal dominant polycystic kidney disease (ADPKD), 192
    clinical diagnosis, 198
    genes, 198
    phenocopy, 199
    testing living donor candidates, 199
Autosomal dominant tubulointerstitial disease
    clinical diagnosis, 199
    genes, 199
    phenocopy, 200
    testing living donor candidates, 200

B

B-cell depleting therapies, 245

C

Canadian Society of Transplantation (CST), 341
Cardiovascular risk
    current recommendation for selection, 151
    measurement, 150
    outcomes data, 151

Chronic kidney disease (CKD)
  diagnostic tools, 191–192
  genetic mechanisms of, 192–194
Compatibility assessment, 233
  ABO incompatibility, 234
  HLA incompatibility (*see* (*see* Human
      leucocyte antigens (HLA)
      incompatibility)
  kidney paired donation (*see* (*see* Kidney
      paired donation (KPD)))
Complement-dependent cytotoxic (CDC)
      crossmatch, 236
Conflict of interest, 25
Congenital abnormalities of the kidney and
      urinary tract (CAKUT), 193

D
Desensitization
  ABMR treatment
    B-cell activating factor/B-lymphocyte
        stimulator inhibitors, 246
    complement inhibitors, 246
    IgG degrading enzyme, 246
    interleukin-6 receptor inhibitor, 246
    proteasome inhibitors, 245
  incompatible living donor transplantation
    B-cell depleting therapies, 245
    plasmapheresis, 244
  kidney paired donation and, 247
Direct acting antivirals (DAAs), 168
Disclosure of information
  dilemma of recommendation, 36
  donor rights and care processes, 34–35
  methods of, 35
  recipient care, rights and processes, 35
  requirements, 31–34
  risks of donation, 35
  shared decision-making models, 36
  US legal standards and guidelines, 31
Donor-derived infections
  classification, 161
  fungal infections
    coccidiodomycosis, 170
    histoplasmosis, 169
  parasitic infections
    chagas disease, 172
    strongyloides, 171
  recommended screening tests, 162–165
  risk factors, 162
  routine infectious screening
    cytomegalovirus, 166
    epstein-barr virus (EBV), 167
    hepatitis B virus, 166, 168–169

  hepatitis C virus, 166, 168–169
  human immunodeficiency virus,
      166, 168–169
  syphilis, 167
  tuberculosis, bacterial infections, 172–173
  viral infections
    west nile virus, 174
    zika virus, 174
Donor-related malignancy
  cancer transmission
    donor with cancer, 178–180
    management, 181
    outcomes after, 182
    risk categories, 177, 178
    screening and evaluation, 175, 176

E
ELPAT Psychosocial Assessment Tool
      (EPAT), 263
End stage kidney disease (ESKD), 25,
      141, 327
  adjusted hazard ration, 191
  apolipoprotein L1 risk variants, 190
  cause of, 191
  diagnostic tools, 191–192
  incidence of, 26, 191
  kidney transplantation for, 190
  risk of, 189, 191
  unknown cause of, 205
End-stage renal disease (ESRD), 303
Enhanced recovery protocols
      (ERP), 227–229
Ethical challenges
  anticipated donor benefits, 331
  APOL1 genetic testing, 337–339
  ethically fraught, 328–329
  informed consent, 329–331
  kidney paired donation, 334–337
  objective risk of harm, 333
  public solicitation
    awareness of organ donations, 340
    Canadian Society of
        Transplantation, 341
    covert organ trafficking, 340
    definition, 339
    Facebook pages, 341
    media coverage, 339
    motives and experiences of kidney
        transplant, 340
    for organ donors, 342
    privacy/publicity management, 341
    transplant program, 341
  values and principles, 327–328

F

Fabry disease
  clinical diagnosis, 204
  GLA gene, 204
  phenocopy, 204
  testing living donor candidates, 205
Fibromuscular dysplasia (FMD), 96
Flow cytometry crossmatch, 236
Focal segmental glomerulosclerosis (FSGS)
  clinical diagnosis, 202
  genes
    primary (glomerular genes), 202
    secondary, 202
  phenocopy, 203
  testing living donor candidates, 203
Follow-up care, 254, 265–267
  center-based initiatives, 319
  collected data on clinical components, 307–310
  communication and integrated care models, 317
  consequences of program compliance with LDF, 316
  data collection, 317–318
  education on health promoting practices, 307
  eGFR-based chronic kidney disease, application of, 311, 312
  ethical principles and outcomes, 304
  international models
    European Living Donation and Public Health project, 311
    European Union Health Programme, 312
    Living Donor Assessment model, 313
    Living Donor Observatory, 312
    Swiss Organ Living Donor Health Registry, 313
  KDIGP Living Donor Guidline recommendation, 307, 311
  LD kidney donation, risks and consequences of, 304
  local donor community outreach, 320
  logistical and financial challenges, 314–316
  medical care, 304–306
  novel smartphone-based mobile health (mHealth) technologies, 318, 319
  OPTN/UNOS "toolbox" recommendations, 320, 321
  policy and practice, United States, 307–311
  psychosocial and socioeconomic impacts, 306
  reimbursement programs for follow-up costs, 315

G

Genetic kidney disease, 196–197
  Alport nephropathy, 200–201
  atypical hemolytic uremic syndrome, 203–204
  autosomal dominant polycystic kidney disease, 198–199
  autosomal dominant tubulointerstitial disease, 199–200
  clinic role, 209–210
  fabry disease, 204–205
  focal segmental glomerulosclerosis, 202–203
  genetic testing
    copy number variant analysis, 195
    next-generation sequencing, 195
    polymerase chain reaction, 194
  by genetic variants, 194
  monogenic and, testing for, 195, 198
  risk variants
    APOL1 gene (*see* (*see APOL1* genotyping))
    sickle cell trait (*see* (*see* Sickle cell trait (SCT)))
  unknown cause of, 205
Global Observatory on Donation and Transplantation (GODT), 4–5, 303
Glomerular filtration rate (GFR)
  KDIGO recommendations for evaluation, 68–71
  kidney failure risk
    after kidney donation, 67
    in general population, 65
    mortality and kidney disease outcomes, 65
  lifetime risk for ESRD, 66, 67
  pathophysiology and measurement
    CKD-EPI equation, 62
    definition, 61
    KDIGO CKD recommendations for evaluation, 61
    mean, 60
    mGFR estimation, 64
    normal range and variability, 60, 61
    sources of error, 63
  recommended steps for estimation, 70
Glucose tolerance
  current recommendation for selection, 146
  measurement, 146
  outcomes data, 146

H

Health-related quality of life (HRQOL)
  outcomes, 254

Health-related quality of life (HRQOL)
outcomes (*cont.*)
and postdonation psychosocial
care, 265–267
and psychosocial outcomes, 267
prevalence, 275
Health Resources and Services Administration
(HRSA), 307
Hematuria
KDIGO recommendations for microscopic
evaluation, 85
kidney failure risk
after kidney donation, 84
Alport syndrome, 82
IgA nephropathy, 83
in general population, 82
of persistent postdonation proteinuria, 84
TBMN disease, 83
microscopic evaluation, 86
pathophysiology and measurement
AUA recommendations for evaluation, 81
normal range and variability, 80
Hepatitis B surface antigen (HBsAg)
testing, 169
Horseshoe kidney, 99
Human leucocyte antigens (HLA)
incompatibility
crossmatch technqiues
anti-human globulin-enhanced CDC
crossmatch, 236
complement-dependent cytotoxic
crossmatch, 236, 237
cPRA calculator, 235
flow cytometry crossmatch, 236
SAB assay, 237
sensitized patients with cPRA, 238
virtual crossmatch, 236
definition, 235
genes classification, 235
Hypertension
accurate blood pressure measurement, 120
algorithm for, 125
ambulatory blood pressure monitoring, 121–123
case studies, 130
contraindications, 127
current recommendations for selection, 149
definition, 119, 121
donor candidates, 126
additional testing for, 126
controlled hypertension history, 125
post-donation follow-up, 126

selection of, 124
special counseling, 129
donor characteristics, 142
ESKD risk, 142
frequency and outcomes of, 148
hypertensive disorders of pregnancy, 126
losartan, 136
masked, 120
measurement, 148
medication, 123
metabolic/cardiovascular risks, 142
nephrectomy impact
cardiovascular risk and kidney
survival, 127–128
on future pregnancies, 128
obesity and, 130
office-based blood pressure assessment, 121–122
postdonation risk of, 129
white coat, 120

I
Ibuprofen, 130
informed consent
independent living donor advocate role, 27
Informed consent, 329–331
bioethical principles, 28
beneficence, 29
of non-maleficence, 29
respect for persons/autonomy, 29
donor care
specific care teams, 27
donor evaluation, 27
donors care
by multidisciplinary team, 26
by physicians support, 27
OPTN regulatory guidelines, 26
WHO guiding principles, 26
elements of, 32, 33
future research questions, 43, 44
comprehension, 45
develop and evaluate interventions, 47
disclosure, 45
priority setting and donor
engagement, 47
satisfaction, 46
standardization, 46
voluntariness, 46
independent living donor advocate
role, 27–28
requirements for, 30
agreement, 39
comprehension, 36

decisional capacity, 30
decision-making, 39
disclosure of information (*see* (*see*
    Disclosure of information))
voluntariness (*see* (*see* Voluntariness))
special considerations
    advance donation, 42
    APOL1 genetic testing, 40–41
    incarcerated donor candidate, 41, 50
    'increased risk' criteria, 43, 51
    misattributed relationship, 40
    nondirected and directed donors with
        limited relationship, 42
    potential donors solicited via social
        media, 42
    vulnerable populations, 41
Interstitial fibrosis and tubular atrophy
    (IFTA), 106

K
KDIGO Clinical Practice Guideline on the
    Evaluation and Care of Living
    Kidney Donors, 11
Kidney
    anatomy
        arterial, 95–96
        assessment of, 93
        horseshoe, 99
        left kidney retro-aortic veins, 97
        renal vein, 97
        ureteral, 99
    biopsy, 102
    development, 95
    factors associated with pre and postdona-
        tion, 100, 101
    function, 93
    functional nephrons, 102
    histology, 94
    implant biopsy, histopathology of
        chronic changes, 105
        CKD progression, 104
        clinical outcomes, 106
        demographic patterns and clinical
            practice, 104
        ESKD, 104
        glomerular hyperfiltration, 108
        nephron hypertrophy, 105
        nephrosclerosis, 105
        obesity and metabolic syndrome, 107
        and postdonation eGFR, 106
        postdonation renal function, 106
        renal parenchyma, 105
        risk factors, 105

subclinical histological abnormali-
    ties, 104
wedge/core biopsy, 107
nutcracker renal vein, 98–99
renal artery stenosis (RAS), 95–96
size and volume, 99–100
stone disease (*see* (*see* Stone disease))
volume
    and GFR, 102
    increasing after donor nephrec-
        tomy, 102–103
    nephron mass, 102
    predonation volume vs. long term
        postdonation, 103
Kidney Coach Program, 353
Kidney Disease Improving Global Outcomes
    (KDIGO), 122, 161, 175
Kidney Disease Improving Global Outcomes
    (KDIGO) Living Donor
    Guideline, 307
Kidney Disease: Improving Global Outcomes
    (KDIGO) Clinical Practice
    Guideline, 283
Kidney paired donation (KPD), 14–16,
    25–26, 334–337
    advanced donation, 240
    blood type O donors, 240
    desensitization and, 247
    donor recipient pair, 240
    family voucher, 241
    quality of donor kidney assessment, 241
        cold ischemia time, 242
        cytomegalovirus seronegative, 242
        donor kidney function and comorbidi-
            ties, 241
        HLA mismatch, 241
        living kidney donor profile index, 242
    scope of, 243
    transplantation types
        kidney donor chains, 239
        multiple-way exchange, 239
        two-way exchange, 239

L
Living Donor Champion program, 353
Living Donor Extended Time (LETO)
    studies, 339
Living donor kidney transplantation
    (LDKT), 25
    between identical twins, 4
    costs, 350
    economic costs of, 350
    follow-up care of donors, 11

Living donor kidney transplantation (LDKT) (*cont.*)
  for racial and ethic minorities, 353–354
  geographic variations and trends in, 4–5
  informed consent process, 7
  institutional culture promoting, 351, 352
  institutional strategies and resources
    candidate and donor education, 361
    electronic living donor screening, 360
    ensuring living donor follow-up, 352–353
    leadership and staffing, 360
    living donor satisfaction, 363
    programmatic support, 360
    robust quality assurance and performance improvement process, 363, 364
    timely evaluation process for all donors, 361
  interventions, reducing financial burden, 352–353
  kidney failure, 94
  kidney paired donation, 14–16
  lack of social support, 351
  with low SES, 350
  nephrectomy, 4, 12
    hand-assisted approach, 12
    intraoperative complications, 13
    laparoscopy, 12
    open approach, 12
    open flank incision, 12
    robotic-assisted laparoscopic radical nephrectomy, 13
    standard laparoscopic approach, 12
    surgical advances, 13
  partnerships with community providers, 364
    partnering with chronic kidney disease management clinics, 365
    physicians/nephrologists, 364
  population-base analyses, 350
  programmatic structure, education, evaluation and care processes, 358, 359
  promotion using social media, 356–357
  rationale for
    chronic kidney disease and kidney failure, 1
    kidney tansplantation vs. chronic dialysis, 2
    living vs. decreased kidney tranplantation, 3, 7
  recipient disparities in access to, 6
  risks of
    donation rates between low vs. high income populations, 10
    gestational hypertension, 10
    medical, surgical, psychosocial, and financial, 9
    online risk assessment tools, 10
  technology, 355
    American Society for Transplantation Live Donor Tool Kit program, 356
    The Big Ask, The Big Give program, 355
    Inform yourself about Living Kidney Donation for Hispanic/Latinos, 356
    Living About Choices in Transplant and Sharing (Living ACTS), 356
    mobile applications, 355
    Providing Resources to Enhance African American Patients Readiness to Make Decisions about Kidney Disease (Prepared) program, 355
    The UNOS Kidney Learning Center (KTLC), 356
    web-based tools, 355
  temporal trends, 6
Living kidney donation
  benefits of, 303
  history of, 25–26
  risks of, 190, 303

M
Medically complex donor candidates, 141
Metabolic syndrome
  current recommendations for selection, 147
  definition, 147
  incidence, 147
  measurement, 147
  outcomes data, 147
  risk factor, 147
Microalbuminuria, 136
Microangiopathic hemolytic anemia (MAHA), 203
Multiple hit hypothesis, living kidney donation, 305–306

N
National Health and Nutrition Examination Survey (NHANES), 142
National Living Donor Assistance Center (NLDAC), 352
Nephrectomy
  enhanced recovery protocols, 227–229
  evaluation
    computed tomography imaging, 292
    education and counseling, 291

evidence-based clinical practice
 guidelines, 291
kidney function assessment, 292
left nephrectomy, 292
magnetic resonance imaging, 292
pre-operative imaging, 292
hand-assisted laparoscopy, 296
intraoperative considerations
 catheter insertion, 226
 endotracheal intubation, 226
 intravascular volume expansion, 226
 mild hypercapnia tolerance, 227
 prophylactic antibiotics, 226
 vasopressors avoidance, 226
laparocopic approach, 227
low risk surgical procedure, 26
natural orifice transluminal surgery, 297
open approach, 293
outcomes, 298
perioperative complications, 220
readmission rates, 220
retroperitoneoscopic approach, 297, 298
robotic-assisted laparoscopy, 296
single site surgery, 297
surgical approaches, advantages and
 disadvantages, 298, 299
transperitoneal laproscopy
 invasive technique, 294
 left kidney dissection, 294, 295
 patient positioning and port placement, 294
transvaginal extraction, 297
Nephrolithiasis, *see* Stone disease

O
Obesity
 current recommendations for selection, 145
 measurement, 143
 outcomes data, 143–144
 risk factor, 144
 weight management post-donation, 145
Office blood pressure measurement, 121–122
Organ Procurement and Transplantation Network
 (OPTN) policy, 121, 161, 220

P
Paired kidney exchange (PKE), *see* Kidney
 paired donation (KPD)
Panel reactive antibody (PRA), 235
Perioperative evaluation
 evidence-based recommendations, 219
 goals of, 219
 history

family, 222
personal, 221
surgical, 222
imaging studies, 223, 224
intraoperative donor nephrectomy
 anesthetic considerations, 225
 catheter insertion, 226
 intravascular volume expansion, 226
 mild hypercapnia tolerance, 227
 prophylactic antibiotics, 226
 vasopressors avoidance, 226
laboratory testing, 222, 223
medical evaluation, 221
physical examination, 222
risk stratification
 assessment of bleeding history, 224
 cardiac, 224
 chronic obstructive pulmonary
  disease, 225
 venous thromboembolism, 225
surgical outcomes, 229
Psychosocial care, 265–267
Psychosocial evaluation
 additional assessment and treatment
  outcomes, 264
 biologically and emotionally related
  donors, 257
 communication with living donor
  transplantation team, 264
 domains, 254–256
 donor selection, objectives for, 253
 goals, 254
 interview
  checklists, 263
  evaluator role and qualification, 259
  logistics, 262
 living kidney donor candidates, 254
 and predonation care, 260–261
 process and predonation care, 259
 prospective donor and transplant candidate,
  relationship between, 256
 prospective donors screening, 259
 psychological pressure experience, case
  study, 258
 team decisions about donor candidacy, 265
 unrelated donors, case study, 257
Psychosocial outcomes
 HRQOL and, 267
 prevalence, 275
 qualitative research, 267–270
 quantitative research
  descriptive findings, 270–273
  prediction of poor donor psychosocial
   and HRQOL outcomes, 273–274
 risk factors, 253

R

Renal and Lung Living Donors Evaluation (RELIVE) Study, 271
Renal artery stenosis (RAS), 95–96
Risk assessment
    genetic factors, 287
    long-term ESKD risk, 284–285
    perinatal factors, 287
    perioperative risk, 284
    postdonation risk, 284
    predonation risk, 283
    risk-benefit approach, 287
    risk factors and health outcomes, 286

S

Scientific Registry of Transplant Recipients (SRTR), 317
Shared decision-making models, 36
Sickle cell trait (SCT)
    CKD risk, 208
    definition, 206
    and malaria, 207
    recommended testing, 209
    role in living donor kidney transplantation, 208
Single nucleotide variants (SNVs), 194
Steroid-resistant nephrotic syndrome (SRNS), 202
Stone disease
    after kidney donation, 111–112
    contraindication, 109
    in donor candidates
        American Urological Association for Evaluation guidelines, 111
        asymptomatic stones, 109
        CKD progression, 109
        imaging studies, 109
        vs. Randall's plaques, 109
        "rule of halves", clinical rule, 110
        surgical intervention, 110
        symptomatic *vs.* radiographic recurrences, 109
    imaging studies, 108
    incidence, 108
    prevalence, 108
Swiss Organ Living Donor Health Registry (SOL-DHR), 313

T

Thrombotic microangiopathy (TMA), 203
Tobacco use
    current recommendation for selection, 150
    measurement, 149
    outcomes data, 149, 150
    risk associated with, 150

V

Virtual crossmatch, 236
Voluntariness, 37
    internally-experienced pressure, 38, 48
    protections against coercion, 38, 49
    protections against undue influence/under pressure, 37, 47
    valuable considerations, 38

W

Wedge biopsy, 107
Wellness and Health Outcomes in the Live Donor (WHOLE-Donor) multicenter study, 127

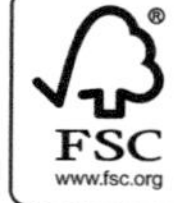